HEALTH CARE IN TRANSITION

FUNDAMENTALS OF LEADERSHIP FOR HEALTHCARE PROFESSIONALS

VOLUME 2

HEALTH CARE IN TRANSITION

Additional books and e-books in this series can be found on Nova's website under the Series tab.

Copyright © 2019 by Nova Science Publishers, Inc.

All rights reserved. No part of this book may be reproduced, stored in a retrieval system or transmitted in any form or by any means: electronic, electrostatic, magnetic, tape, mechanical photocopying, recording or otherwise without the written permission of the Publisher.

We have partnered with Copyright Clearance Center to make it easy for you to obtain permissions to reuse content from this publication. Simply navigate to this publication's page on Nova's website and locate the "Get Permission" button below the title description. This button is linked directly to the title's permission page on copyright.com. Alternatively, you can visit copyright.com and search by title, ISBN, or ISSN.

For further questions about using the service on copyright.com, please contact:
Copyright Clearance Center
Phone: +1-(978) 750-8400   Fax: +1-(978) 750-4470   E-mail: info@copyright.com.

NOTICE TO THE READER

The Publisher has taken reasonable care in the preparation of this book, but makes no expressed or implied warranty of any kind and assumes no responsibility for any errors or omissions. No liability is assumed for incidental or consequential damages in connection with or arising out of information contained in this book. The Publisher shall not be liable for any special, consequential, or exemplary damages resulting, in whole or in part, from the readers' use of, or reliance upon, this material. Any parts of this book based on government reports are so indicated and copyright is claimed for those parts to the extent applicable to compilations of such works.

Independent verification should be sought for any data, advice or recommendations contained in this book. In addition, no responsibility is assumed by the Publisher for any injury and/or damage to persons or property arising from any methods, products, instructions, ideas or otherwise contained in this publication.

This publication is designed to provide accurate and authoritative information with regard to the subject matter covered herein. It is sold with the clear understanding that the Publisher is not engaged in rendering legal or any other professional services. If legal or any other expert assistance is required, the services of a competent person should be sought. FROM A DECLARATION OF PARTICIPANTS JOINTLY ADOPTED BY A COMMITTEE OF THE AMERICAN BAR ASSOCIATION AND A COMMITTEE OF PUBLISHERS.

Additional color graphics may be available in the e-book version of this book.

Library of Congress Cataloging-in-Publication Data

ISBN: 978-1-53615-729-1

Published by Nova Science Publishers, Inc. † New York

HEALTH CARE IN TRANSITION

FUNDAMENTALS OF LEADERSHIP FOR HEALTHCARE PROFESSIONALS

VOLUME 2

STANISLAW P. A. STAWICKI
MICHAEL S. FIRSTENBERG
AND
THOMAS J. PAPADIMOS
EDITORS

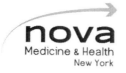

CONTENTS

Preface		ix
Introduction	The Leadership Journey is a Life-Long Quest *Stanislaw P. A. Stawicki, Thomas J. Papadimos* *and Michael S. Firstenberg*	xi
Chapter 1	Leadership in Health-Care: From Theory to Practical Application *Derek M. Tang, Ankita Bassi, Alec Gayner,* *Gregory S. Domer, Jay Fisher, Timothy Oskin,* *Michael S. Firstenberg, Thomas J. Papadimos* *and Stanislaw P. A. Stawicki*	1
Chapter 2	Interviewing for a Leadership Position: Key Aspects and Considerations *Jacqueline Seoane, Ronya Silmi* *and Stanislaw P. A. Stawicki*	49
Chapter 3	The Benefits of Inclusive Leadership among Healthcare Professionals *Erick Alexanderson, Carlo Angello Sanchez* *and Aloha Meave*	67

Chapter 4	Reflections on FLEX: A Professional Development Program for Women Faculty of the School of Medicine at Case Western Reserve University (CWRU-SOM) *Elizabeth Fine Smilovich, Phyllis A. Nsiah-Kumi and Marion J. Skalweit*	**95**
Chapter 5	Medical Leadership Skills: Exploring the Executive Function-Dysfunction Spectrum *CJ Maron, Alfred DiGregorio and Stanislaw P. A. Stawicki*	**111**
Chapter 6	Resilience in Leadership *Richard Martin and Manish Garg*	**133**
Chapter 7	Leadership in Complex Medical Systems with Limited Resources: Social and Economic Considerations *Rodolfo A. Neirotti, Luiz F. Caneo and Aida L. Ribeiro Turquetto*	**147**
Chapter 8	Managing Change in Healthcare: The Rise of Electronic Medical Records *Veronica Sikka, Raaj Popli and Naazli Shaikh*	**185**
Chapter 9	Pitfalls of Academic Affiliations: Health Center at a Crossroad *Thomas J. Papadimos, James P. Hofmann, Steven J. Margolis and Andrew B. Casabianca*	**197**
Chapter 10	Creating a Culture of Curiosity to Improve Quality and Patient Safety *Dianne McCallister*	**219**

Contents

vii

Chapter 11   Aviation and Cardiac Surgery:
Review of Their Relationships. Implication on
Complexity Theory and Ethical Considerations   **231**
*Roberto Battellini, Michael S. Firstenberg
and Mauricio Perez-Martinez*

Chapter 12   Setting Up a Hospice and Palliative Care
Program at a University Health Network:
Turning Challenges into Opportunities   **255**
*Ric Baxter, John R. Interrante, Gregory S. Domer,
Timothy Oskin, Michael S. Firstenberg
and Stanislaw P. A. Stawicki*

Chapter 13   Training the Next Generation of Surgeons:
Leadership for Mentors and Mentees   **281**
*Alexander P. Nissen, Juan B. Umana-Pizano,
Jacqueline K. Olive and Tom C. Nguyen*

Chapter 14   Crisis Leadership: A Practical Perspective   **299**
Daniel del Portal and Manish Garg

About the Editors   **313**

Index   **317**

Related Nova Publications   **341**

PREFACE

Welcome to *Fundamentals of Leadership for Healthcare Professionals, Volume 2*. The editors are proud to present our readers with a significantly expanded book, featuring 14 chapters by a distinguished group of 40 academic authors with decades of collective leadership experience. Based on the success of Volume 1, the current book in our series seeks to expand into important new areas. This includes diverse topics such as resilient leadership; electronic medical record implementations; interviewing for leadership positions; effective management in the low-resource setting; academic affiliations; crisis leadership; care quality and patient safety; the importance of diversity in health-care; complexity theory and ethics; change management; exploration of the executive function-dysfunction spectrum; and many other related concepts. The current tome begins with an introductory chapter that provides an in-depth overview of various theoretical aspects of leadership, including the most commonly encountered leadership styles. Throughout the book the authors focus on practical relevance of the topics being discussed, presenting 'lessons learned' and stressing the importance of flexible, authentic, servant leadership. The editors hope that Volume 2 of the *Fundamentals of Leadership for Healthcare Professionals* will be equally, or perhaps even more successful than Volume 1, and that it will provide an excellent springboard for Volume 3 in this important and unique book series!

Sincerely,

Stanislaw P. A. Stawicki MD, MBA, FACS,
Michael S. Firstenberg MD, FACC,
and
Thomas J. Papadimos MD, MPH, FCCS
The Editors

INTRODUCTION: THE LEADERSHIP JOURNEY IS A LIFE-LONG QUEST

Stanislaw P. A. Stawicki, Thomas J. Papadimos and Michael S. Firstenberg

I. INTRODUCTORY REMARKS

Welcome to the second volume of *Fundamentals of Leadership for Healthcare Professionals*. Due to the success of the original book, published in 2018, we decided to turn *The Fundamentals* into a multi-volume series with the phenomenal support of NOVA Scientific Publishers. We are also delighted to inform the reader that our Editorial team has expanded to include Professor Thomas Papadimos.

With nearly 1,200 published scholarly works including more than 25 books, as well as more than 30 years of combined leadership experience, this Editorial team and co-authors are fully dedicated to applying our collective knowledge, experience and skills to help address one of the most pressing crises in modern health-care: *the crisis of leadership*. With increasing demand on our health-care systems and constant changes as a function of evolving payment models, patient (and community) expectations, growing emphasis on quality initiatives, and an ever evolving reliance on high-end technological solutions for electronic medical records and clinical management tools, there is an increasing need for the sustained supply of both greater quantity and higher quality leaders. Although many areas of health-care administration can be managed well without intimate involvement of health-care professionals (e.g., physicians, nurses, advanced practitioners, and other allied health experts); significant proportion of operational aspects of health-care do require ongoing and proactive involvement of individuals whose patient-facing efforts are the true cornerstone of why hospitals and clinics exist. However, the interactions between health-care providers – including very complex and dynamic power-relationships and human resource challenges – require strong leadership to navigate through divergent perspectives that have emerged since the outdated and paternalistic model of "the doctor is always right" has transitioned into a more pluralistic one.

While the perfect roadmap for developing effective health-care leaders can be elusive, our understanding of required core competencies continues to evolve – and without a doubt, a strong clinical background is critical foundation for a sufficient understanding of the issues that challenge healthcare systems at all levels. Throughout this book, the authors utilize case- and experience-based models of presenting relevant (and commonly encountered) leadership vignette scenarios. Based on shared practical experiences, each chapter then presents further insight to leadership qualities and behaviors best suited to addressing the particular situation, conflict, or crisis from the perspective of a good health-care leader. Today's health systems and their leaders face multiple challenges and competing priorities in their daily decision making and governing process. Thus, despite attempts to reform the U.S. health-care system, the medically uninsured and under-insured are still among us; the cost of health-care services continues to increase; divided government and its effect on funding availability creates perpetual anxieties and persistent uncertainty; the shift from "pay for service" to "pay for performance" (i.e., focus on outcomes and quality) compensation and reimbursement models highlights the disconnect between medical training and subsequent provider practice;

Introduction xiii

the growing dependence on technology that leads to continuous concerns about individual privacy; the opioid crisis that may in part be due to the drive to improve patient experience scores, persists despite massive efforts to reverse it; and public health emergencies of international concern (including emerging infectious diseases) become increasingly prevalent, to name only a few concerns.

Training healthcare leaders to be insightful, inclusive, empathetic, and display emotional intelligence is vitally important – especially when our communities and increasing number of human lives, participate in rapidly growing health and insurance networks. The days of the self-centered, narcissistic, and dictatorial style of leadership are over, and those who continue to attempt to "impose" rather than genuinely lead, no longer belong within the fabric of modern health-care. This takes us to the logical realization that leadership is a life-long quest, where the leader never quite arrives at the finish line. Instead, he or she needs to focus on evolving and adapting in order to create new perspectives to solve complex problems. In this new paradigm, the re-calibration of one's financial, performance/quality, and other goals should be accompanied by a mandatory re-evaluation of one's ability to empathize, create shared value, and serve. Concepts like "burnout" and "mental health hygiene" should be as important as "profit margin", "hospital ranking" or "performance points". Finally, one must never forget that no human being should ever be considered a "resource", "commodity", or "health encounter", and above all human dignity must be preserved at all levels of every health-care organization.

II. VOLUME 2: WHAT'S NEW AND UNIQUE

The current volume of *Fundamentals of Leadership for Healthcare Professionals* discusses a number of important topics in a unique and practical fashion. Although each chapter contains fair amount of theoretical knowledge, the authors devote significant amount of focus toward sharing personal experiences, lessons learned, and the identification of important opportunities that are collectively intended to help our readers grow and develop in their quest to become better leaders. The leadership vignettes and problems presented – some hypothetical and some based on actual experiences – without a doubt will resonate to anyone familiar with health-care systems as the scenarios discussed are often characterized by common themes and recurring patterns of individual and institutional behaviors.

Volume 2 of *The Fundamentals* begins with a comprehensive and insightful discussion of health-care governance in the context of commonly encountered leadership styles and qualities of successful leaders. This discussion is further expanded to touch upon the importance of the often-underappreciated aspects of leadership interviews and onboarding process. Richly referenced, the chapter highlights the importance of recruiting, developing, and supporting leaders within modern health-care organizations.

The book then transitions into the topic of interviewing for leadership position. Here, the authors discuss the critical importance of pre-interview preparations, realistic and honest assessment of one's abilities and the overall fit between the candidate and the organization, as well as the need for effectively demonstrating one's positive attributes in a humble yet sufficiently assertive fashion. The information provided is a must-have for both organizations and interviewees engaged in the process of mutual evaluation and compatibility assessment.

The importance of inclusiveness and collaborative approaches in the workplace cannot be overstated. Throughout the entire Volume 2 of *The Fundamentals* we present diverse perspectives on introducing and ensuring equal voice for all stakeholders, regardless of one's age, gender, ethnic or religious background, or any other unique characteristic. Emphasis is placed on respectful and egalitarian approaches, including the focus on fostering empathy and flexibility throughout professional interactions. Clearly, team-based care at all organizational levels is becoming more established as an effective leadership approach – including the development and maintenance of strong relationships between clinical and non-clinical leaders. The strategy of mutual respect and inclusion has been demonstrated to reduce overall costs (e.g., favorable legal liability

Introduction xv

and employee turnover profile); improve outcomes (reduced length of stay, readmissions); enhance care quality and patient experience (e.g., fewer adverse events and improved patient satisfaction scores).

Among the most unique aspects of the current book is the chapter dedicated to the topic of executive function-dysfunction spectrum. Here, the authors discuss various domains that are critical to effective leadership functioning, from cognitive flexibility and attentional control to self-monitoring and emotional/impulse control. The authors discuss strategies that may help guide organizations in designing functional teams that are complementary in terms of synergy and effectiveness based on individual member strengths, self-awareness, team-based collaboration, and value creation. Emphasis is placed on the importance of team approach in health-care leadership. The chapter on resilience in leadership then follows, with a discussion that greatly complements other contributions in the second volume of *The Fundamentals*.

Presentation on leadership in complex medical systems is another unique feature of the current book. Various aspects of systemic complexity are outlined, focusing on the critical impact of resource availability, as is often encountered in low-resource environments, and the closely associated concepts of social and economic welfare. This chapter also represents a valuable summation of our understanding how a successful executives carry out the institutional mission effectively under challenging – and often adverse – conditions. Moreover, the authors present various characteristics of resilient leaders.

Of note, a number of additional topics that are both important and unique are included in the current volume of *Fundamentals of Leadership for Healthcare Professionals*. Throughout this book, the authors emphasize the importance of practical application of theory to promote leadership effectiveness. This includes demonstrations of how staying true to time-proven, fundamental ethical principles can make a leader more effective in facilitating successful organizational outcomes. Using these principles as one's guideposts will help ensure that a leader will remain true to self, his or her team(s), as well as the organization and its mission.

The Editors feel that is important to embrace more recent developments in health-care. For instance, a modern health-care leadership compendium would not be complete without mentioning some of the key technological advances that are shaping the future of medicine. Consequently, Volume 2 of *The Fundamentals* discusses the emergence of electronic medical records, including the change management associated with organizational implementations of such technological improvements.

Relevant to long-term viability of the entire health-care system is the educational infrastructure that trains future generations of medical and allied health professionals. Given the rapidly changing and increasingly challenging economic climate of health-care, our educational systems are experiencing significant financial stresses that threaten some of the smaller and less profitable schools of medicine and allied health. Of special concern is the maldistribution of educational resources, away from smaller communities and toward larger urban centers. To help address this problem, some academic medical centers are forming affiliations with larger, sometimes private institutions, in order to maintain financial viability. Such affiliations are discussed in the current volume of *The Fundamentals*.

Sustainability of a culture of safety in a health system is of utmost importance, especially when the increasingly competitive "pay for performance", value-driven paradigms come in direct conflict with existing (and often pervasive and long-standing) institutional cultures that are not sufficiently flexible to quickly adapt to these new realities. In this context, leadership vignettes are presented to help demonstrate how a culture of curiosity can improve the quality of care and enhance critical thinking. This is followed by a comparison of key safety aspects of aviation and cardiac surgery in order to highlight complexity and uncertainty in attempting to successfully avoid mishaps and create the level of perfection expected by the public. The aviation industry, long known for its emphasis on developing and encouraging a culture of safety, is providing an important "zero defect" blueprint for the health-care sector. In the current volume of *The Fundamentals*, the authors highlight the importance of

Introduction

xvii

translating the lessons of airline safety into sustainable culture of safety across our clinics, hospitals, and pharmacies.

Organizational design tends to be an overlooked, yet critically important aspect of institutional growth. In an excellent example of creative institutional leadership, the authors discuss the intricacies involved in setting up a hospice program at a large, university-based health network, and make the important point that an effective leader must actively engage and bring together governmental and private sector insurers, professional and regulatory organizations, as well as civic leaders to crystallize a clear and concise plan of providing optimal and sustainable care to an inherently vulnerable patient population.

Physicians and surgeons must be able to quickly and flexibly adapt to changing environments, and to effectively share their experiences across consecutive generations of health-care professionals. Of great importance to establishing leadership continuity will be the development and sustained presence of effective mentorship. In this particular content area, the authors discuss the critical importance of mentor-mentee relationship in the context of surgical training.

And lastly, a practical perspective on crisis leadership is presented. In modern health-care setting, a crisis can occur at any time – and the implications can be both substantial and unpredictable. Not only are lives at stake, but the reputation and financial stability of an institution can change with a singular event or an evolving problem that goes undetected, or worse yet – left unaddressed. Crisis management, a topic that can fill entire volumes, has unique nuances in the world of health-care. We are proud to incorporate a full chapter dedicated to this area in the current volume of *The Fundamentals*.

CONCLUDING REMARKS

The Editors and chapter authors hope that the second volume of *Fundamentals of Leadership for Healthcare Professionals* provides the reader with an expanded source of experiences, knowledge, and the corresponding practical considerations. It is our goal to continue this important health-care leadership book cycle well into the future, with the intent of expanding the content matter well beyond the foundational leadership topics and skills. The readers' input, feedback, and contributions are both welcome and valued. Our plans for upcoming volumes of *The Fundamentals* include "focus issues" that are dedicated to specific areas of health-care leadership across a broad range of topics, from human resource management to public speaking skills. The authors hope that the reader will find the material presented to be of value, and a basis for generating discussions among stakeholders as to what constitutes good and effective leadership in health-care.

In: Fundamentals of Leadership … ISBN: 978-1-53615-729-1
Editors: S. P. A. Stawicki et al. © 2019 Nova Science Publishers, Inc.

Chapter 1

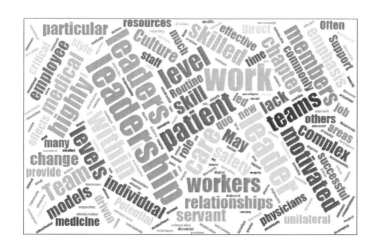

LEADERSHIP IN HEALTH-CARE: FROM THEORY TO PRACTICAL APPLICATION

Derek M. Tang[1], Ankita Bassi[2], Alec Gayner[2], Gregory S. Domer[3], Jay Fisher[3], Timothy Oskin[3], Michael S. Firstenberg[4], Thomas J. Papadimos[5] and Stanislaw P. A. Stawicki[2],*

[1]Medical School of Temple University / St. Luke's University Hospital Campus, Bethlehem, Pennsylvania, US
[2]Department of Research & Innovation, St. Luke's University Health Network, Bethlehem, Pennsylvania, US

---

* Stanislaw P. Stawicki, MD, MBA, FACS, FAIM; Chair & Network Medical Director of Department of Research & Innovation, St. Luke's University Hospital Campus, Bethlehem, Pennsylvania; E-mail: stanislaw.stawicki@sluhn.org; stawicki.ace@gmail.com.

[3]Heart & Vascular Center, St. Luke's University Health Network, Bethlehem, Pennsylvania, US
[4]Department of Surgery (Cardiovascular), The Medical Center of Aurora, Aurora, Colorado, US
[5]Department of Anesthesiology, The Ohio State University Wexner Medical Center, Columbus, Ohio, US

ABSTRACT

Effective leadership in a healthcare organization requires a practical approach supported by a sound theoretical basis. Successful organizations rely on efficient teamwork between individuals, divisions, and departments through communication and coordination that results in patient safety, high quality care, and, therein, trust in the healthcare system as a whole. However, healthcare in the early 21st century has a conundrum, a paucity of high quality leaders. While leadership does not require a specific position or title, it does require certain qualities in an individual, an appropriate style of leadership for a particular situation, and an understanding of an organization's phase of growth in order to foster the knowledge and skills required for dynamic institutional change. Recruiting a good leader (from the organization's perspective) or acquiring a leadership position (from an individual's perspective) requires successful navigation of the interview process and an understanding as to where the organization is in regard to its phase of growth. Once in place, the ultimate test to a leader and the organization, will involve behavioral challenges in the workplace where negligent hiring, retention, and promotion of employees unsuitable for specific roles continues to be a problem. Here we highlight the important application of competent and practical leadership that leads to the necessary patient outcomes and quality of care that will take an organization from acceptable to exceptional.

1. INTRODUCTION

Health-care delivery paradigms continue to evolve at a rapid pace, with new approaches to care, dynamically changing patient expectations, and highly complex value-quality relationships [1-3]. Of paramount importance within this fluid environment are the growing importance of team approaches and the multidisciplinary nature of modern health-care models [4, 5]. Patient management paradigms have grown reliant on teamwork that closely integrates disciplines including but not limited to nursing, primary care and specialty physicians, social workers, pharmacists, occupational and physical therapists, administrative experts, and many others [4, 6]. With the presence of increasingly complex levels of cumulative expertise across diverse and interrelated domains, it is critical that the responsibility for accountability and effective communication is preserved [7-9]. The continuum of team-based care also introduces the challenges associated with facilitating the development of efficient and well-structured networks in hospital and clinic settings, including the presence of providers and staff from various disciplines and educational environments [9-11]. The overall magnitude of such challenges is evidenced by the persistence of medical error among the leading causes of death in the U.S. [12]. Coupled with the finding that approximately 80% of medical error can be attributed to teamwork failure [13, 14], the need for more refined health-care leadership cannot be understated.

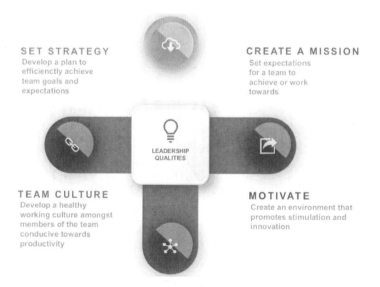

Figure 1. Several key attributes that are essential for effective leadership in a team-based setting.

The changing environment of modern health-care prompted numerous institutions to focus on developing universal measures to improve both quality and safety of patient care, as well as the associated leadership competencies [15, 16]. For example, the Institute of Medicine highlights six measures designed to improve healthcare systems, including patient safety, effectiveness, timeliness, efficiency, equity, and focus on the patient [17]. Recent exploration of organizational culture, team dynamics, and leadership has revealed that topics such as communication and coordination still require significant improvements to not only provide safer and higher quality care, but also strengthen patient trust in the health-care system as a whole [16, 18]. This is further compounded by the fact that many providers report a lack of exposure to leadership experiences and positions during their medical training [19-22].

Historically, health-care decisions regarding patient management have been dictated at the individual level, forging not only the way care is delivered but also how it is perceived within an organizational culture [23, 24]. Driven by the well-intended desire to provide exceptional patient care, this paradigm has unintentionally led to the emergence of the so-called "blame culture" rather than much more effective communication and collaboration strategies [25, 26]. Among the most important contributors to the modern health-care conundrum is the paucity of high quality leaders, especially those with adequate understanding of both medical and operational aspects of running a contemporary medical institution [16, 27, 28]. Moreover, quantitative research into successful leadership attributes and their applications within medicine still lags behind [19], with other high-stakes, high-performance fields such as the military, aviation, and finance actively cultivating and adopting evidence-based leadership approaches into everyday practice [29, 30]. Despite vast differences in subject matter, commonly accepted, shared principles associated with high quality leadership continue to have substantial utility across modern health-care settings (Figure 1).

Leadership does not necessarily require a specific title or position within an organization. Consequently, it can be defined as one's ability to generate constructive influence at any level of an organization, from grassroots initiatives to major strategic realignments [16]. The terms "managing up" and "managing down" contain an implied understanding that leadership is synonymous with a significant degree of flexibility from leaders, and that leadership is not confined to the executive suite [16, 31]. Versatility in management skills, which will be discussed throughout this book, has become mandatory in the perpetually evolving modern health-care environment. As our health-care systems transform into leaner, much more efficient entities, lessons from the past should guide our understanding of what is absolutely critical to organizational success – dramatic increase in collaborative cross-communication as opposed to instituting mutual accountability for actions or processes that may not always be communicated effectively [31].

Empiric experience strongly suggests that improving patient care and outcomes begins at the level of individual treatment teams [32]. Yet those teams rely on unconditional support from upper management to execute their goals and objectives [33]. Consequently, the overall leadership culture within a particular organization can largely be derived from leadership traits embraced by upper management, especially when goals and visions are embraced by all stakeholders [33-36]. Conversely, suboptimal leadership at top levels of management can yield varying and often unpredictable degrees of efficacy with respect to administration at the individual team and departmental levels [33, 37, 38]. What may ultimately result is the potential for exacerbation of preexisting problems within areas or teams responsible for the practical implementation of organizational plans [39, 40]. One way of fostering constructive change within health-care institutions is the eight-step process of change described by Kotter [41]. Under such paradigm, established comfort zones (e.g., areas of institutional "complacency") are deconstructed, guiding coalitions are formed, vision(s) is/are created, teams are empowered to act on the vision, improvements are incrementally consolidated, and change is embraced and institutionalized into new approaches [31, 41].

This second volume of *Fundamentals of Leadership for Healthcare Professionals*, a reflection of the success of the first volume [16], will provide a broader perspective on key aspects of health-care leadership, highlighting both favorable and deleterious qualities of individuals, teams, and institutions. The qualities that define a successful leader are both nuanced and broad-ranging. However, there exists a definable set of fundamental characteristics that each leader should embrace, regardless of what position they occupy or organization they serve. These transcendental qualities and traits are covered in this chapter and throughout this book cycle. While health-care leadership presents its own challenges, most qualities that identify a successful leader in business apply to medicine and related fields. This collected work represents an aggregation of ideas from sociology, medicine, and published experiences that cumulatively demonstrate key attributes and help construct a primer for those wishing to pursue a career in health-care leadership. Our discussion will begin with an overview of the qualities of a successful leader, followed by a review of primary leadership styles and characteristics. We will then touch upon some of the less commonly discussed, but equally important aspects of health-care leadership, such as leader interviews.

2. QUALITIES OF A SUCCESSFUL LEADER

2.1. Sincere Enthusiasm

Often forgotten in the minute-to-minute complexities and multiple tasks associated with a leadership position is the importance of genuine interest and passion for the assignment [42, 43]. Motivation (or lack thereof) tends to be contagious across organizations [44]. When the leader is motivated to improve the quality of the institution, their enthusiasm becomes a critical tool that helps generate the required momentum to create an environment conducive of achieving both individual and team goals [45, 46]. An unmotivated or apathetic leader will be less likely to maintain the required level of intensity within an organization, may foster underachievement, and can ultimately prove to be a detriment to the institution [47, 48]. More importantly, beyond the extroverted, "surface level" enthusiasm and projected confidence, a leader's motivation must be genuine [49, 50]. The leader's authenticity becomes apparent very quickly to their team and the institution, with manifestations of self-less (versus selfish) behaviors, and the ability to stand up for "what's right" whilst knowing that there will be some disagreement and/or complaints [51, 52]. An apathetic leader is content with the *status quo*, comfortable at maintaining the level the institution is currently at, whereas a truly motivated leader is constantly looking for constructive change and genuine betterment [53, 54].

2.2. Excellent Communication Skills

The way a leader communicates with both their teams and top organizational management is of critical importance [33, 55]. Inherent to the top-down structure of the vast majority of companies, most leaders are not "the tip of the hierarchy" and are much more likely to have other managers within their so-called "reporting chain", thus relying on others to effectively execute the intended organizational strategy [56, 57]. Consequently, most leaders are the direct bridge between upper level management and their employees [58, 59]. Thus, the leader must communicate the meaning and the impact of any large scale projects or institutional changes in terms of each department's responsibilities and operations, while also relating back employee issues or feedback to upper management [60-62]. The key and foundation to any successful communication is bilateral (or multilateral) respect among parties that participate in dialogue. A leader must show a degree of deference to his or her supervisor(s) to demonstrate respect for organizational hierarchy [63, 64]. At the same time, he or she must also be able to bring difficult issues to the attention of their supervisors, even when such communication might contain difficult topic(s) [63-65]. When communicating with their teams, leaders must show utmost respect for others, especially when relaying messages of those that report to them in a way that is non-judgmental, accurate and appropriately prioritized [66, 67]. A leader should be highly proficient at listening to staff in addition to communicating tasks that need to be completed or given priority. At the same time, the leader must be flexible and adaptable, maintaining the same relationship with their direct supervisors, listening to their requests and direction, while communicating problems, concerns and goals to their teams and individual team members [68-70].

2.3. Networking

Networking for leaders means creating trust-based symbiotic and synergistic relationships with others, both within the organization and externally, including teams, peers, as well as senior leaders [71, 72]. One's peers tend to have similar interests and goals, which facilitates sharing of ideas, coaching, and other forms of productive collaboration [73-75]. Collaboration with peers is a simple and intuitive idea, but tends to be underutilized across most professional communities, including health-care leadership [75-77]. Just as physicians and provider teams collaborate when approaching difficult diagnoses, leaders should embrace peer-to-peer collaboration on issues of interest to all stakeholders, thus allowing different perspectives to amalgamate into a productive solution [78-80]. Forming relationships with more senior leadership furthers a manager's reach within the organization; each senior leader provides unique experience-based wisdom and guidance [81, 82]. Senior leaders have more than likely been in the position (or situation) the manager may be in, and can offer valuable insight that one may not be able to readily obtain from others within the institution [82-84]. Further, a relationship with senior leadership is imperative for future projects and organizational value creation. Extramural networking is equally important and provides an excellent opportunity for managers and leaders to share information, create strategic collaborations, and foster inter-institutional partnerships [85-87].

2.4. Self-Awareness

Self-awareness is essential to success in leadership. As one advances through the organization, on must learn to reflect on one's feelings, thoughts, and actions, recognizing his or her own opportunities for improvement, and forming a team of trusted advisors who will support him or her through constructive and honest feedback [88-90]. A leader should be in a constant state of introspection, analyzing where they excel, what they need to work on, and who they should recruit to make a more complete and effective team [91-93]. This is especially applicable at the highest levels of leadership – the knowledge of self, as well as the acute awareness of various "blind spots" greatly increases the leader's effectiveness and credibility [94-97]. Further, a leader should always provide honest and unrestricted feedback to the institutional leadership in areas of significant expertise, especially when organizational well-being could be at stake [98, 99]. A seasoned leader must be willing to put their hand up, and communicate difficult issues so that the institution can be best prepared to tackle any potential crises and other challenges [100-102]. Finally, it may be better for all stakeholders to allow others to take over as a leader under certain scenarios, such as in situations where unforeseen personal or organizational circumstances render the current leader ineffective [103, 104].

2.5. Flexibility

Flexibility is a required (and expected) characteristic for leaders, especially in the health-care sector [105, 106]. It is imperative that leaders in medicine remain open to new ideas, innovations, adapt to new circumstances, and are able to relate across different personality styles [89, 107]. A "hard-headed", stubborn leader is unlikely to garner sufficient support from his or her team, and their actions/behaviors may put a ceiling on new ideas and/or collaborations [108-110]. It is critical for leaders to understand that even small change or idea may have a disproportionate effect on members of his or her team, or across the entire organization [111, 112]. In this way a leader may see an idea as a small, beneficial change, but a team member downstream will perceive its implementation as a very drastic change in their day-to-day functioning [112, 113]. At the same time, the downstream team member stands to benefit from a flexible leader who is willing to hear and consider the employee's concerns, work together on mutually beneficial solutions, and minimizing any unintended impacts of institutional change [114, 115].

2.6. Decisiveness

It is important for health-care leaders to be open to new ideas and accommodate different perspectives, but a leader's job is to make the final decision [116-118]. Not infrequently, a leader is tasked with deciding or choosing between competing – or even outright conflicting – paths or projects [119, 120]. So while a leader should be flexible, they must also be able to "put their foot down" and make crucial decisions with confidence. A "wishy-washy" leader that constantly vacillates between paths for the institution doesn't command confidence and can create a confusing work environment [121, 122].

2.7. Loyalty and Integrity

It is well known that institutions value employees who demonstrate high levels of loyalty [123]. The same can be said about leaders and their teams. For example, loyalty between a leader and their team, especially when facing adversity, serves to demonstrate that someone "has their backs" [69, 124-127]. Under such circumstances, team members feel safe, protected, and consider their leader trustworthy. When a department feels like a well-functioning team, it facilitates productive conversation without fear of rejection or punishment from upper leadership [127-129]. Open conversation opens the door for constructive change and allows the leader to keep their finger on the pulse of their team. Additionally, a leader with integrity repeatedly proves to team members that what is said can be equated with what is meant, and vice-versa. Furthermore, the team is more likely to observe that the leader presents one attitude around them and another to other groups, thus feeling more confident that "what they see is what they get". Loyal and highly ethical leaders are those whose actions project trust, not only in their leadership, but also within the organization [130-132].

2.8. Persistence

One of the most important qualities of a good leader is a relentless drive to accomplish goals and implement a vision [133, 134]. Such persistence, when coupled with team vision and institutional support, can produce truly impressive results [45, 135, 136]. It has been reported that as many as 40% of newly appointed executives fail in the first 18 months [137, 138]. The message is clear – although long-term vision and goals are important, a newly appointed leader should not neglect to focus on short-term "wins", building team morale, and foster mission-critical individual and group confidence [139]. Of course, this does not mean that one should blindly commit to new ideas or distractions without retro-/introspection. Rather, one must balance short- and long-term objectives by maintaining persistent focus on long-term initiatives while creating organizational traction and building momentum [140-142].

3. MODELS/STYLES OF LEADERSHIP

As with other areas of organizational life, the "one-size-fits-all" model does not apply to leadership. Companies tend to take on specific "behavioral characteristics" that reflect their leaders' approach to team building, coordination, and motivation. These leadership styles have been studied extensively, with a number of specific patterns that emerge as a result of social scientific inquiry [143-145]. Our subsequent discussion will outline major leadership models/styles, with a corresponding summary in Table 1. To provide an orderly overview, we have organized items in an alphabetical fashion.

Table 1. Overview of contemporary leadership models/styles

Style	Description	Characteristics	Pitfalls
Authoritarian (autocratic)	Unilateral communication and direct supervision of team members with sole emphasis on efficiency to achieve a specific goal	Routine work that is static in nature (i.e., does not require innovation or change in direction) or emergency situations	May create a climate of fear within the team; Discourages motivation; High employee turnover
Democratic (participative)	Shared decision-making between leaders and team members with guidance from leaders	Goals that require innovation and increased team morale to enhance productivity; Members are eager to discuss and share resources	Can be associated with wasted resources and/or incomplete or abandoned projects
Laissez-Faire (delegative)	Decisions made largely by individual team members. Leaders provide resources and guidance when requested	Highly skilled, trusted, and motivated workers	Requires consistent feedback to team members; Well suited for highly skilled/motivated groups/members
Paternalistic	Culture of work built on close, personal relationships to establish trust and increase productivity	Team members are able to communicate and work together seamlessly in and out of the work environment. Useful in projects that require long-term commitments	Difficult to maintain in work climate of high-turnover or better opportunities; Tension between workers with perceptions of others being favored
Servant	An ideology which places emphasis on the success of employees/followers	Useful in building and attracting highly skilled and motivated individuals through brand awareness and appreciation of staff	Requires investment in time and resources to build; May not be optimal for company or team undergoing change
Situational	A model based on the ability to transition between leadership styles based on employee willingness and skill level	Situations with dynamic levels of employee skill and motivation	Requires leaders with experience and ability to quickly adapt to multiple leadership styles
Transactional	Productivity driven by rewards and punishment	Routine work with areas for improved productivity by means of extrinsic motivation	See "Authoritarian"
Transformational (charismatic)	Works to improve or innovate upon pre-existing work models. Not fixated on maintaining *status quo*	Work that requires innovation and new strategies for progression	Can adversely embolden leaders; Potential for decreased productivity

3.1. Authoritarian

Also known as autocratic, this style of leadership is often described as the prototypical leadership model imagined by many, and is defined by a clear distinction between leader supervision and their subordinates bounded by strictly professional relationships [144]. Perhaps more pragmatic in nature, authoritarian leaders place priority on organizational and process efficiency. Communication within this leadership modality tends to be primarily unidirectional, with leaders taking a supervisory role over followers. Control and decision-making capabilities are commonly restricted to the leadership role and are not subject to flexibility or negotiation [146-148]. Consequently, some studies have found that this particular leadership style may be associated with a climate of fear and abuse amongst workers, with associated high employee turnover and low morale/motivation [149, 150]. Despite having an overall predilection for adverse workplace culture, this leadership style's priority on efficiency and inopportunity for dissent often make it beneficial in crisis or emergency situations [151].

3.2. Democratic

Also termed participative, this leadership approach is grounded in shared decision-making processes between leaders and their teams/followers [152, 153]. While leadership roles still assume responsibility for any final team decisions, many members within an organization provide input before any final determination is made [154-156]. Priority and status as the leader are de-emphasized within this style of leadership, primarily in an attempt to foster trust between managers, their peers, and working teams in general [157]. Characterized by participatory decision-making, democratic leadership shares many benefits common to both transformational and transactional leadership approaches [158, 159]. Specifically, this approach places emphasis on creativity and promotes a culture that aims to incorporate all members of a team towards decisions and achieving goals [160, 161]. Social equality is a cornerstone of the democratic leadership approach and requires a great deal of respect, transparency and fairness in the leader-team interaction [162, 163]. Efforts to create an environment that makes key stakeholders feel valued and supports their full engagement toward shared goals and strategy can be a powerful motivator of productivity, well beyond financial compensation and other traditional factors [164-166]. In addition to increasing efficiency and productivity, such environments have been shown to also foster improved team morale and individual skill set development [166-168]. Unlike some of the other leadership styles, democratic leadership may not be best suited in situations that are time-sensitive or call for crisis management. Because shared decision making processes require time – and sometimes a prolonged dialogue – projects may be at risk of stalling or abandonment [169-171].

3.3. Laissez-Faire

This type of leadership, roughly translating to "let do", is also identified by some authors as delegative leadership [172, 173]. Leaders who utilize this technique relinquish many of the managerial aspects of their formal title, leaving decision making largely at the discretion of the follower(s) [174]. The work place is governed by near complete autonomy although laissez-faire leaders also make effort to be available when necessary. Leaders provide resources necessary for task or goal achievement, while management and decision-making are considered secondary roles. Occasional oversight of individual performance with guided input from leadership positions can often increase productivity without the need for micromanagement [175]. Self-governance can be both an advantage and disadvantage for a leader who employs the laissez-faire approach, and is largely dependent on the skill set and motivation of members within the team/working group. Consequently, team members working under laissez-fire leader should optimally be experienced, flexible, and adept at their craft while also holding a strong sense of self-motivation. Such character qualities must also be associated with a sense of mutual trust between the leader and his/her team to ensure efficient performance. Teams that lack individual members with such attributes are likely to falter, which may be further compounded in the presence of a leader who does not provide timely feedback to the group [176, 177]. Of note, a laissez-faire leadership pattern may also emerge in the setting of a leader who lacks the charisma or managerial skills to effectively build authority or respect over staff, usually resulting in poor outcomes [105, 144].

3.4. Paternalistic Leadership

As implied by the name, paternalistic leadership aims to instill a family-like dynamic in the workplace, primarily by leader-follower conduct similar to that of a parent-child relationship [178-180]. Desired endpoints of the paternalistic relationship include absolute trust, full commitment to the leader's vision, with only limited and very controlled dissent from followers [179-181]. A successful leader using this particular approach will have the ability to create strong bonds with employees, resulting in lasting commitment and decreased rates of turnover within a team [182, 183]. The presence of a personal bond means that team dynamics often extend beyond the professional workplace, and into the personal lives of leaders and followers alike. One potentially deleterious byproduct of paternalistic leadership is the potential for actual or perceived favoritism and the creation of "in-groups" consisting of employees who are "more loyal" to their leader than those in the "out-group" [184, 185]. While paternalistic leaders require the charisma necessary to navigate the complexity of multiple employee relationships, it is also imperative they hold organizational prowess and technical credibility. Finally, one must note that contemporary workplaces are less amenable to paternalistic leadership styles given the inherently higher rates of turnover across many industries, including health-care. This is because over the past few decades employees became much less inclined to engage in commitments inherent to the paternalistic leader-follower dynamic, and thus much more likely to seek better opportunities elsewhere. As a consequence, the paternalistic leadership model is becoming more isolated to smaller companies and/or teams [186].

3.5. Servant Leadership

In a way, this type of leadership follows a similar philosophy to both democratic and transformational leaderships, and may well represent a natural evolution of the latter two styles [187-189]. One differentiating tenet of the servant leader is the emphasis on importance of "the other" as opposed to the self-centeredness and well-being of the leader or the company [190]. For the servant leader, his or her leadership role tends to be intentionally diminished in many capacities. The servant leader strives to provide employees with all necessary resources for success. Such dedication to employee (as well as customers) has several intended benefits, many of which are supported heavily by research [191, 192]. Both brand and external perceptions of the company tend to be superior for organizations that embrace the servant leadership approach. This, in turn has the positive by-product of attracting greater talent and reducing company turnover rates, especially so for highly skilled workers [193, 194]. It is therefore not surprising that servant leadership model is becoming more prominent given the aforementioned benefits. However, this approach to leading requires significant time and investment before the ultimate gains can be realized.

3.6. Situational Leadership

Leaders are not forced to remain within the confines of a single style of leadership, and many indeed choose to diversify their approaches based on specific circumstances, teams, employees or customers [195]. The situational leadership approach provides the leader with a diversified repertoire of responses that help facilitate customization and personalization of the professional interaction [196]. This is somewhat similar to the so-called distributed leadership, where the "distributed perspective" is based on the ease with which one can reconcile concepts and approaches simultaneously representing "many things to many people" [197]. Consequently, some of the most effective leaders become experts in adopting certain leadership approaches in accordance with the needs of a particular situation [198, 199]. Because the situational leadership model does not endorse a unified approach or style, it is defined by the leader's willingness to be fluid in one's leadership approach, adapting (a.k.a., "flexing") readily to the environment or culture of work at hand [199, 200]. Originally introduced as the "life cycle theory of leadership", Hersey and Blanchard developed a model that placed emphasis on fluidity as a leader [196]. Within this theoretical paradigm, leadership approaches were governed by the situation, skillset and engagement of the workforce, as well as the characteristics of the task at hand. Based on these parameters, leaders may choose to utilize highly individualized approaches that are optimized to the particular situation:

Direct: Employees lack skill but are engaged and willing to contribute/work;
Coach: Employees are mildly skilled but lack engagement;
Support: Employees are highly skilled but lack confidence or willingness to work;
Delegate: Employees are both highly skilled and engaged/willing to work.

Because of the shifting nature required to navigate this leadership role, it takes significant experience as a leader across multiple styles to effectively enforce [196, 201].

3.7. Transactional Leadership

This type of leadership shares some of the attributes held by autocratic leaders, albeit to a somewhat lesser extent [202, 203]. Sustaining the *status quo* in terms of organizational structure and performance is often the main objective of a transactional leader [203, 204]. Similar to the more autocratic analogues, this method of leadership is defined by direct supervision of subordinate performance to identify areas of error or deviation (e.g., opportunity for improvement) as a means to increase productivity towards a static goal [205, 206]. As implied by the nomenclature, this category of leadership is driven by immediate reward (or punishment) as it relates to productivity. In contrast with autocratic leadership, transactional approaches allow for increased efficiency towards primary endpoints through simultaneous use of extrinsic motivators (i.e., rewards) with established routines and fairly rigidly set rules [207, 208]. Transactional approaches also tend to be most relevant to, and effective in, situations of crisis. *Bureaucratic leadership* follows suit in many aspects where stringent enforcement of rules and boundaries are applied meticulously to individual worker and/or team routine. This style of leading is often reserved for occupations that involve significant safety precautions (e.g., the handling of hazardous materials in a laboratory or industrial setting) [176, 209, 210].

3.8. Transformational Leadership

Charisma is the image the leader projects toward people around them, both within the organization and externally, encompassing management and team members alike [211, 212]. While it is important for the leader to be respected, the presence of charisma goes "beyond respect" and establishes a deeper (e.g., emotional) bond between the leader and his/her followers [88, 213, 214]. In his book, *Give and Take*, Adam Grant presents three management styles, one of which is given the monomer "giver" [215, 216]. A giver selflessly offers their time and energy without expecting anything in return. In turn staff and peers feel compelled, on their own, to work to their fullest potential for the leader. Thus, a kind, courteous, supportive, and understanding leader passively demands the best from their staff without the need to be an authoritarian.

Leadership in Health-Care 19

A work culture defined by innovation and dynamic growth mandates transformational, or charismatic, leaders. Such leaders are able to motivate their followers so as to instill a sense of "greater purpose" and generate strong inspiration amongst advocates. Schultz and Schultz [207] delineate transformational leaders with the following three attributes:

Willingness to take risk and use unconventional strategies to spark inventive thinking;
Stimulation of followers intellectually;
Individualized relationships with followers.

Charismatic leadership not only can be associated with enhanced organizational productivity, but often the ability to surpass stated expectations. However, teams governed using this type of leadership run the risk of ruin as the personality of the leader often serves as a pillar of confidence with respect to the organization itself. Furthermore, because this leadership style mandates bold personalities, follower discord can appear unpredictably, and quickly result in intra-organizational conflict and subsequent collapse [217, 218].

4. LEADERSHIP RECRUTEMENT: THE CRITICAL IMPORTANCE OF THE INTERVIEW PROCESS

Although internal development of top talent within organizations is very important, it is neither possible nor advisable to replace every leader with internally promoted candidates [219-221]. When evaluating external talent for potential leadership roles within an institution, the interview process takes on a critical role. After all, bringing in a new manager/leader carries significant risks that an organization may not be willing (or able) to undertake [221, 222].

Interview preparation is a vital part of the process, both for the organization and the leadership candidate. Mutually important, prior research by all stakeholders not only demonstrates good intentions and openness, but also establishes a solid foundation from which to build mutual understanding. Key participants should consider reviewing pertinent information/materials (e.g., curriculum vitae, financial reports, internet-based info, third-party experiences, etc.); planning questions based on this research; and brainstorm ways in which potential synergies can be created. Both parties should be honest and transparent in terms of disclosing other potentially competing offers.

From an institution's perspective, most will avoid hiring someone who is not informed regarding the business, goals and objectives, or the organization's impact on the greater community. Lack of preparation may make the interviewee appear disengaged. Likewise, perceived lack of interest from the institution may come across as insincere. An organization will likely be looking for an employee who is informed, active, and enthusiastic about bettering the company's future, especially in a leadership position. Finally, one must keep in mind that among the principal characteristics of an effective leader are integrity and preparation. Preparing for an interview, good knowledge of relevant background information, and demonstration of high integrity all help increase the odds that the interviewee becomes highly desirable from an institution's perspective.

4.1. Researching the Organization

Conducting research on the company and its mission is a crucial step in interview preparation. One should approach the interview process with a clear understanding of the business model, which includes the ability to anticipate relevant questions and/or concerns. Among the simplest ways to gather information is through an online search. Another source of "must know" relevant and important information is the company's website. Most company websites feature their mission statement, product(s), team(s), etc.

To further one's research, one can review press releases from the company or review articles written about the company. Additionally, to gain a better understanding of the organization's relationships within its market niche, one can review information about local, regional, and national competitors. This may highlight important differences between the institution one is interviewing with, and similar locally active business entities. Of importance, when researching the organization, one must ensure that sources being consulted are credible. Misinformation regarding the institution can be quite damaging, not only to the company but also to the interviewee, who may come across as inappropriate or ill prepared, especially in the context of a leadership position.

When interviewing for a leadership position, it is also vital to be able to concisely present how exactly one expects to lead in a manner that contributes to the fulfillment of the institution's mission. Knowing the organization's historical background can also be beneficial, and the interviewee will be wise to comment on the institution's accomplishments and points of pride. At the same time, one should either request (or attempt to find) recent company-specific information for insight on current performance and projected growth. If possible, the interviewee should prepare a brief conceptual plan to present to the interviewer demonstrating their previous research while also offering/proposing some innovative ideas. Demonstrating that one has taken time to learn about the organization is a great way to make a good impression, provided that any information or recommendations are both accurate and synergistic. It can also be beneficial to become familiar with the interviewer and their role in the institution before the interview. This information is often listed on the company's website, including both the professional title/position and the scope of responsibilities. Additionally, publically accessible professional social media pages (e.g., LinkedIn [223, 224]) may be great sources to learn more about key individuals and their qualifications, while also noting any connections in common. Taken together, the above measures help demonstrate that as a leader, the interviewee will strive to direct the team toward more successes.

Along with collecting information on the institution and its mission, it is also necessary to analyze the specific job position one is applying for. If asked, "Why should you be picked for this position?", one must have a sufficient understanding of the associated duties/responsibilities. While answering this question, character traits and ideas that exemplify the position's requirements must be included. Whilst analyzing the job description, one must also evaluate their own strengths and weaknesses to see if they align with the scope of the position. If the interviewee perceives specific skill or knowledge deficiency in one area, she or he should clearly indicate that they might need assistance in that particular domain for some time before taking charge on their own. A reasonable institution will not expect someone to fulfill every single responsibility tasked to the job position, especially in highly complex areas of leadership. It is recognized that it is better to hire someone that is open about their strengths (and weaknesses) and provide adequate assistance, than expecting unreasonable levels of performance and thus risking systemic failure [225].

It is also essential to examine the hierarchy of the institution and to determine where the open position would fit in the company's organization. For a leadership position, it is imperative to not only familiarize oneself with other leaders in the institution, but also to become aware of all the other strata of reporting within the company's hierarchy. Familiarity with the tasks and jobs throughout the entire reporting structure puts into perspective the type of leadership that will need to be exercised [226, 227]. Furthermore, it is vital to not only understand the tasks of other leaders, but also the tasks of key teams/functional units. Armed with such knowledge, one can interweave one's ideas and creativity into the conversation as he or she answers the interviewer's questions. From an institution's perspective, a leader that realizes the impact he or she has on the entire company's hierarchy, truly represents what it means to be a leader.

Questions are an inevitable aspect of an interview. However, an interview is a two-sided event. Not only is the institution trying to see if the candidate is suitable for the team, but in return, one also must ask pertinent questions regarding the company. To seem engaged and enthusiastic about the position, one should also bring appropriate questions to ask the interviewer based on the collected research. These questions can be about the position advertised, your future boss, or the company. More vague and broader questions can be asked towards the end to leave the interviewer with a strong lasting impression. Questions about current management can be asked. This would demonstrate both engagement and good understanding of the company, especially when interviewing for a leadership position. Yes or no questions should be avoided, as well as questions that can easily be answered by taking a look at the company's website. Also, it is a better idea to avoid personal questions (e.g., salary, health insurance, vacation time, etc.) during this stage. A big part of being a leader is thinking about the whole team. Thus, questions should be aimed around the idea of how to create synergies for the company and how to manage and motivate the whole team to work towards a specific goal (or set of objectives) [228]. One has to keep in mind that relatively detailed questions are more likely to be asked during leadership interviews. For example, many institutions ask applicants what they *would do* versus what they *previously did*. Asking these types of questions will be more likely to reveal the interviewee's important personality or behavior traits while prompting him or her to think fast when facing a specific situation – a trait that is highly valued by institutions [229]. Most interview questions for prospective leaders look for soft skills in candidates that may reflect their leadership styles. Soft skills reflect one's behavior/personality rather than credentials [230, 231]. These scenario type questions can range from all aspects of leadership to collaboration – how would one manage a team to achieve goals, motivate their coworkers, approach challenges and conflicts, and reach decisions. Questions could highlight a variety of personality traits, including, but not limited to, motivation, delegation, communication, and integrity [232]. Below is a list of sample leadership interview questions asked to candidates [232]:

Two employees left from your team just before the deadline on a big project. How would you change your leadership style to meet the deadline?

How do you monitor the performance of individual team members?

In what specific ways do you motivate your team?

How do you make decisions about the compensation of team members?

How would you describe your leadership style?

Another important aspect of preparing oneself for an interview would be to either experience the services, product(s) or other output(s) the institution provides or interact with others that have had the experience. This can be done by speaking with others or reading reviews online about the experiences. One should note both the positives and negatives found in such reviews. During the interview, the positives should be stressed, while the negatives can be briefly mentioned as having the potential to be improved. Lastly, necessary documents should be gathered to bring along on the day of the interview. Although for a leadership position most attention will be focused on interviewee's soft skills, it is still a good idea to bring along a couple extra copies of the resume. Additionally, a list of references, with name and contact information, is also helpful for the institution.

5. Phases of Organizational Growth: What "Gets us There" Depends on Circumstances

One of the most critical aspects of effective leadership is the understanding that the knowledge and skills required to succeed at different phases of organizational growth change dynamically [206]. In fact, distinct phases of sequential growth have been described, depending on the overall maturity of an organization [233]. This paradigm appears to apply to both institutions and individual departments/units within institutions. Newly founded organizations or departments/units tend to grow through creativity, with the introduction of novel protocols and procedures, as well as a great deal of simultaneous organizational learning

[206, 233]. This phase tends to end with the so-called "crisis of leadership" whereby the owner takes control, creating potential problems and constraints.

The second phase of organizational development is called "growth through direction" and follows the "crisis of leadership" [233]. Here, a new senior leadership team takes responsibility for directing the company's strategy and existing managers assume more functional (rather than leadership) responsibilities. Predictably, this growth phase tends to end with the so-called "crisis of autonomy" associated with tensions between the new top management and existing managerial staff [234].

The third phase of growth is termed "growth through delegation" and emerges as a response to the "crisis of autonomy" [206, 235]. The associated institutional behavior includes the gradual delegation of authority to lower-level managers across all functions and linking their management performance to pre-defined, contribution-reward incentive structures [206]. This, in turn, enables each department or unit to expand more rapidly and to fulfill both own and organizational needs more nimbly. However, almost inevitably various levels of management end up in mutual competition for control and resources, resulting in the so-called "crisis of control" [235].

The most common way to solve this problem is through re-establishing a more optimal balance between centralized control and decentralized functions [236]. This new regime, called "growth through coordination" entails the top management taking on the role of coordinating various divisions and motivating managers to take a companywide perspective. However, as we evolve into other stages of organizational growth, another crisis typically emerges. For this phase of growth, the typical hurdle is called "crisis of red tape" and results from management's failure to coordinate increasingly complex processes [206].

When organizations reach the "crisis of red tape" phase, critical decisions must be made regarding the subsequent course of action, with options ranging from restructuring of established units to divestment of areas that are not critical to the company's core business [237, 238]. Regardless of what course of action is taken, the most important aspect of any change is the need for ongoing planned process of change as a means of improving the organization's effectiveness in achieving its goals through appropriate problem solving and hardwired self-improvement cycles [239]. A wise leader will follow others' advice, collect required information, synthesize the best available evidence, and then act in accordance with organizational success and well-being [101, 240].

6. BEHAVIORAL CHALLENGES IN THE WORKPLACE: THE ULTIMATE LEADERSHIP TEST

It has been once said that one is not a proven leader until one has effectively mastered the art of managing individuals with significant behavioral issues [241-243]. Although admittedly the most effective way of preventing problems that arise with the so-called "problem employees" is screening during the interview process, no approach or system is perfect in this regard [244, 245]. Within this broader context, negligent hiring, retention, and promotion of employees who are not suitable for a specific role, continues to be a significant problem [244-246]. Given the emphasis on technical competencies, employers are more likely to find themselves onboarding and ultimately supporting a category of managers/leaders who have previously been termed "technical tyrants" [247]. These individuals are exceedingly good at various technical aspects of their work, but their inability to be flexible or to effectively lead others results in stifled employee/team growth and development, and may eventually lead to the emergence of a hostile work environment [247]. An associated finding of a toxic leader may be the presence of the so-called "dark triad" of Machiavellianism, narcissism, and psychopathy [248, 249]. Workplace bullying is among the most prominent signs of a toxic leader, often combined with deferential treatment of superiors and derogatory treatment of peers and subordinates [250]. It is critical for organizations to identify difficult employees early, to institute appropriate corrective action(s) and to provide ample opportunity/support for positive change, and then appropriately re-assign or transition such individuals out of their department or even the current organization, as indicated [250, 251].

On the opposite side of the spectrum, employees with excellent interpersonal skills, but little to no technical (e.g., "hard") skills, can also represent a challenge to organizations [252]. Although such individuals are less likely to contribute to a toxic workplace, their lack of technical knowledge or skills can be frustrating to those around them. Consequently, employers should quickly identify what skills are needed, provide required training, and create a time-limited framework for either improvement or transitioning out of the department/organization [253].

CONCLUSION

Both literature and experience show that the health-care industry is a perpetually evolving field, mandating dynamic operational processes and improved methodological approaches to eliminate both active and latent factors associated with failure modes [12, 13, 15, 17]. The presence of excellent management and leadership is required to ensure proficient organizational function and excellent patient outcomes [19, 20, 254]. Consequently, health-care institutions must actively work to improve leadership through training, strengthening, and appropriate diversification [255]. This introductory chapter, as well as this second volume of *Fundamentals of Leadership for Healthcare Professionals,* are intended to highlight the importance and application of leadership in modern health-care, emphasizing the critical importance of focus on patient outcomes and quality of care. The health-care leadership journey starts with recruiting and rewarding the best and the brightest to join institutional teams, ensuring that appropriate technical skills and knowledge can be provided to those with excellent "soft skills" who desire to serve as compassionate and empathetic leaders of tomorrow.

REFERENCES

[1] Leebov, W. and M. Clara Jean Ersoz, *The health care manager's guide to continuous quality improvement.* 2003: iUniverse.

[2] Scheurer, D., et al., The value equation: enhancing patient outcomes while constraining costs. *The American journal of the medical sciences,* 2016. **351**(1): p. 44-51.

[3] Jones, P., *Design for care: Innovating healthcare experience.* 2013: Rosenfeld Media.

[4] Reeves, S., et al., *Interprofessional teamwork for health and social care.* Vol. 8. 2011: John Wiley & Sons.

[5] Drinka, T.J. and P.G. Clark, *Health care teamwork: Interdisciplinary practice and teaching.* 2000: Greenwood Publishing Group.

[6] Mitchell, P. and R. Golden, *Core principles & values of effective team-based health care.* 2012: National Academy of Sciences.

[7] Guirdham, M., *Communicating across cultures at work.* 2011: Macmillan International Higher Education.

[8] Rosen, B., A. Israeli, and S. Shortell, *Accountability and responsibility in health care: Issues in addressing an emerging global challenge.* 2012: World Scientific.

[9] Drinka, T.J. and P.G. Clark, *Healthcare Teamwork: Interprofessional Practice and Education: Interprofessional Practice and Education.* 2016: ABC-CLIO.

[10] Porter-O'Grady, T. and K. Malloch, *Evidence-Based Practice and the Innovation Paradigm: A Model for the Continuum of Practice Excellence.* Leadership for Evidence-Based Innovation in Nursing and Health Professions, 2016: p. 1.

[11] Fried, B., S. Topping, and A.C. Edmondson, *Teams and team effectiveness in health services organizations. Shortell and Kaluzny's Healthcare Management:* Organization Design and Behavior, 2011: p. 121.

[12] Makary, M.A. and M. Daniel, Medical error-the third leading cause of death in the US. *BMJ,* 2016. **353**: p. i2139.

[13] Joint Commission. *Sentinel event data: root causes by event type,* 2004-2015. 2016 [cited 2018 Nov 21]; Available from: https://www. jointcommission.org/ assets/ 1/ 18/ Root_ Causes_ by_ Event_ Type_2004-2015.pdf.

[14] Stawicki, S.P., et al., Natural history of retained surgical items supports the need for team training, early recognition, and prompt retrieval. *The American Journal of Surgery,* 2014. **208**(1): p. 65-72.

[15] Kohn, L.T., J. Corrigan, and M.S. Donaldson, *To err is human: building a safer health system.* 2000, Washington, D.C.: National Academy Press. xxi, 287 p.

[16] Stawicki, S.P.A. and M.S. Firstenberg, *Fundamentals of leadership for healthcare professionals.* 2018, New York: Nova Medicine & Health. xvii, 269 pages.

[17] Berwick, D.M., T.W. Nolan, and J. Whittington, The triple aim: care, health, and cost. *Health Aff (Millwood),* 2008. **27**(3): p. 759-69.

[18] Bisognano M, K.C., *Pursuing the Triple Aim: Seven Innovators Show the Way to Better Care, Better Health, and Lower Costs.* 2012, Somerset, New Jersey: John Wiley & Sons.

[19] Collins-Nakai, R., Leadership in medicine. *Mcgill J Med,* 2006. **9**(1): p. 68-73.

[20] Jefferies, R., et al., Leadership and management in UK medical school curricula. J Health Organ Manag, 2016. **30**(7): p. 1081-1104.

[21] Spurgeon, P., et al., Do we need medical leadership or medical engagement? *Leadersh Health Serv (Bradf Engl),* 2015. **28**(3): p. 173-84.

[22] Turner, A.D., S.P. Stawicki, and W.A. Guo, Competitive Advantage of MBA for Physician Executives: A Systematic Literature Review. *World journal of surgery,* 2018. **42**(6): p. 1655-1665.

[23] Emanuel, E.J. and L.L. Emanuel, Four models of the physician-patient relationship. *JAMA,* 1992. **267**(16): p. 2221-6.

[24] Kenney, C., *Transforming health care: Virginia Mason Medical Center's pursuit of the perfect patient experience.* 2016: Productivity Press.

[25] Armstrong, J.H., Leadership and team-based care. *Virtual Mentor,* 2013. **15**(6): p. 534-7.

[26] Manser, T., Teamwork and patient safety in dynamic domains of healthcare: a review of the literature. *Acta Anaesthesiol Scand,* 2009. **53**(2): p. 143-51.

[27] Reinertsen, J.L., Physicians as leaders in the improvement of health care systems. *Annals of Internal Medicine,* 1998. **128**(10): p. 833-838.

[28] Burns, J.P., Complexity science and leadership in healthcare. *Journal of Nursing Administration,* 2001. **31**(10): p. 474-482.

[29] QICT, F., *Doing What Counts for Patient Safety: Federal Actions to Reduce Medical Errors and their Impact.* 2000, US Department of Health and Human Services: Washington, DC.

[30] Stawicki, S., et al., *Fundamentals of patient safety in medicine and surgery.* 2014, New Delhi: Wolters Kluwer Health (India) Pvt Ltd.

[31] Ryan, J.J., *Strategy transformation and change: changing paradigms in Australian Catholic health and aged care.* 2001, Curtin University.

[32] McFadden KL, H.S., Gowen III CR., The patient safety chain: Transformational leadership's effect on patient safety culture, initiatives, and outcomes. *Journal of Operations Management,* 2009. **27**(5): p. 390-404.

[33] Hambrick, D.C. and P.A. Mason, Upper echelons: The organization as a reflection of its top managers. *Academy of management review,* 1984. **9**(2): p. 193-206.

[34] Krause, D.E., D. Gebert, and E. Kearney, Implementing process innovations: The benefits of combining delegative-participative with consultative-advisory leadership. *Journal of Leadership & Organizational Studies,* 2007. **14**(1): p. 16-25.

[35] Ogawa, R.T. and S.T. Bossert, Leadership as an organizational quality. *Educational administration quarterly,* 1995. **31**(2): p. 224-243.

[36] Edmondson, A., Psychological safety and learning behavior in work teams. *Administrative science quarterly,* 1999. **44**(2): p. 350-383.

[37] Hackman, J.R. and C.G. Morris, Group tasks, group interaction process, and group performance effectiveness: A review and proposed integration. *Advances in experimental social psychology,* 1975. **8**: p. 45-99.

[38] Schyns, B. and J. Schilling, How bad are the effects of bad leaders? A meta-analysis of destructive leadership and its outcomes. *The Leadership Quarterly,* 2013. **24**(1): p. 138-158.

[39] Shambach, S.A., *Strategic leadership primer.* 2004, Army War Coll Carlisle Barracks PA.

[40] Naseer, S., et al., Perils of being close to a bad leader in a bad environment: Exploring the combined effects of despotic leadership, leader member exchange, and perceived organizational politics on behaviors. *The Leadership Quarterly,* 2016. **27**(1): p. 14-33.

[41] Kotter, J.P., *Leading change: Why transformation efforts fail.* 1995.

[42] Boris-Schacter, S. and S. Langer, *Balanced leadership: How effective principals manage their work.* 2006: Teachers College Press.

[43] Davis, S., *Pearls of Leadership Wisdom: Lessons for Everyday Leaders.* 2012: BookBaby.

[44] Shapiro, A., *Creating contagious commitment: Applying the tipping point to organizational change.* 2010: Strategy Perspective.

[45] Katzenbach, J.R. and D.K. Smith, *The wisdom of teams: Creating the high-performance organization.* 2015: Harvard Business Review Press.

[46] Dutton, J.E., *Energize your workplace: How to create and sustain high-quality connections at work.* Vol. 50. 2003: John Wiley & Sons.

[47] Alderman, M.K., *Motivation for achievement: Possibilities for teaching and learning.* 2013: Routledge.

[48] Fabritius, F. and H.W. Hagemann, *The Leading Brain: Powerful Science-Based Stratagies for Achieving Peak Performance.* 2018: Penguin.

[49] Cameron, K., *Practicing positive leadership: Tools and techniques that create extraordinary results.* 2013: Berrett-Koehler Publishers.

[50] Drucker, P.F., *HBR's 10 Must Reads Leader's Collection (3 Books)*. 2014: Harvard Business Review Press.

[51] Gallagher, D. and J. Costal, *The self-aware leader: A proven model for reinventing yourself*. 2012: American Society for Training and Development.

[52] Wheaton, C.E., *At Your Service: Lessons in Leadership*. 2009: Dorrance Publishing.

[53] Gilley, J. and A. Maycunich, *Beyond the Learning Organization: Creating a Culture of Continuous Growth and Development through State-of-the-Art Human Resource Practices*. 2000: Basic Books (AZ).

[54] Cran, C., *The Art of Change Leadership: Driving Transformation in a Fast-Paced World*. 2015: John Wiley & Sons.

[55] Goleman, D., What makes a leader. *Organizational influence processes*, 2003: p. 229-241.

[56] Dive, B., *The accountable leader: Developing effective leadership through managerial accountability*. 2008: Kogan Page Publishers.

[57] Moore, S.A., *Practices of Relational Leadership in Action Learning Teams*. 2014: Tilburg University.

[58] Day, D.V., Leadership development: A review in context. The *Leadership Quarterly*, 2000. **11**(4): p. 581-613.

[59] Laschinger, H.K.S., et al., Leader behavior impact on staff nurse empowerment, job tension, and work effectiveness. *Journal of nursing administration*, 1999. **29**(5): p. 28-39.

[60] Buchanan, D., et al., No going back: A review of the literature on sustaining organizational change. *International Journal of Management Reviews*, 2005. **7**(3): p. 189-205.

[61] Alvesson, M. and S. Sveningsson, Good visions, bad micro-management and ugly ambiguity: contradictions of (non-) leadership in a knowledge-intensive organization. *Organization studies*, 2003. **24**(6): p. 961-988.

[62] DiFonzo, N. and P. Bordia, *A tale of two corporations: Managing uncertainty during organizational change*. Human Resource Management: Published in Cooperation with the School of Business

Administration, The University of Michigan and in alliance with the Society of Human Resources Management, 1998. **37**(3-4): p. 295-303.

[63] Yang, J., Z.X. Zhang, and A.S. Tsui, Middle manager leadership and frontline employee performance: Bypass, cascading, and moderating effects. *Journal of Management Studies*, 2010. **47**(4): p. 654-678.

[64] Rizzo, J.R., R.J. House, and S.I. Lirtzman, Role conflict and ambiguity in complex organizations. *Administrative science quarterly*, 1970: p. 150-163.

[65] Zeithaml, V.A., L.L. Berry, and A. Parasuraman, Communication and control processes in the delivery of service quality. *The Journal of Marketing*, 1988: p. 35-48.

[66] Bendaly, L. and N. Bendaly, *Improving healthcare team performance: The 7 requirements for excellence in patient care.* 2012: John Wiley & Sons.

[67] Phillips, A., *Communication and the Manager's Job.* 2002: Radcliffe Publishing.

[68] Fullan, M., *Leading in a culture of change.* 2001: John Wiley & Sons.

[69] Kouzes, J.M. and B.Z. Posner, *Credibility: How leaders gain and lose it, why people demand it.* Vol. 244. 2011: John Wiley & Sons.

[70] Heifetz, R.A., A. Grashow, and M. Linsky, *The practice of adaptive leadership: Tools and tactics for changing your organization and the world.* 2009: Harvard Business Press.

[71] Warren, O.J. and R. Carnall, Medical leadership: why it's important, what is required, and how we develop it. *Postgraduate Medical Journal*, 2011. **87**(1023): p. 27-32.

[72] Kemp, C.R., *Trust-the key to leadership in network centric environments.* 2003, Army War Coll Carlisle Barracks PA.

[73] Bollinger, A.S. and R.D. Smith, Managing organizational knowledge as a strategic asset. *Journal of knowledge management*, 2001. **5**(1): p. 8-18.

[74] Glatthorn, A., Cooperative professional development: Peer-centered options for teacher growth. *Educational leadership*, 1987. **45**(3): p. 31-35.

[75] Showers, B. and B. Joyce, The evolution of peer coaching. *Educational leadership*, 1996. **53**: p. 12-16.

[76] Bouncken, R.B. and A.J. Reuschl, Coworking-spaces: how a phenomenon of the sharing economy builds a novel trend for the workplace and for entrepreneurship. *Review of Managerial Science*, 2018. **12**(1): p. 317-334.

[77] Eysenbach, G., Medicine 2.0: social networking, collaboration, participation, apomediation, and openness. *Journal of medical Internet research*, 2008. **10**(3).

[78] Prahalad, C.K. and V. Ramaswamy, *The future of competition: Co-creating unique value with customers.* 2004: Harvard Business Press.

[79] Gould, L.J., et al., Clinical communities at Johns Hopkins Medicine: An emerging approach to quality improvement. *The Joint Commission Journal on Quality and Patient Safety*, 2015. **41**(9): p. 387-AP1.

[80] Ramaswamy, V. and F.J. Gouillart, *The power of co-creation: Build it with them to boost growth, productivity, and profits.* 2010: Simon and Schuster.

[81] George, B., *Authentic leadership: Rediscovering the secrets to creating lasting value.* 2003: John Wiley & Sons.

[82] McCauley, C.D., et al., *Experience-driven leader development: Models, tools, best practices, and advice for on-the-job development.* 2013: John Wiley & Sons.

[83] Pfeffer, J., *Managing with power: Politics and influence in organizations.* 1992: Harvard Business Press.

[84] Kotter, J.P., *John P. Kotter on what leaders really do.* 1999: Harvard Business Press.

[85] Roussos, S.T. and S.B. Fawcett, A review of collaborative partnerships as a strategy for improving community health. *Annual review of public health*, 2000. **21**(1): p. 369-402.

[86] Whelan, E., et al., Creating employee networks that deliver open innovation. *MIT Sloan Management Review,* 2011. **53**(1): p. 37.

[87] Lazzarotti, V., R. Manzini, and E. Pizzurno. Managing innovation networks of SMEs: A case study. In *Engineering Management Conference, 2008. IEMC Europe 2008. IEEE International.* 2008. IEEE.

[88] Gardner, W.L., et al., "Can you see the real me?" A self-based model of authentic leader and follower development. *The Leadership Quarterly,* 2005. **16**(3): p. 343-372.

[89] Goleman, D., R.E. Boyatzis, and A. McKee, *Primal leadership: Unleashing the power of emotional intelligence.* 2013: Harvard Business Press.

[90] Roberts, L.M., et al., Composing the reflected best self-portrait: Building pathways for becoming extraordinary in work organizations. *Academy of Management Review,* 2005. **30**(4): p. 712-736.

[91] Bennis, W.G. and R. Townsend, *On becoming a leader.* Vol. 36. 1989: Addison-Wesley Reading, MA.

[92] Northouse, P.G., *Leadership: Theory and practice.* 2018: Sage publications.

[93] LaFasto, F. and C. Larson, *When teams work best: 6,000 team members and leaders tell what it takes to succeed.* 2001: Sage.

[94] McDonald, M.J., *Voice and volume of leader self-awareness.* 2009.

[95] Shiner, M., *7 Leadership Blind Spots: Adult Development, Emotional Intelligence, and Leadership Effectiveness among Biotech R&D Leaders.* 2015.

[96] Bell, A., *Great leadership: What it is and what it takes in a complex world.* 2006: Davies-Black Publishing.

[97] Fairholm, G.W., *Mastering inner leadership. 2001:* Greenwood Publishing Group.

[98] Weick, K.E., The collapse of sensemaking in organizations: The Mann Gulch disaster. *Administrative science quarterly,* 1993: p. 628-652.

[99] Furnham, A., *The elephant in the boardroom: The causes of leadership derailment.* 2016: Springer.

[100] Boin, A., E. Stern, and B. Sundelius, *The politics of crisis management: Public leadership under pressure.* 2016: Cambridge University Press.

[101] Crosby, B.C. and J.M. Bryson, *Leadership for the common good: Tackling public problems in a shared-power world.* Vol. 264. 2005: John Wiley & Sons.

[102] Maxwell, J.C., *The 21 indispensable qualities of a leader: Becoming the person others will want to follow.* 2007: Thomas Nelson.

[103] Fairholm, M.R. and G. Fairholm, Leadership amid the constraints of trust. *Leadership & Organization Development Journal,* 2000. **21**(2): p. 102-109.

[104] Trevino, L.K., L.P. Hartman, and M. Brown, Moral person and moral manager: How executives develop a reputation for ethical leadership. *California management review,* 2000. **42**(4): p. 128-142.

[105] Bass, B.M., Two decades of research and development in transformational leadership. *European journal of work and organizational psychology,* 1999. **8**(1): p. 9-32.

[106] Millward, L.J. and K. Bryan, Clinical leadership in health care: a position statement. *Leadership in Health Services,* 2005. **18**(2): p. 13-25.

[107] Schwartz, R.W. and C. Pogge, Physician leadership: essential skills in a changing environment. *The American journal of surgery,* 2000. **180**(3): p. 187-192.

[108] Stowell, S.J. and M.M. Starcevich, *Win Win Partnerships: Be on the Leading Edge with Synergistic Coaching.* 1996: Cmoe.

[109] Burke, R.J., Why leaders fail: Exploring the darkside. *International Journal of Manpower,* 2006. **27**(1): p. 91-100.

[110] Schafer, J.A., The ineffective police leader: Acts of commission and omission. *Journal of Criminal Justice,* 2010. **38**(4): p. 737-746.

[111] Peterson, R.S., et al., The impact of chief executive officer personality on top management team dynamics: one mechanism by

which leadership affects organizational performance. *Journal of Applied Psychology,* 2003. **88**(5): p. 795.

[112] Benn, S., M. Edwards, and T. Williams, *Organizational change for corporate sustainability.* 2014: Routledge.

[113] Smeds, R., Managing change towards lean enterprises. *International Journal of Operations & Production Management,* 1994. **14**(3): p. 66-82.

[114] Ellison, S.D. and D.W. Miller, Beyond ADR: working toward synergistic strategic partnership. *Journal of Management in Engineering,* 1995. **11**(6): p. 44-54.

[115] Lewis, S., *Positive psychology at work: How positive leadership and appreciative inquiry create inspiring organizations.* 2011: John Wiley & Sons.

[116] Saaty, T.L., *Decision making for leaders: the analytic hierarchy process for decisions in a complex world.* 1990: RWS publications.

[117] Russ, F.A., K.M. McNeilly, and J.M. Comer, Leadership, decision making and performance of sales managers: A multi-level approach. *Journal of Personal Selling & Sales Management,* 1996. **16**(3): p. 1-15.

[118] Janis, I.L., *Crucial decisions: Leadership in policymaking and crisis management.* 1989: Simon and Schuster.

[119] Badaracco, J. and R.R. Ellsworth, *Leadership and the Quest for Integrity.* 1989: Harvard Business Press.

[120] Reeleder, D., et al., Leadership and priority setting: the perspective of hospital CEOs. *Health Policy,* 2006. **79**(1): p. 24-34.

[121] Wood, M., The fallacy of misplaced leadership. *Journal of Management Studies,* 2005. **42**(6): p. 1101-1121.

[122] Haskew, L., Leadership is personal. *The bulletin of the National Association of Secondary School Principals,* 1964. **48**(291): p. 177-181.

[123] Kouzes, J.M. and B.Z. Posner, *The leadership challenge.* Vol. 3. 2006: John Wiley & Sons.

[124] Patterson, J.L., G.A. Goens, and D.E. Reed, *Resilient leadership for turbulent times: A guide to thriving in the face of adversity.* 2009: R&L Education.

[125] Sipe, J.W. and D.M. Frick, *Seven pillars of servant leadership: Practicing the wisdom of leading by serving.* 2015: Paulist Press.

[126] Boone, L.W. and S. Makhani, Five necessary attitudes of a servant leader. *Review of Business,* 2012. **33**(1): p. 83.

[127] Renesch, J., *Leadership in a new era: Visionary approaches to the biggest crises of our time.* 1994: Cosimo, Inc.

[128] Walker, D.H. and K.D. Hampson, Developing cross-team relationships. *Procurement strategies: A relationship based approach,* 2003: p. 169-203.

[129] Maccoby, M., *The leaders we need: And what makes us follow.* 2007: Harvard Business Press.

[130] Walumbwa, F.O., et al., Linking ethical leadership to employee performance: The roles of leader–member exchange, self-efficacy, and organizational identification. *Organizational Behavior and Human Decision Processes,* 2011. **115**(2): p. 204-213.

[131] Bass, B.M. and P. Steidlmeier, Ethics, character, and authentic transformational leadership behavior. *The leadership quarterly,* 1999. **10**(2): p. 181-217.

[132] Mayer, R.C., J.H. Davis, and F.D. Schoorman, An integrative model of organizational trust. *Academy of management review,* 1995. **20**(3): p. 709-734.

[133] Kirkpatick, S.A. and E.A. Locke, Leadership: do traits matter? *Academy of Management Perspectives,* 1991. **5**(2): p. 48-60.

[134] Bass, B.M. and B.J. Avolio, Transformational leadership and organizational culture. *Public administration quarterly,* 1993: p. 112-121.

[135] Collins, J.C. and J.I. Porras, Building your company's vision. *Harvard business review,* 1996. **74**(5): p. 65-&.

[136] Suchman, M.C., Managing legitimacy: Strategic and institutional approaches. *Academy of management review,* 1995. **20**(3): p. 571-610.

[137] Crainer, S. and D. Dearlove, Death of executive talent. *Management review*, 1999. **88**(7): p. 16.

[138] McCauley, C.D. and E. Van Velsor, *The center for creative leadership handbook of leadership development*. Vol. 29. 2004: John Wiley & Sons.

[139] Augustine, A., *The First 100 Days on the Job: How to plan, prioritize and build a sustainable organisation*. 2017: Routledge.

[140] Cross, J., *Informal learning: Rediscovering the natural pathways that inspire innovation and performance*. 2011: John Wiley & Sons.

[141] Cawood, S. and R.V. Bailey, *Destination profit: Creating people-profit opportunities in your organization*. 2006: Davies-Black Publishing.

[142] Pollins, B.F., *Awakening Your Organization*. 2017: Book Venture Publishing LLC.

[143] Zhang, X.-a., et al., Getting everyone on board: The effect of differentiated transformational leadership by CEOs on top management team effectiveness and leader-rated firm performance. *Journal of Management*, 2015. **41**(7): p. 1898-1933.

[144] Bass, B.M. and R.M. Stogdill, *Bass & Stogdill's handbook of leadership: Theory, research, and managerial applications*. 1990: Simon and Schuster.

[145] Nahavandi, A., The art and science of leadership, Ltd. 2006: Pearson Education.

[146] Bradshaw, M.A., *Organizational leadership and its relationship to outcomes in residential treatment*. 2007: Indiana Wesleyan University.

[147] Pauquet, A., *Emotional intelligence as a determinant of leadership potential*. 1998, University of Johannesburg.

[148] Nawaz, Z. and I. Khan_ PhD, Leadership theories and styles: A literature review. *Leadership*, 2016. **16**: p. 1-7.

[149] Salin, D.H., H., *Organizational Causes of Workplace Bullying*, Bullying and Harassment in the Workplace: Developments in Theory, Research, and Practice. 2010.

[150] Fink-Samnick, E., The New Age of Bullying and Violence in Health Care: Part 3: Managing the Bullying Boss and Leadership. *Prof Case Manag,* 2017. **22**(6): p. 260-274.

[151] Sfantou, D.F., et al., Importance of Leadership Style towards Quality of Care Measures in Healthcare Settings: A Systematic Review. *Healthcare (Basel),* 2017. **5**(4).

[152] Ojokuku, R., T. Odetayo, and A. Sajuyigbe, Impact of leadership style on organizational performance: a case study of Nigerian banks. *American Journal of Business and Management,* 2012. **1**(4): p. 202-207.

[153] Bolden, R., Distributed leadership in organizations: A review of theory and research. *International Journal of Management Reviews,* 2011. **13**(3): p. 251-269.

[154] Korsgaard, M.A., D.M. Schweiger, and H.J. Sapienza, Building commitment, attachment, and trust in strategic decision-making teams: The role of procedural justice. *Academy of Management journal,* 1995. **38**(1): p. 60-84.

[155] Carson, J.B., P.E. Tesluk, and J.A. Marrone, Shared leadership in teams: An investigation of antecedent conditions and performance. *Academy of management Journal,* 2007. **50**(5): p. 1217-1234.

[156] Katzenbach, J.R. and D.K. Smith, *The discipline of teams.* 2008: Harvard Business Press.

[157] Kaner, S., *Facilitator's guide to participatory decision-making.* 2014: John Wiley & Sons.

[158] Avolio, B.J. and B.M. Bass, *Developing potential across a full range of Leadership Tm: Cases on transactional and transformational leadership.* 2001: Psychology Press.

[159] Aldoory, L. and E. Toth, Leadership and gender in public relations: Perceived effectiveness of transformational and transactional leadership styles. *Journal of Public Relations Research,* 2004. **16**(2): p. 157-183.

[160] Woods, P., *Democratic leadership in education.* 2005: Sage.

[161] Wellman, J., Leadership behaviors in matrix environments. *Project Management Journal,* 2007. **38**(2): p. 62-74.

[162] Frisch, B., *Who's in the Room?: How Great Leaders Structure and Manage the Teams Around Them*. 2011: John Wiley & Sons.

[163] Vandekerckhove, T. and J. Giovagnoli, *Distributed Leadership: Potential & Implementation through self-managed teams*. 2015.

[164] Macey, W.H., et al., *Employee engagement: Tools for analysis, practice, and competitive advantage*. Vol. 31. 2011: John Wiley & Sons.

[165] Kaplan, R.S., et al., *The strategy-focused organization: How balanced scorecard companies thrive in the new business environment*. 2001: Harvard Business Press.

[166] Ram, P. and G.V. Prabhakar, The role of employee engagement in work-related outcomes. *Interdisciplinary Journal of Research in Business*, 2011. **1**(3): p. 47-61.

[167] Woods, A.P., Democratic leadership: drawing distinctions with distributed leadership. *International Journal of Leadership in Education*, 2010. **7**(1): p. 3-20.

[168] Leana III, C.R. and H.J. Van Buren, Organizational social capital and employment practices. *Academy of management review*, 1999. **24**(3): p. 538-555.

[169] Gastil, J., *A Definition and Illustration of Democratic Leadership*. Sage journals, 1994.

[170] McManus, J., *Leadership: Project and human capital management*. 2006: Elsevier.

[171] De Bruijn, H. and E. Ten Heuvelhof, *Process management: why project management fails in complex decision making processes*. 2010: Springer Science & Business Media.

[172] Cruz, M.C., *Generation Y workplace needs and preferred leadership styles*. 2014: Pepperdine University.

[173] Bentley, K.L., *An investigation of the self-perceived principal leadership styles in an era of accountability*. 2011.

[174] Wren, K., *Social Influences* 2013: Routledge.

[175] Abdul Qayyum Chaudhr, H.J., Impact of Transactional and Laissez Faire Leadership Style on Motivation. *International Journal of Business and Social Science*, 2012. **3**(7).

[176] Rose Ngozi Amanchukwu, G.J.S., Nwachukwu Prince Ololube, A Review of Leadership Theories, Principles and Styles and Their Relevance to Educational Management. *Scientific & Academic Publishing*, 2015. **5**(1): p. 6-14.

[177] Glube, R., *Leadership decision making: an empirical test of the vroom and yetton model.* 1978.

[178] Martínez, P.G., Paternalism as a positive form of leader–subordinate exchange: Evidence from Mexico. Management Research: *Journal of the Iberoamerican Academy of Management,* 2003. **1**(3): p. 227-242.

[179] Mansur, J.A., *On paternalistic leadership fit: exploring cross-cultural endorsement, leader-follower fit, and the boundary role of organizational culture.* 2016.

[180] Zankovsky, A. and C. von der Heiden, *Style 7.1+: Paternalist (To Assign and to Manage), in Leadership with Synercube.* 2016, Springer. p. 95-111.

[181] Erben and Guneser, G.a.A., The Relationship Between Paternalistic Leadership and Organizational Commitement:Investigating the Role of Climate Regarding ethics. *Journal of Business Ethics,* 2008. **82**(4): p. 960.

[182] Mowday, R.T., L.W. Porter, and R.M. Steers, *Employee—organization linkages: The psychology of commitment, absenteeism, and turnover.* 2013: Academic press.

[183] Rousseau, D.M., Why workers still identify with organizations. Journal of Organizational Behavior: T*he International Journal of Industrial, Occupational and Organizational Psychology and Behavior,* 1998. **19**(3): p. 217-233.

[184] Den Hartog, D.N., Ethical leadership. *Annu. Rev. Organ. Psychol. Organ. Behav.* 2015. **2**(1): p. 409-434.

[185] Kramer, R.M., Trust and distrust in organizations: Emerging perspectives, enduring questions. *Annual review of psychology,* 1999. **50**(1): p. 569-598.

Leadership in Health-Care 43

[186] Aycan, Z. Paternalism: Towards Conceptual Refinement and Operationalization in Indigenous and Cultural Psychology. *International and Cultural Psychology.* 2006, Springer: Boston.

[187] Flemming, P.L., *A study of the relationship between transformational leadership traits and organizational culture types in improving performance in public sector organizations: A Caribbean perspective.* 2009: Capella University.

[188] Washington, R.R., C.D. Sutton, and H.S. Feild, Individual differences in servant leadership: The roles of values and personality. *Leadership & Organization Development Journal,* 2006. **27**(8): p. 700-716.

[189] Chen, K.C.-C., *An exploratory case study of servant leadership in Taiwan Mennonite churches.* 2002.

[190] Sendjaya, S.S., James C, Servant Leadership: Its Origin, Development, and Application in Organizations. *Journal of Leadership & Organizational Studies,* 2002. **9**(2): p. 60-64.

[191] Cameron, K., *Positive leadership: Strategies for extraordinary performance.* 2012: Berrett-Koehler Publishers.

[192] Maxwell, J.C., *The 21 irrefutable laws of leadership: Follow them and people will follow you.* 2007: Thomas Nelson.

[193] Kashyap, V.R., Santosh Servant leadership, employer brand perception, trust in leaders and turnover intentions: a sequential mediation model. *Review of Managerial Science,* 2014. **10**(3): p. 440-454.

[194] Becker, G.S., Investment in human capital: A theoretical analysis. *Journal of political economy,* 1962. **70**(5, Part 2): p. 9-49.

[195] Wren, J.T., *The leader's companion: Insights on leadership through the ages.* 2013: Simon and Schuster.

[196] Hersey, P. and K.H. Blanchard, *Situational leadership.* 1977: California American University, Center for Leadership Studies.

[197] Spillane, J.P., *Distributed leadership.* Vol. 4. 2012: John Wiley & Sons.

[198] Zaccaro, S.J., et al., Leadership and social intelligence: Linking social perspectiveness and behavioral flexibility to leader effectiveness. *The Leadership Quarterly,* 1991. **2**(4): p. 317-342.

[199] Graeff, C.L., The situational leadership theory: A critical view. *Academy of management review,* 1983. **8**(2): p. 285-291.

[200] Hersey, P.a.B., K. H., *Management of Organizational Behavior: Utilizing Human Resources* 3rd ed. 1977, New Jersey: Prentice Hall.

[201] Hersey, P., K.H. Blanchard, and W.E. Natemeyer, Situational leadership, perception, and the impact of power. *Group & Organization Studies,* 1979. **4**(4): p. 418-428.

[202] Alas, R., K. Tafel, and K. Tuulik, Leadership style during transition in society: Case of Estonia. *Problems and Perspectives in Management,* 2007. **5**(1): p. 50-60.

[203] Gleeson, D. and D. Knights, Reluctant leaders: An analysis of middle managers' perceptions of leadership in Further Education in England. *Leadership,* 2008. **4**(1): p. 49-72.

[204] Bass, B.M., *A New Paradigm for Leadership: An Inquiry into Transformational Leadership.* 1996, State Univ of New York at Binghamton.

[205] Lyons, J.B. and T.R. Schneider, The effects of leadership style on stress outcomes. *The Leadership Quarterly,* 2009. **20**(5): p. 737-748.

[206] Kumviboul, P., *Perception of employees of organizational factors towards performance effectiveness: A case study of Siam Makro Public Company Limited.* 2005.

[207] Schultz & Schultz, D., *Psychology and work today.* 2010, New York: Prentice Hall.

[208] Burke, W.W., *Organization change: Theory and practice.* 2017: Sage Publications.

[209] Chandler, G.E., *The relationship of nursing work environment to empowerment and powerlessness.* 1986, College of Nursing, University of Utah.

[210] Huber, G.A., *The craft of bureaucratic neutrality: Interests and influence in governmental regulation of occupational safety.* 2007: Cambridge University Press.

[211] Barbuto Jr, J.E., Motivation and transactional, charismatic, and transformational leadership: A test of antecedents. *Journal of Leadership & Organizational Studies,* 2005. **11**(4): p. 26-40.

[212] Shamir, B., R.J. House, and M.B. Arthur, The motivational effects of charismatic leadership: A self-concept based theory. *Organization science,* 1993. **4**(4): p. 577-594.

[213] Conger, J.A. and R.N. Kanungo, *Charismatic leadership in organizations.* 1998: Sage Publications.

[214] Wasielewski, P.L., The emotional basis of charisma. *Symbolic Interaction,* 1985. **8**(2): p. 207-222.

[215] Grant, A.M., *Give and take: A revolutionary approach to success.* 2013: Penguin.

[216] Grant, A., In the company of givers and takers. *Harvard business review,* 2013. **91**(4): p. 90-97.

[217] Hazaz Abdullah Alsolami, K.T.G.C., Abdulaziz Awad M. Ibn Twalh, Revisiting Innovation Leadership. *Open Journal of Leadership,* 2016. **5**(2).

[218] Leadership Types, in *The New Penguin Business Dictionary,* G. Bannock, Editor. 2003, Penguin.

[219] Bernthal, P. and R. Wellins, Trends in leader development and succession. *People and Strategy,* 2006. **29**(2): p. 31.

[220] Rothwell, W., *Effective succession planning: Ensuring leadership continuity and building talent from within.* 2010: Amacom.

[221] Inman, M., *The journey to leadership: A study of how leader-academics in higher education learn to lead.* 2007, University of Birmingham.

[222] Manderscheid, S.V., New leader assimilation: An intervention for leaders in transition. *Advances in Developing Human Resources,* 2008. **10**(5): p. 686-702.

[223] Russell, M.A., *Mining the Social Web: Data Mining Facebook, Twitter, LinkedIn, Google+, GitHub, and More.* 2013: "O'Reilly Media, Inc.".

[224] Zukas, J.A., et al., *Impact dynamics.* Vol. 452. 1982: Wiley New York.

[225] Branham, L., *The 7 hidden reasons employees leave: How to recognize the subtle signs and act before it's too late.* 2012: Amacom.

[226] Armstrong, M. and T. Stephens, *A handbook of management and leadership: A guide to managing for results.* 2005: Kogan Page Publishers.

[227] Ladkin, D., *Rethinking leadership: A new look at old leadership questions.* 2010: Edward Elgar Publishing.

[228] Doyle, A. *Best questions to ask in a job interview.* 2018 December 17. 2018]; Available from: https://www.thebalancecareers.com/questions-to-ask-in-a-job-interview-2061205.

[229] Taylor, P.J. and B. Small, Asking applicants what they would do versus what they did do: A meta-analytic comparison of situational and past behaviour employment interview questions. *Journal of Occupational and Organizational Psychology,* 2002. **75**(3): p. 277-294.

[230] Pierre, G., et al., *STEP skills measurement surveys: innovative tools for assessing skills.* 2014.

[231] Sams, D.A., *An analysis of leadership beliefs and practices of 25 TESOL leaders.* 2010.

[232] Workable. *Leadership interview questions.* 2017 December 17, 2018]; Available from: https://resources.workable.com/leadership-interview-questions.

[233] Jones, G.R., *Organizational theory, design, and change: Texts and cases.* 2012: Pearson Higher Ed.

[234] Whetten, D. and K. Cameron, *Developing Management Skills: Global Edition.* 2014: Pearson Higher Ed.

[235] Rothwell, W.J. and R.L. Sullivan, *Practicing organization development: A guide for consultants.* Vol. 27. 2005: John Wiley & Sons.

[236] Brown, D.R. and D.F. Harvey, *An experiential approach to organization development.* 2011.

[237] Sutherland, J. and D. Canwell, *Key concepts in strategic management.* 2004: Macmillan International Higher Education.

[238] Morris, M.H., D.F. Kuratko, and J.G. Covin, *Corporate entrepreneurship & innovation.* 2010: Cengage Learning.

[239] Lussier, R.N., *Human relations in organizations: Applications and skill building.* 2010: McGraw-Hill.

[240] Komives, S.R., N. Lucas, and T.R. McMahon, *Exploring leadership: For college students who want to make a difference.* 2009: John Wiley & Sons.

[241] Sussman, L. and J. Kline, Who Are The Difficult Employees? Psychopathological Attributions Of Their Co-workers. *Journal of Business & Economics Research,* 2007. **5**(10).

[242] Young, N.K., J. Williamson, and J. Deeken, Tact and tenacity: dealing with difficult people at work. *The Serials Librarian,* 2002. **42**(3-4): p. 299-304.

[243] Rosen, M.I., *Thank you for being such a pain: Spiritual guidance for dealing with difficult people.* 1999: Harmony.

[244] Minuti, M., Employer liability under the doctrine of negligent hiring: Suggested methods for avoiding the hiring of dangerous employees. *Del. J. Corp. L.,* 1988. **13**: p. 501.

[245] Lienhard, R., Negligent retention of employees: An expanding doctrine. *Def. Counsel J.,* 1996. **63**: p. 389.

[246] Calvasina, G.E., R.V. Calvasina, and E.J. Calvasina, Making more informed hiring decisions: Policy and practice issues for employers. *Journal of Legal, Ethical and Regulatory Issues,* 2008. **11**(1): p. 95.

[247] Frisina, M., The tyrany of the "technically competent competitor". *Influential Leader,* 2014. **2014**(40): p. 1-2.

[248] Paulhus, D.L. and K.M. Williams, The dark triad of personality: Narcissism, Machiavellianism, and psychopathy. *Journal of research in personality,* 2002. **36**(6): p. 556-563.

[249] Jonason, P.K., S. Slomski, and J. Partyka, The Dark Triad at work: How toxic employees get their way. *Personality and individual differences,* 2012. **52**(3): p. 449-453.

[250] Lubit, R.H., *Coping with toxic managers, subordinates... and other difficult people: Using emotional intelligence to survive and prosper.* 2003: FT Press.

[251] Liff, S., *Improving the Performance of Government Employees: A Manager's Guide.* 2011: Amacom.

[252] Laker, D.R. and J.L. Powell, The differences between hard and soft skills and their relative impact on training transfer. Human Resource *Development Quarterly,* 2011. **22**(1): p. 111-122.

[253] Carnevale, A.P., *Workplace basics: The essential skills employers want. ASTD best practices series: Training for a changing work force.* 1990: ERIC.

[254] Berghout, M.A., et al., Medical leaders or masters?-A systematic review of medical leadership in hospital settings. PLoS One, 2017. **12**(9): p. e0184522.

[255] Robyn Clay-Williams, K.L., Luke Testa, Zhicheng Li, Jeffrey Braithwaite, Medical leadership, a systematic narrative review: do hospitals and healthcare organisations perform better when led by doctors? *BMJ Open,* 2017.

In: Fundamentals of Leadership ...
Editors: S. P. A. Stawicki et al.
ISBN: 978-1-53615-729-1
© 2019 Nova Science Publishers, Inc.

Chapter 2

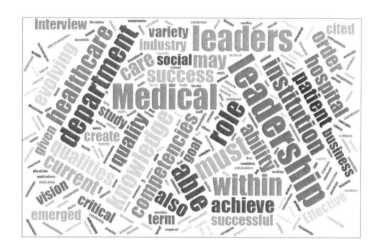

INTERVIEWING FOR A LEADERSHIP POSITION: KEY ASPECTS AND CONSIDERATIONS

Jacqueline Seoane[1], Ronya Silmi[1] and Stanislaw P. A. Stawicki[2],*

[1]Medical School of Temple University/St. Luke's University Health Network, Bethlehem, Pennsylvania, US
[2]Department of Research & Innovation, St. Luke's University Health Network, Bethlehem, Pennsylvania, US

---

* Corresponding Author's E-mail: stawicki.ace@gmail.com.

ABSTRACT

Effective leadership is critical to the functioning of any successful organization, especially in a highly complex sector such as the health-care industry. Considered to be leadership competencies, certain traits emerged as key determinants of compatibility, synergy creation and ultimate success between the prospective leadership candidate and the organization. These core competencies include one's knowledge of the role and the institution, the ability to create and project a vision, emotional intelligence, and organizational orientation. When viewed in the context of a leadership job interview, the presence of these qualities allows all stakeholders to determine if a successful "match" can be made for a long-term, sustainable professional relationship. Although our discussion focuses on physician-leaders, principles outlined herein apply to all those who may be seeking professional advancement that involves leadership interviews.

Keywords: interviewing skills, health-care recruitment, leadership interviews, leadership qualities

1. INTRODUCTION

Effective leadership is the cornerstone of organizational success, and is especially critical in the fast-paced, rapidly evolving health-care industry. During the past century, a lot has changed in how our clinics and hospitals are managed, from focus on patient safety and quality of care, employee wellness, advancements in workflow management, to applications of modern information management and economics concepts [1-5]. The composition of health-care leadership cadre is likewise evolving. In the 1930's, physicians accounted for about 35% of hospital leadership in the United States. However, over the past several decades, health administration has seen a significant decline in physician leaders (including prospective physician candidates) [6], with today's figure standing at only approximately 4% [7]. The de-emphasis of physician leadership has several important implications, including the perceived lack of inclusion, loss of empowerment, and lower levels of organizational engagement [8-12].

One theory as to why such decline in physician participation in leadership has occurred is the growing complexity of health-care systems, especially with the parallel increases in the complexity of clinical patient care [13-15]. The continuous and highly dynamic interactions between professional groups, departments, specialties, and external stakeholders make effective leadership exceedingly challenging [16-18]. Most health administration strategies are developed using a business model that is later applied to health-care institutions. In addition, the evolving role of hospital administration often falls out of a typical physician's scope of practice due to the political, economic, social, and technological factors involved [19], each of which require a unique skillset well beyond the standard medical education curriculum. As a result, the qualities that make an exceptional physician do not always translate into effective leadership ability, as required within the context of health-care management [20].

As suggested above, the gradual shift in hospital administration may be linked to the lack of leadership training in medical school and residency programs, with emphasis placed on medical knowledge and patient care, as opposed to business administration training [21]. In addition, the constraints of an administrative position prevent physicians from incorporating meaningful patient interactions into their practice as patient care takes secondary role to the leadership position [22-24]. Ultimately, physicians must determine in what capacity they would pursue a career as a hospital administrator, whether this is in the position of department chairman or residency director/coordinator.

Modern health-care leaders and leadership teams should optimally incorporate both the qualities of an experienced clinician and those of a highly effective administrator [25, 26]. Consequently, physicians should be encouraged to take on active leadership roles within their institutions, with the primary goal of improving organizational performance which includes the quality of patient care, patient safety, as well as the focus on cost-effectiveness [19, 27]. Individual leadership style should represent a blend of the clinician leader's individual personality and the departmental or institutional culture, all while devoting themselves to ensuring the highest level patient care [18, 28]. In this chapter, we present two unique healthcare leadership perspectives. In both vignette-based scenarios, highly qualified, experienced physicians are applying for leadership roles within their respective institutions. Our goal is to provide an overview of key competencies that are essential to the success of an applicant looking to advance his or her career in an administrative role (Figure 1). Additionally, we discuss a variety of leadership styles and specific nuances associated with each style so that both prospective applicants and current leaders may find this chapter helpful as a reference for guiding their current and future practices.

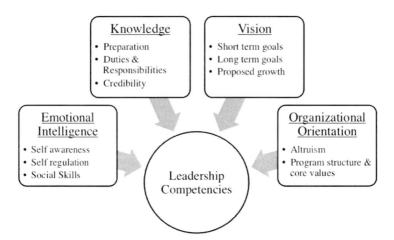

Figure 1. Key leadership competencies important to consider for both potential applicants and organizations during the leadership interviewing process.

2. LEADERSHIP VIGNETTE #1

Dr. G. Smith is a general surgeon for a major urban hospital and has been in practice for the last twelve years. Following his undergraduate education at a top state university, he pursued a career in medicine at a Patriot League institution. Upon completion of his residency, Dr. Smith finalized his training with an additional fellowship in trauma and critical care at a nearby teaching hospital. He continued on as faculty during which time he conducted clinical research in the field of trauma and critical care. With his extensive experience in both surgery and research, Dr. Smith is applying for the Program Director position for the general surgery residency at a major academic center in Eastern Pennsylvania. During his interview with the Chairman of surgery, Dr. Smith was asked about his plan for the Residency Program and how he hoped to improve the Department of Surgery. Unfortunately, due to his lack of preparedness, he was unable to effectively communicate his view of the strengths and weaknesses of the program. Furthermore, he provided a generic design that lacked vision for the future growth of the both the residency program and the Department as a whole. Despite his many years of teaching experience, excellent international reputation, and numerous publications, Dr. Smith was not offered the position as Program Director.

2.1. Skill Set

Effective leaders possess a collection of traits that enable them to guide a team of individuals in order to achieve a common goal [29]. While these traits may vary slightly depending on the task, there are a core set of qualities that are essential and required in all positions of leadership (Figure 2) [29-31]. Taylor et al. conducted a qualitative, structured interview based study with the goal of understanding the specific leadership competencies required by physicians within an institution. Four qualities emerged from this study that proved to be significant for individuals seeking a leadership role: (1) Emotional Intelligence, (2) Knowledge, (3) Plan or "vision", (4) Organizational Orientation [32]. While these four competencies are explained individually in this discussion, their relationship is far more complex and dynamic in practice (Figure 3). Individuals in leadership roles often possess all of these qualities to a varying degree, and differ in their ability to utilize them when placed in a leadership position.

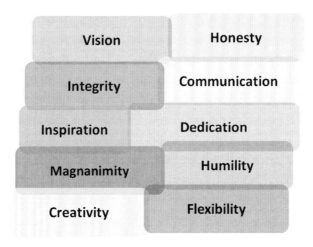

Figure 2. List of important leadership traits and characteristics; Note that this listing is not comprehensive, with additional characteristics including innovation, open-mindedness, delegating, trustworthiness, feedback, positivity, responsibility, and motivation.

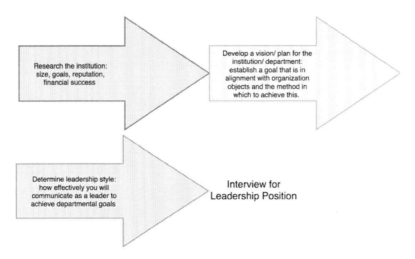

Figure 3. Proposed sequence of preparatory steps ahead of an interview for a leadership position. It is important for potential candidates to possess requisite knowledge, skills, vision, and the ability to demonstrate sensitivity toward institutional culture and values.

A. *Emotional intelligence:* Emotional intelligence, or "people-skills," consists of an individual's ability to communicate their

Interviewing for a Leadership Position 55

viewpoint effectively to their peers in a clear and respectful manner. According to the study by Taylor et al, it was the most cited quality of both aspiring and current physician leaders. This competency encompasses a variety of qualities including self-awareness, self-regulation, motivation, empathy, and social skills [32].

Persons with self-awareness have the ability to recognize and understand his or her own feelings, beliefs, and motivations. This individual is able to acknowledge personal strengths and weaknesses, collaborate with their peers, and compromise during conflict in order to achieve a common goal. They must be able to self-regulate their behavior, free of judgment or bias, and execute a rational and thoroughly planned decision. Leaders should be motivated, and have the passion and persistence to succeed. Additionally, they should have the ability to instill their drive to succeed into those around them [32]. Medical leaders should have the skills to communicate effectively with their clinical team and manage relationships between participants to ensure optimal patient care.

B. *Knowledge*: The overall theme of knowledge in the medical setting encompasses both insight about the department and institution, as well as and medical knowledge within the physician's discipline. This includes the roles and responsibilities of the position available and how the applicant plans to fulfill this role given their experiences. Medical leaders in a managerial role must have a clear understanding of growth constraints, department budgets, technology implementation, etc. within their institution in order to utilize their finances efficiently. However, credibility in a clinical role was also cited as a significant quality, as medical leaders must make informed decisions regarding their patients and the colleagues within their department [27].

Preparation for a leadership role can also be included under this theme. Interviewers are searching for applicants that are able to learn how a program operates and utilize his or her experience within the clinical setting to advance their respective departments and institution as a whole while enhancing patient care [32].

C. *Plan or "vision":* The health-care system is constantly evolving and future leaders are expected to have a sense of direction when navigating through this change. Applicants should share their institutional vision for success and growth, but must also be able to propose a strategy to achieve this within their respective department if given the appropriate means and financial support. Potential candidates should be able to propose short-term and long-term goals for the program and describe a course of action to achieve them. These individuals are able to communicate their strategies clearly to colleagues. Medical leaders constantly analyze and reevaluate their departments to identify strengths and weaknesses in order to create a solution that both optimizes patient care and is cost-effective.

D. *Organizational orientation:* Organizational orientation is described as a thorough understanding of the history, structure, and values of an institution [32]. While it is important for an applicant to have their own set of beliefs and values, it is essential that they also have a profound understanding of the institution's values. When selecting an individual for a leadership role, senior administrators are searching for an individual that will uphold the values of the institution above one's own personal opinion when it is appropriate. By creating this network of like-minded individuals that share core values, an institution is able to achieve results that would otherwise be unattainable due to lack of support [19].

3. VIGNETTE #2

Dr. E. Q. Sawyer is board certified emergency physician with fellowship training in toxicology, who is applying for a Fellowship Program Director position. Currently, she is a faculty member at a community hospital that has seen significant growth over the past 5 years. Throughout her 15 years of practice, Dr. Sawyer has been a prolific researcher having produced multiple protocols on improving emergency response to chemical attacks. Prior to interviewing for the position, Dr. Sawyer extensively researched the hospital network. While the Fellowship had a well-known regional reputation, she hoped to expand the research within the Department to establish the program as a major academic institute. Through her research of the institution, it was evident that the hospital shared her goal of expansion as it had recently acquired three nearby regional hospitals. During her interview, Dr. Sawyer discussed her vision of the program as well as her leadership style with administrators and staff. Using an adaptation of a democratic and transformational leadership style, she explained how she would encourage residents, fellows and staff to provide input on improvements that could be made within the Fellowship and the Department. Impressed with her plan for the Fellowship Program, Dr. Sawyer was offered the position of Program Director.

3.1. Leadership Styles

Leadership style is defined as the approach used to motivate followers to a shared goal. While there is no "one size fits all" approach to achieve this, prior to interviewing for an administrative position within an institution, it is useful to understand the different leadership styles and determine which may be adapted to lead effectively [33, 34]. One's chosen leadership style should take into consideration the institution, groups, and individuals involved. The six commonly referenced leadership styles are as follows: transactional, autocratic, bureaucratic, laissez-faire, transformational/charismatic, and democratic/participative [35-37]. Of note, experienced leaders may be able to "flex" between different leadership styles, depending on the exact circumstances, goal/task, and personal/team characteristics [38-40].

Under the guise that team members agree to follow their leader, the transactional model is based on stringent goals and objectives for the followers. In this model, institutions pay for the compliance and effort of its team members. Based on pre-determined "transactional exchange" system, rewards and positive reinforcement are provided or mediated by the leader [41]. It is not expected within this model that subordinates think innovatively or contribute to the structure of performance incentives. Instead the transactional leader works to define clear objectives and criteria for team members to follow.

An extreme form of transactional leadership, autocratic leadership, allows the leader to have complete decisional control over subordinates' work-related activities. In an authoritarian model, all decisions are made by a single individual (or entity). The efficiency of this relies on quick implementation of decisions that are made [42]. Autocratic leaders, as the primary authority, set a clear direction and monitor progress closely. If in crisis, this model is efficient as decisions are usually made without significant dissent. Otherwise, the lack of consideration in regard to staff opinions and ideas denotes an ineffective leader-subordinate relationship.

Bureaucratic leaders tend to rely on stringent rules and clearly defined positions within institutions. Weber, a German sociologist, describes this model on strict hierarchy that is formalized by leaders. Promotion is based on the ability of oneself to conform to the rules and regulations mandated by the organization. Due to the focus on structure, there is an unfortunate loss of flexibility, creativity, and innovation [43]. It is an impersonal model of leadership that focuses on the performance and productivity of the work accomplished and not on subordinates. Effectively bureaucratic leaders are able to produce consistent quality of work, when expectations are clearly defined and followers are comfortable in their position.

French for "let it be", the laissez faire leadership style allows teams to work self-directed with freedom to complete their assignments largely on

Interviewing for a Leadership Position 59

their own conditions. Leaders provide access to resources and make themselves available if subordinates are in need of advice [42]. The success of this overall approach is dependent of the self-directed productivity of team members. Providing subordinates with autonomy within their position/scope of practice has the possibility of increasing job performance; however, leaders who do not regularly communicate with staff risk a loss of productivity due to poor managerial direction. Ultimately, this model is designed for leaders to abdicate responsibilities and defer decisions.

The transformational or charismatic style of leadership is directed to motivate both individuals and teams beyond required expectations. This is achieved by a transformational leader's adoption of innovation and implementing a close supervisory relationship [41]. This increases intrinsic motivation of the team as there is a mutual respect for the value and importance of institutional goals. Furthermore, this model encourages staff to contribute in the decision-making process and invites suggestions that will bring about desired change. In doing so, staff becomes highly invested in the success of the organization.

While subordinates are encouraged to participate in the decision-making process in the democratic leadership model; ultimately, the final decision is dependent on the leader. Nevertheless, this paradigm is able to encourage team members to be highly engaged in projects and trust that their contributions are appreciated. Thus, staff members are motivated beyond financial means [42]. Utilizing this leadership style is time intensive as it requires strategizing a plan and filtering multiple inputs before executing a decision. It is troublesome to utilize this style in times of crisis because valuable time is lost before goals and a plan are established.

3.2. Factors Affecting Leadership Style

Before an aspiring leaders can determine which leadership style they will adapt in their administrative position, there are multiple factors that determine which particular approach will be the most effective. Aspects that should be considered include size of institution, decision-making expectations, and goal congruence. These contributing factors should be considered prior to interviewing for a position as they define the vision the applicant may have for the institution / department / unit.

Most organizations have the tendency to grow, whether it's through the expansion of existing departments or acquisition of an existing institution. An applicant for a leadership position must consider the ramifications of how the institution's development coincides with their own vision and how this will impact their leadership model. Similar to the second vignette, considering and including expansion plans within one's vision demonstrates to the interviewers that one is prepared for the ramifications of a future expansion. With the continual evolution of health-care, there are multiple facets that contribute to the complexity of managing a health-care organization. Decision makers must consider government regulations, technological advancements, ethical nuances, and technical implications prior to the execution of a proposed plan. Thus, sound decision making is a fundamental process at the core of an organization's success. An effective leader is evaluated based on the quality of decisions that they are able to make. An applicant should not shy away from discussing their decision-making paradigm during an interview. This will demonstrate that the applicant is likely to be an effective leader, which in turn leads to favorable outcomes through the implementation of strategic decisions [44].

Goal congruence is defined as the shared goals of individuals and their institution. With this in mind, institutions will ensure support and resources in order to support the achievement of said goals. Prior to an interview, understanding the goals of the department, institution, and employees is crucial. For an individual applying to be a program director, as in the vignettes, the physician should consider not only their goals for the program but also the institution's and residents' goals for their program. Different leadership styles may be adapted depending on the degree of goal congruency within the institution.

While interviewing, applicants should be forthcoming regarding their preferred leadership style and addressing the factors that influence his or

Interviewing for a Leadership Position

her particular leadership approach. Effectively discussing the ways in which one plans to integrate and encourage staff to contribute to a shared goal of the institution shows well-placed ambition to the interviewer and further supports that this is a career goal rather than a hierarchy/position-motivated transition, with the ultimate goal of a better or more desired position rather than a pre-defined leadership outcome. For an administrative position, a candidate should convey that while it may be necessary to take charge quickly in an emergency, ultimately, decisions will be made in the best interest of the department and institution as a whole [45].

SYNTHESIS & CONCLUSION

The evolution of health-care is shifting towards an increasingly complex system that demands well-trained, highly qualified medical leaders. Currently, many medical programs include leadership training with other themes such as "professionalism" or "communication skills" [19]. However, the current level of leadership training in medical school is insufficient to develop skilled leaders needed to run these growing, complex organizations [7]. Strategies geared towards targeting these deficiencies include dual degree-granting (i.e., MD-MBA) programs, residency and specialized fellowship training. In addition, leadership development programs have been proposed in an attempt to close the gap between clinicians and non-clinician hospital administrators [6].

More and more physicians are expected to take on administrative roles in addition to their clinical duties. As a result, two major categories of medical leaders have emerged; there are physicians who have trained and intentionally applied to leadership roles and then there are those that were informally required to take on leadership roles within their practice [6, 27]. Regardless of how they have obtained their role, medical leaders are tasked with the responsibility of optimizing patient care, improving patient safety, and enhancing overall quality while managing an institution in a cost-effective manner. This has resulted in physicians taking on managerial roles that they are ill equipped for and lack the training needed to be successful. Thus, a more comprehensive and fundamentally better approach is needed to set health-care provider leaders up for success.

It is crucial for current and prospective applicants to prepare for the duties and responsibilities of their potential role as leaders. Prior to interviewing for a leadership position within an institution, a physician should thoroughly investigate the organization / department / unit that he or she will be potentially joining. This includes the size, structure, financial strength, and members of executive teams. It is essential that the applicant take into consideration the plan and vision of the institution and how their proposed plans coincide with the organization. The applicant should be able to reflect on their own goals and values to ensure this position is appropriate fit. Applicants are expected to be knowledgeable in not only their area of specialty but also the laws and regulations of the state and federal government related to their position.

During an interview, potential candidates should display appropriate leadership qualities, as outlined both here and the introductory chapter of this book. These include the short-term and long-term goals for the program and plan to achieve these goals. Applicants should have a clear understanding of the roles and responsibilities of the position and clarify any aspect of the position that remains unclear. Displaying laxity in an interview, as demonstrated in the first vignette, shows the interviewer at least some degree of disregard for the position and may be perceived as dismissive.

In summary, it is critically important for the interviewee to be appropriately assertive and to be willing to discuss key topics openly. Honest and authentic projection of one's qualities, strengths, and weaknesses, without exaggerations or insincere projections of "fake confidence" will combine to create a positive impression of a capable leader who is caring, empathetic and passionate. The ability to effectively share/communicate one's vision for the institution as well as conveying the style (or styles) of leadership one utilizes to inspire others is also very important.

REFERENCES

[1] Graban, M., *Lean hospitals: improving quality, patient safety, and employee satisfaction*. 2011: CRC Press.

[2] Finkler, S.A., C.T. Kovner, and C.B. Jones, *Financial management for nurse managers and executives*. 2007: Elsevier Health Sciences.

[3] Lee, R.H., *Economics for healthcare managers*. 2009: Health Administration Press Chicago, IL.

[4] Zelman, W.N., et al., *Financial management of health care organizations: an introduction to fundamental tools, concepts, and applications*. 2009: John Wiley & Sons.

[5] Haux, R., et al., *Strategic information management in hospitals: an introduction to hospital information systems*. 2004: Springer Science & Business Media.

[6] Ackerly, D.C., et al., Training the next generation of physician–executives: an innovative residency pathway in management and leadership. *Academic Medicine*, 2011. **86**(5): p. 575-579.

[7] Gunderman, R. and S.L. Kanter, Perspective: educating physicians to lead hospitals. *Academic Medicine*, 2009. **84**(10): p. 1348-1351.

[8] Guthrie, M.B., Challenges in developing physician leadership and management. *Frontiers of Health Services Management*, 1999. **15**(4): p. 3.

[9] Burchell, R.C., H.L. Smith, and N.F. Piland, *Reinventing Medical Practice: Care Delivery that Satisfies Doctors, Patients, and the Bottom Line*. 2002: Medical Group Management Assn.

[10] Kaissi, A., *A roadmap for trust: enhancing physician engagement*. Canadian Policy Network, 2012.

[11] Snell, A.J., D. Briscoe, and G. Dickson, From the inside out: the engagement of physicians as leaders in health care settings. *Qualitative Health Research*, 2011. **21**(7): p. 952-967.

[12] Whitlock, D.J. and R. Stark, Understanding physician engagement-and how to increase it. *Physician leadership journal*, 2014. **1**(1): p. 8.

[13] Frankel, A.S., M.W. Leonard, and C.R. Denham, Fair and just culture, team behavior, and leadership engagement: The tools to achieve high reliability. *Health services research,* 2006. **41**(4p2): p. 1690-1709.

[14] Weberg, D. *Complexity leadership: A healthcare imperative.* in *Nursing Forum.* 2012. Wiley Online Library.

[15] Kernick, D., Complexity and healthcare organisation. *Complexity and healthcare: An introduction,* 2002: p. 93-121.

[16] Denis, J.-L., L. Lamothe, and A. Langley, The dynamics of collective leadership and strategic change in pluralistic organizations. *Academy of Management journal,* 2001. 44(4): p. 809-837.

[17] Ginter, P.M., W.J. Duncan, and L.E. Swayne, *The strategic management of health care organizations.* 2018: John Wiley & Sons.

[18] Mannion, R., H. Davies, and M. Marshall, *Cultures for performance in health care.* 2004: McGraw-Hill Education (UK).

[19] Warren, O.J. and R. Carnall, Medical leadership: why it's important, what is required, and how we develop it. *Postgraduate Medical Journal,* 2011. **87**(1023): p. 27-32.

[20] Al-Sawai, A., Leadership of healthcare professionals: where do we stand? *Oman medical journal,* 2013. **28**(4): p. 285.

[21] Turner, A.D., S.P. Stawicki, and W.A. Guo, Competitive Advantage of MBA for Physician Executives: A Systematic Literature Review. *World journal of surgery,* 2018. **42**(6): p. 1655-1665.

[22] Hopkins, M.M., D.A. O'Neil, and J.K. Stoller, Distinguishing competencies of effective physician leaders. *Journal of Management Development,* 2015. **34**(5): p. 566-584.

[23] Kaplan, K. and D.L. Feldman, Realizing the value of in-house physician leadership development. *Physician executive,* 2008. **34**(5): p. 40-46.

[24] Stoller, J.K., Developing physician-leaders: a call to action. *Journal of General Internal Medicine,* 2009. **24**(7): p. 876-878.

[25] Mitchell, P. and R. Golden, *Core principles & values of effective team-based health care.* 2012: National Academy of Sciences.

[26] Musson, D.M. and R.L. Helmreich, Team training and resource management in health care: current issues and future directions. *Harvard Health Policy Review,* 2004. **5**(1): p. 25-35.

[27] Berghout, M.A., et al., Medical leaders or masters?—A systematic review of medical leadership in hospital settings. *PloS one,* 2017. **12**(9): p. e0184522.

[28] Drinka, T.J. and P.G. Clark, *Health care teamwork: Interdisciplinary practice and teaching.* 2000: Greenwood Publishing Group.

[29] George, B., et al., Discovering your authentic leadership. *Harvard business review,* 2007. **85**(2): p. 129.

[30] Kouzes, J.M. and B.Z. Posner, *Credibility: How leaders gain and lose it, why people demand it.* Vol. 244. 2011: John Wiley & Sons.

[31] Gibb, C.A., The principles and traits of leadership. *The Journal of Abnormal and Social Psychology,* 1947. **42**(3): p. 267.

[32] Taylor, C.A., J.C. Taylor, and J.K. Stoller, Exploring leadership competencies in established and aspiring physician leaders: an interview-based study. *Journal of general internal medicine,* 2008. **23**(6): p. 748-754.

[33] Pearce, C.L., The future of leadership: Combining vertical and shared leadership to transform knowledge work. *Academy of Management Perspectives,* 2004. **18**(1): p. 47-57.

[34] Bolden, R., et al., *A review of leadership theory and competency frameworks.* 2003, Centre for Leadership Studies, University of Exeter.

[35] Murari, K., *Impact of leadership styles on employee empowerment.* 2015: Partridge Publishing.

[36] Gray Sr, T.A., *Leading in Cyclical Environments: An Examination of North American Executive Leadership Styles in Global Semiconductor Organizations.* 2013, University of Charleston-Beckley.

[37] Goleman, D., R. Boyatzis, and A. McKee, *Primal leadership: Realizing the power of emotional intelligence.* 2002, Boston: Harvard Business School Press.

[38] Cashman, K., *Leadership from the inside out: Becoming a leader for life*. 2017: Berrett-Koehler Publishers.

[39] Sydow, J., L. Lindkvist, and R. DeFillippi, *Project-based organizations, embeddedness and repositories of knowledge*. 2004, Sage Publications Sage CA: Thousand Oaks, CA.

[40] Dearborn, K., Studies in emotional intelligence redefine our approach to leadership development. *Public Personnel Management,* 2002. **31**(4): p. 523-530.

[41] Aarons, G.A., Transformational and transactional leadership: Association with attitudes toward evidence-based practice. *Psychiatric services,* 2006. **57**(8): p. 1162-1169.

[42] Amanchukwu, R.N., G.J. Stanley, and N.P. Ololube, A review of leadership theories, principles and styles and their relevance to educational management. *Management,* 2015. **5**(1): p. 6-14.

[43] Santrock, J., *A topical approach to life-span development, 3E*. Ch, 2007. **5**: p. 192.

[44] Weddle, J., *Levels of Decision Making in the Workplace*. Retrieve March, 2013. **13**: p. 2014.

[45] Harolds, J.A., Tips for a physician in getting the right job, Part VI: some possible interview questions for an executive position. *Clinical nuclear medicine,* 2014. **39**(1): p. 49-51.

In: Fundamentals of Leadership ...
Editors: S. P. A. Stawicki et al.

ISBN: 978-1-53615-729-1
© 2019 Nova Science Publishers, Inc.

Chapter 3

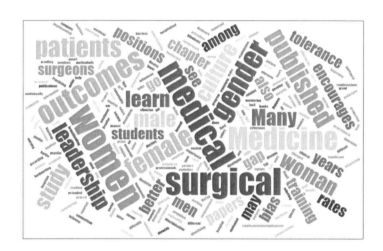

THE BENEFITS OF INCLUSIVE LEADERSHIP AMONG HEALTHCARE PROFESSIONALS

Erick Alexanderson[1], MD, Carlo Angello Sanchez[2], MD and Aloha Meave[3], MD

[1]Chair of Nuclear Cardiology Department, Instituto Nacional de Cardiología Ignacio Chavez, Mexico City, Mexico and Department of Physiology, National Autonomous University of Mexico, Mexico City, Mexico

[2]Social Service in Nuclear Cardiology Department, Instituto Nacional de Cardiologia Ignacio Chavez, Mexico City, Mexico and Universidad Anahuac Mexico, Mexico State, Mexico

[3]Chair of Cardiovascular Magnetic Resonance Unit, Instituto Nacional de Cardiologia Ignacio Chavez, Mexico City, Mexico

ABSTRACT

Have you ever heard about inclusiveness in your workplace? Today our society is changing worldwide and that´s the focus of this chapter. The enrolment of women in universities has increased, but leadership positions are still occupied mostly by men. While recently there might be more diversity, clearly there is a need for more inclusiveness, and women have to have a role in making important organizational decisions. Doing this has showed better outcomes across multiple domains, including patient care, family well-being, economic benefits and improved mental health. This important trend is currently evolving. Thus, there needs to be opportunitieis to define and create opportunities. The obvious question is "How different might the world be if women had been included from the start?"

Keywords: diversity, inclusive approaches, medical leadership, mentorship, surgical leadership, women leaders

1. INTRODUCTION

As health-care professionals, we have responsibilities that go beyond being good clinicians and providing good quality patient-care. In this chapter you will learn about the importance of inclusiveness, the role women need to play in medicine, the economic implications locally and worldwide, and what is being done in developed and developing countries. We will also discuss movements that currently occupy media headlines, such as #MeToo or initiatives such as "Mujeres en Medicina" - a sorority term - and others. The statistics are surprising when you explore the salary gap and employment/unemployment gap between female and male doctors in relation to leadership positions. Furthermore, you will learn about mentoring and how it influences medical students during their training.

Of note, for the purposes of this chapter, the term diversity is not only referring to inclusivity in terms of gender, but also to sexual orientation, ethnicity, race, and religious beliefs. We will only have better outcomes if we create a culture of tolerance and respect. Being young brings an opportunity to learn and develop skills. In Mexico, there exists only one university which has a medical leadership program that encourages and equips students with the leadership experiences and tools to transform society and to make a positive impact. After reading this chapter you will have a broader understanding of this topic with reference to published peer-reviewed papers, books, online Technology, entertainment, design (TED) talks and personal experiences.

2. THE EVOLVING ROLE OF WOMEN IN MEDICINE

In recent years, the rates of enrolment into medical programs have changed remarkably with more women choosing to study medicine. Over the years, there have been many papers published that have clearly demonstrated that women have proved their capacity to succeed in social medicine, medical practice and science. Nevertheless, women have had to face a popular prejudice that is irrational and unfair. Practicing medicine is hard for everyone, and involves working extended hours, nightshifts, retaining a lot of information, and sometimes you will have to go without eating or sleeping. For women, it's particularly harder when they have to stand up against those biases [1].

Erica Baker posted on industrywide diversity and inclusion on the social code-hosting site GitHub. In the report she wrote, "...Diversity numbers remain stagnant... Resolution: This failure is still in progress." Another impediment to progress as Joelle Emerson says is that "If you focus on trying to raise awareness, you probably won´t see a ton of impact. If you train people on actions they can take, that will have an impact" there is more focus on raising awareness about unconscious bias rather than educating employees about actions they can take to combat this bias [2].

There are some publications where we can see the different outcomes among women and men who perform a medical or surgical procedure. For example, a study published in 2017 reported that patients treated by female surgeons had a small but statistically significant decrease in 30-day mortality and similar surgical outcomes compared those treated by male surgeons. It was suggested that in clinical practice this difference exists because female doctors are more likely to use a centered approach and follow evidence-based guidelines compared with male clinicians, whereas surgeons are more technical and there is less difference between male and female surgeons – as such, these results and findings might not apply to surgical specialties. There was another study by Lou et al. where they show that women perform better in tests of theoretical surgical knowledge having higher scores compared with men [3].

Women who undertake a surgical career, experience barriers during their medical training and practice. There are many deterrents for women considering a surgical specialty, such as sex discrimination, workload, surgical culture and lifestyle. Many female surgical mentees had difficulty identifying mentors because of the lack of women in leadership positions in surgery. It may be more difficult for women to enter a surgical specialty and those who are accepted into medical programs tend to be more skilled, motivated and hardworking [3].

In another study published in Journal of the American Medical Association (JAMA) Internal Medicine, there was a comparison of hospital mortality and readmission rates for Medicare patients treated by male and female physicians showing lower mortality and readmissions in elderly hospitalized patients treated by female internists. This suggests that there are important clinical implications for patient outcomes according to the differences in practice terms between men and women. Knowing these differences would help improving quality of care of all patients.

When we consider salaries between male and female physicians, we can see higher salaries among male physicians. These arguments include career interruptions for childrearing, higher rates of part-time employment, and greater tradeoffs between home and work responsibilities among women [4]. Our task is to address this, it is a great opportunity to solve it, what we can do first is change our mind culture, avoiding gender bias, set facilities for the employees such as breastfeeding areas, nursing spaces, food, follow-up, and implementing programs that encourages conversations about gender tolerance and how being more inclusive those hospitals can be more productive having better outcomes and a "happier

The Benefits of Inclusive Leadership among Healthcare ... 71

place to work". We have to avoid gender blindness and be more gender smart as it is portrayed on the advertising company Saatchi & Saatchi [5].

When considering women's skills, they might be more intuitive, more emphatic, more attentive to detail, better listeners, or even kinder [6]. Is it true? Well, some qualities that makes one a better doctor is that of being a unique human being, committed to making a difference in the lives of your patients, together with excellent medical training. Humankind will serve your patients even better. I encourage you, the young student, to discover over the years how powerful your own personal and unique way of communicating with your patients can be. Pay attention, because authentic and compassionate communication can as effective as any drug.

Have you heard about #MeToo movement? This started in the digital domain of social media with the primary goal of demonstrating the widespread prevalence of sexual assault and harassment in the workplace, and believe it or not, it is ubiquitous [7]. Many female physicians have "horror stories" to tell. Now there is a term that is in vogue which is *sorority*, it has its origins during 17th century with the formation of the Adelphean Society Alpha Delta Pi and this emerged because a Latin professor thought that the term fraternity was no appropriate for ladies. It all began to accomplish women´s rights and equality, despite the difficulties women overcome every obstacle and attained their goals [8]. Surprisingly in 2017 for the first time, more than half of medical school entrants were women. It means that all of them are young students, trainees, and junior faculty members, and it seems quite away for them taking a role as Deans, Chairs, or Search Committee members. Our duty is not just being equally in enrollment, it is inclusiveness and enlisting allies, and educating our trainees, students and patients moving forward to a workplace where women can be more involved and can have input in important decisions. There is an example where Sheryl Sandberg on a TED talk entitled *"Why we have too few women leaders",* she says that she was on a three-hour meeting, and after two hours, she had needed to use the restroom, and in attempt to find the rest room, she needed to ask for directions as the group had just moved to a high-end New York private office. A male replied and said she was the first women invited to pitch a deal in that office or maybe the only one who had to go to the bathroom since no one knew where the female bathroom was. This makes new generations question what we can do as individuals. What are the messages we need to tell ourselves and what can we learn from this? What are the messages we tell the women that work with and for us? What are the messages we are telling our daughters? [9].

One of the big problems is that women have to be more confident, they deserve better than now, and it will be better. There is another example Sandberg mentions on her TED talk, it should be easier just to say to women that have to "Believe in themselves and negotiate for themselves". As health professionals I want to invite you to reach what seems to be impossible, I would like to share a phrase once told to me by a friend: "Those who try the absurd achieve the impossible." So, never let yourself down, never doubt yourself, give you that value you know you have, because as a human being that is always looking for the welfare of your patients, you have to know how important you are. Be courageous, fight against adversities, and use them as your weapon, take advantage of these great learning opportunities, and visualize yourself in a better world enriched by diversity and inclusiveness for your children."

It is surprising how many male colleagues had to join to recognize the necessity and how they engage in ending gender bias. This is not least and ultimately, because there are sexual orientation, skin, religion, nationality, or appearance prejudice, and this will be review later [7].

By way of example of Michael Kimmel´s TED talk *Why gender equality is good for everyone, men included*; a child and his father had a car accident and unfortunately the dad passed away. When the child was taken to the emergency room, the physician sees the boy and says "Oh, I can´t treat him, that´s my son." What do you think immediately? You may be flummoxed, but the doctor was her mom! If you thought of another reason it is ok, but the reason for this is because we tend to think of a man when we refer to a doctor. This will change over time [10].

Have you ever wondered about university enrollment and which specialists are chosen by woman? Well, this varies in every country as demonstrated by the results published by the National Institute of Statistic

The Benefits of Inclusive Leadership among Healthcare ... 73

and Geography (INEGI) and the Association of American Medical Colleges (AAMC). It will help you to support gender equity studies and to understand the progress of women's representation in a variety of medical school positions. For example, the AAMC published that among women there were 46% applicants, 47% matriculating students, 46% residents, 38% faculty, 21% full professor and 16% deans. This study may inspire female doctors, who might be more talented, to aim for top positions in clinical research, excellent education, or taking decisions in health-care centers. This study also shows the top 10 specialties for women residents in 2013-14 representing n = 44,592/52,521 being in the next order for the total number [11]:

83% Obstetrics and Gynaecology, 71% Pediatrics, 55% Family Medicine, 55% Psychiatry, 54% Pathology, 43% Internal Medicine, 38% Surgery, 38% Emergency Medicine, 37% Internal Medicine Subspecialties and 37% Anesthesiology [11]. In Mexico this may vary a bit, but what remains almost the same are surgical and internal medicine subspecialties.

INEGI published on 2015 that from every 100 doctors, 64 are men and 36 women. From this just 82 from 100 are economically active, representing 86.1% men and 75.4% women. The statistics also showed how many female and male doctors are in every state, for example in Durango there are 59 and 41 doctors, female and male respectively in a population of 100, meanwhile in Sonora there are just 12 women out of 100 doctors. It is astonishing how just 2 states have more female doctors (Durango and Guerrero), and the other 30 states have a big prevalence of male doctors. In addition, the data also showed that there are more men involves with subspecialties, working in business health sector, occupying a dean or head position whilst women tend to remain working as general doctors or educators [11].

The difference between women and men that studied medicine and stay at home is higher among females. We can see in graphics that women work less than 35 hours or get absent at work during a week rather than men, and vice versa. Something else we can analyze is that there are more women that are subordinate (86.8%) and remunerated workers in relation to men (72.7%), they are more employers or workers on their own, for this reason men have less work benefits [11].

When categorized by income, men are shown to have more than 5 salaries and women would have less than this, but it could vary depending if they are self-employed or not [11].

Mexico has proportionately fewer female health-care providers, lagging behind other countries in the region. This highlights important messages to policy makers and emphasizes the need to make gender equality a critical part of human capital development because there is a strong correlation between countries gender gap and its economic performance. The enrollment of women in medical school in Mexico is about 60%, but in spite of this we do not find women in decision-making positions [12, 13]. We therefore decided to perform a survey among our female residents doing specific questions and the results were as follows:

Female residents considered that empowerment starts at home, 70% have had a lack of confidence, 69% had a mentor during their training, 53% did not respond when unfair acts happened, 73% had felt discriminated because of being a women, 93% had felt uncomfortable about inappropriate comments against women, 53% were harassed at hospital. We can see that besides of this, a third keep quiet, two thirds asked for respect and 3.5% have denounced authorities [14]. These results were presented at the 66th Annual Scientific Meeting & Expo American College of Cardiology 2017 in Washington, DC [14].

In Mexico our traditions, cultural values, and religious beliefs and practices are being misused to curtail women rights to entrench sexism and defend misogynist practices. At this moment in time we need to be thinking from a gender perspective, thinking about opportunities, social roles and interactions. The solution for our Mexican women and girls is empowering them to protect their rights and make sure they can reach their full potential.

There is still a lot to be done and we have a long way to go. A Mexican success story, Teresita Corona, was the first woman to be elected as Vice-president in 150 years by the National Academy of Medicine. She is also on the list of the 300 most influential leaders of 2018 in Mexico [15,16,17].

What is the situation of women in leadership positions? While they are obtaining administrative positions in the Dean´s Office, nonetheless the percentage is still low compared to men, with emphasis on assistant dean positions because it has remained around 46 percent [11]. What is on our hands is changing the way of thinking of new generations, you may question how is it going to be possible? Schools should provide increased resources to help support the advancement of women and attract them to careers in academic medicine. Other ways in which you could start this is near your workplace in order to recruit, retain and advance women faculty are [11]:

- Start a mentoring program.
- Contact and advocate for school's office of women.
- Include men in the conversation about how to mentor and advance women.
- Listen, make a plan, organize and execute.
- Provide resources to invest on women leaders.
- Support women faculty leaders.
- Provide unconscious bias sensitivity for search committees and promotion and tenure committees and make sure there are women participants on those committees.
- Provide mentoring and coaching programs for women faculty.
- Sponsor women into programs.
- Find out what women think about the culture and climate at your institution.
- Do an analysis about salary, administrative burden, lab space and see if it is equitable in relation to other centers or schools.
- Support your local groups on campus and empower women to support, mentor, and sponsor each other.

As said by the Stanford Medicine´s Office of Faculty Development and Diversity, we have to be committed to fostering faculty development and leadership opportunities for women faculty. If we do nothing, this discrepancy can have a negative impact on patient care, teaching and research [11].

Taking note on what Barbara Fivush, Associate Dean for Women in Science and Pediatrics Director Johns Hopkins University School of Medicine, Mexico, Latin America and the rest of the world needs to increase the number of women in leadership roles in order to optimize the success of academic medicine going forward. Our task is to ask for institutional support, if we do not do that, we will stay stagnant. Furthermore, a negative economic and financial impact occurs when there is a loss of women in academic centers. Doing this we can contribute to have a wider and diverse balanced leadership team, enriched by a lot of points of view. This requires a lot of effort and conscious that will be crucial but possible [11].

Women in Mexico have an important role, and they already exist some movements leaded for empower women who wants to make a positive change. One example of this is one conference celebrated on October 2018, called *"Mujeres en Medicina,"* it took part at the National Institute of Cardiology, where nearly 400 people attended, and they talked about topics such as leadership and mentoring, economic impact, inclusiveness of women with a business sight, sexual harassment and violence. Many young students had participated and got involved in those topics that were performed on panel discussions, it is one of the first steps we all are doing to have a more inclusive world, that will be inherited to the young ones [18].

"Mujeres en Medicina" was created and had 8 goals:

1. Networking
2. Leadership and excellence
3. Mentoring
4. Stop gender discrimination in health-care institutions
5. Stop harassment in health institutions

6. Promote and motivate the diversity in management positions.
7. Support female young doctors so that they can succeed in both, personal life and professional work.
8. Seek for equality in both genders and unprotected women [18].

3. MENTORING: WHAT EVERYONE SHOULD DO

Being a mentor is an important key of success for new mentees generations. We can encourage them to be better and improve their skills, identifying intelligence and give them new opportunities in the health-care field, no matter if they have a different profile or a mix of them. Those who train in medicine can pursue at least 4 types: clinical care, education, research, or administration [19].

Our role as a mentor is to pursue those young minds, guide them through their way and help them to reach their goals besides every adversity they could face and overcome it. As a health-care professional you can have a specific duty with your mentees, you can provide initial ideas, infrastructure, financial support, and supervision while the mentees perform the daily work [19].

I have been a busy person my whole life, surround by the talent of my students, many of them from different schools, female, male, foreign students, and some of them continued their studies overseas or have been distinguished for their personal career, having no doubt that they continue to inspire new students in different medical fields. You may define yourself by one of 4 types or archetypes of mentorship listed below [20]:

Archetype 1: The Traditional Mentor

Defined by a formal, dynamic and reciprocal relationship in work environment between themselves and a mentee aimed at promoting the career growth of both. Mentors usually give feedback on papers, projects, scholarships, and career milestones.

Archetype 2: The Coach

A coach teaches people how to improve in a particular skill or subject. Coaches focus on performance related to a specific issue rather than growth multiple dimensions.

Archetype 3: The Sponsor

Sponsors use their influence in a field to make mentees more visible. Visibility may include recommendations. They risk their reputations when recommending junior colleagues.

Archetype 4: The Connector

Connectors are multipliers that link up with the world. They are master networkers who have extensive social and political capital accrued from years of academic success.

Nonetheless, one can fulfill multiple roles for different personalities in distinct positions. Summing this up means that the mentor guides, the coach improves, the sponsor nominates, and the connector empowers [20].

There are many publications where you can see the data about who has had a mentor and how it influences mentees. Somehow it is concerning that less than 50% and, in some cases, fewer than 20% of faculty members had a mentor [21]. Unfortunately, there is not enough evidence about the details, it urges to make an implementation among new generations during the time they are acquiring knowledge. That is not enough, because you have to see them putting on practice the skills they have acquired during their training. At the end of this studies some of them rated departmental mentoring as the most important resource and support, identified mentor guidance as important personal development or as the most important aspect of training experience. Furthermore, they have had some outcomes such as increasing confidence in professional development, education and administration. All of this gave them a career-enhancing, likelihood of achieving promotion, aid in career advancement and were actively advised and fostered their independent career goals intermittently [21].

As mentors have their classification, mentees have two phenotypes which are divided in conflict averse and confidence lacking, listed below [22]:

The Benefits of Inclusive Leadership among Healthcare ... 79

- Conflict averse types
- The Over-committer: Lacks the ability to say no.
- The Ghost: Appears extremely enthusiastic and energetic but disappears without trace and without notice.
- The Doormat: Is on the receiving end of a manipulative mentor.
- Confidence lacking types
- The Vampire: Requires constant attention and supervision, leaving mentors drained and empty.
- The Lone Wolf: Assertive, self-motivated, and determined; prefers working alone; believes mentorship is not a necessity.
- The Backstabber: Rarely fails, but when this does occur, makes excuses or assigns blame to others rather than to personal missteps [22].

The relationship between mentors and mentees is bidirectional and critical to academic success [22].

4. DIVERSITY AMONG HEALTH-CARE CENTERS

Talking about diversity means a lot, it could be about equally, men, woman, transgender, youthfulness, agedness, black, white, Asian or Latin. We all are humans, raised in different cultures, traditions, way of thinking, and values. Vernā Myers is on personal mission to disrupt *status quo.* She is author of the best-selling books *Moving Diversity Forward: How to Move from Well-Meaning to Well-Doing* and *What If I Say the Wrong Thing? 25 Habits for Culturally Effective People,* Vernā has touched over 1,000,000 people through her speeches, appearances and transformative message of power and possibility. Her inspiring TED talk, "How to Overcome Our Biases? Walk Boldly Toward Them," offers three ways any person can become an active participant in countering bias in ourselves and in others to create a more just world. All of this is seen on her website, enriching our way of thinking [23, 24].

For the last two decades, Vernā and her team have helped eradicate barriers of race, gender, ethnicity and sexual orientation at elite international law firms, Wall Street, Fortune 500 companies, and other powerhouse clients with the aim of establishing a new, more productive and just status quo. Appealing is the Vernā quote where she says: "Diversity is being invited to the party. Inclusion is being asked to dance" [23].

The first time I watched Vernā on her TED talk I said to myself, it is actually happening around us, it is not in the past, we are not talking about 20 or 50 years ago, we are talking about 2018 where this macho culture, racism, and sexual orientation lead us to make jokes that cause dignity destruction, which also means human person destruction, because both are synonyms. Immanuel Kant used to say that a person is someone, not something [25].

When we talk about diversity, color skin could be a topic some may ignore or say that no longer exists but for McGowen- Hare she feels something is missing. If we do not address racial diversity it will change partially. At the end they will be just half men and half women, but 100 percent white. She aims for little ones to inspire them to say they want to be where she is right now, not thinking about skin color as a limitation [2].

Impressive is Sanberg´s message about not having to choose between being great employees or being great mothers or fathers, husbands, wives, sons and daughters. Arguing companies to be more attuned to their employees emotional and personal needs [2].

Diversity nowadays is having more acceptance and tolerance. Over the years a more open-minded culture will exist. Those bias will vanish over the years; it will change if we educate our society creating a culture of tolerance and respect. Parents should teach this at home and will be put in practice on our workplaces.

5. OPPORTUNITIES WITHOUT BOUNDARIES

Expanding our horizons is vital since the early beginning. When I entered the faculty of medicine my aims and expectations were high and in certain way unattainable. I should say that I was doing right since the begging, with excellent grades at high school, and good experiences for someone my age. When I was reaching for overly ambitious, I fell down and it was hard to start again, from the bottom. I took some bad decisions through this way; I may regret a bit. But hey! If I would not fail, I would not have learnt. My parents always let me decide on my own but of course giving me examples and analogies of life, and I thank to them because they made me self-confident, trusting in me and pushing me to be a better person.

I had a privileged education where leadership was encouraged from the beginning. I still remember those inspiring and motivational words I received from my Deans and Council President. I was sitting next to one of my best friends and we both said, "I will be there one day". Over the years I joined many different councils and got involved during my college years. It was kind of difficult in the beginning, because almost everyone used to know someone who had invited them to be part of the council and I knew no one. One day a good friend told me we were enrolled to compete for the next student society, it was the opportunity to win, by that time I knew a few from the first council I joined, many of them were part of this societies from the beginning, it was my first time.

Suddenly my friend told me she had to give up the project and I got by myself. I had no previous experience on that, and I said to myself, I've had theoretical classes and workshops about entrepreneurship, negotiation, debate, strategic planning and team work before.

It was two or three weeks before it all started, we need to have sponsorships, a year program, and, of course, people on our side. During those days I made a plan, I need to be inclusive and invite people like me that has never been part of this councils, I started to search for the right team, it all came good, I started a quest for people experience, I watched videos on internet and I looked for my notes.

The competition had previously planned their campaign for almost a year before. I was the head of the team and I had to motivate them, I did not know how I did it but when I realize our team was bigger and bigger, a lot of people joined our project. The election day came, I also had support for other careers, it was few minutes past midnight and then a lot of cheers were claiming for both teams, rumors and whispers were heard, we all were nervous, our team was very animated, we were supporting each other and when all the board had to climb the stairs, the vote counters started to clap this famous song of Queen-We will rock you, the adrenaline was on her top, votes were the same, it was one for them and one for us, we could not believe we had the same number of votes, at the end unfortunately we lost for a little difference of nearly 20 votes among approximately 500 votes.

Now I can say it was a fortune for us, we learned a lot during those 3 weeks, we meet a lot of people, we supported one another, during that year the university council invited me to join them and I said yes, I learned from them and next year I decided with my team to try one more time, it was our year.

At the beginning people told us, the reach is too high to achieve. You better try your best. I talked with my team and I told them: "team, we are all good, the only one we have to show our best is ours". It definitely was our best year, we made things that were not made before and today are still remembered by the youngest generations, some of them were replicated.

Since then I knew the real meaning of transcend. I learned that term on every class of humanities. I felt good about it, inspiring new leaders and sharing our experience was marvelous. That year I invited a lot of people to join, we were the voice and I wanted to hear them, we did meetings to hear everyone, no matter if the where part of this for the first time, I knew there was talent of everyone, they just needed to be heard and be pushed. Every member used to vote, and the board was made up by 3 women and 2 men - including me. I used to listen everyone individually about how they feel or about their ideas, because that diversity of people enriched me, doing my last year at university one of the best things ever happened to me.

I later founded a medical society among my friends, and I was chief intern in the hospital where I made my medical practices during a year. I can sum up this whole story in a single word and it is, try.

Being young is an opportunity to fail and learn, in order to create a better world, a more inclusive and participative decision making. The future is in the decisions that the young ones will decide, they have to learn about a new culture, where equality is not enough, it is important to take a sit and speak louder about our thoughts, giving point of view and be listened through the walls.

If you want to succeed in life you have to build a clear plan of what has to be done in order to achieve a goal and make that happen as Yonatan Zunger said [2].

6. A MESSAGE TO THE YOUTH

I had been a teacher for more than 35 years and I feel committed to teach and mentor the future doctors in training. This has been the result of more than 2000 students who have gone through the classrooms where I have had the pleasure of sowing knowledge as well as seeing several of them who are currently practicing their profession or reaching another stage in their lives and careers [26].

My work as a Professor of Physiology in an uninterrupted way dates from 1980 to date, except for the time I was training at Harvard and UCLA. I remember when I had the opportunity in front of very admirable doctors to present a physiology seminar which was an important pillar in my life and training as a doctor [26], so I think we should all have a professional sphere that involves teaching, clinical practice and research, which will contribute to the medical development of our country. We have very talented new generations.

I feel satisfied day by day watching young enthusiastic students who are committed to their career, and that in the future will stand out for their academic merits and skills acquired in their academic training. Several years ago, I was a student, I had great goals and aspirations, so I want to invite you to be persistent and constant in your study. Medicine is an infinite path of opportunities for learning, be authentic and seek to transcend positively in everything you do.

Wojcicki made Google what it is nowadays, one of the most respected, innovative, and powerful brands on earth. When she was at her office she was really focused and prioritizing. Avoiding problematic projects and forgetting about things that were growing slowly. She did not have time for that. She was focused on big ideas and get them done now [2].

If you want to have results, you need to work daily, nothing is going to come by itself. One of the keys to success is dedication and a positive attitude towards every result.

7. MEXICO AND LATIN AMERICA TODAY

What is next? Felicia Marie Knaul, who is the Director for Advanced Study of the Americas at the University of Miami, on her video streaming talked about *"Valuing the invaluable: The contributions of women to health and the economy in Mexico."* In contribution with his teamwork Hector Arreola- Ornelas, Julio Rosado and Oscar Mendez. She says that these outcomes are performed in an adverse context, she published *Women and Health: the key for sustainable development* on 2015 in Lancet under the leadership of Ana Langer who is a Professor of the Practice of Public Health and Coordinator of the Dean's Special Initiative on Women and Health and Afaf Meleis who is a Professor of Nursing and Sociology and Dean Emerita [15, 27, 28, 29].

What is our aspiration about women in health-care centers? Virtuous or vicious circle? Julio Frenk who was the Former Secretary of Health of Mexico and is currently dean of the Harvard School of Public Health, said today that universal health coverage is far more than a fashionable trend; and I cite him "Only by strengthening health systems and social protection will we be able to overcome the triple burden of disease that our countries are facing," he said. He called for a "paradigm change," in which "health is no longer viewed as a service that is delivered but rather as a basic right, which makes it universal [30]."

His publications for the Pan American Health Organization said that lowering poverty and pushing economic income through the family will have better healthcare outcomes. Adverse socio-economic means results in worse health for men, women and children - if they are not healthy, they work less, and human capital is sub- optimal by not having equally opportunities from a lack of economic growth and education. As a result, there is a tremendous impact that results in more poverty that turns into less human and health development, that will lead us to poor women, unhealthy and without rights turning into health-care facilities, unstable to prevent illness and death. All of this is a downward spiral of chronic illness and socio-economic deterioration. If we aspire to reserve this downward circle we need to offer more health care facilities to the population, kids will learn more and eventually adults will be more productive leading to a world with equally opportunities, improving our economy, which results in more money and resources to invest in health and human development having more healthy and educated women providing more health services, that hereupon will positively resulting in overall greater health and less illness [15].

Women in Mexico are changing health rather than men because they contribute with actions that are not remunerated in spite of gender and opportunities inequality such as women have more home duties, and also dedicate time for professional life [15].

Some of the recommendations made in the study made by Ana Langer, Afaf Meleis and Felicia Knaul where [15, 27]:

1. Expand and equalize maternity and paternity leave in extension and coverage.
2. Offer licenses for women and men to care for sick family members who require palliative care.
3. Strengthen and expand the proactive benefits of the labor market and social security for families that lack social security coverage.
4. Implement a transformative educational policy with gender perspective in medical education and training of health professionals.

5. Strengthen the regulatory framework of health professionals, especially the majority of women, to prevent feminization from leading to inequality.
6. Seek greater representation of women in positions of responsibility and decision making in the health sector [15, 27].

We all should share the pharmaceutical company Merck KGaA vision in which textually says: "The Healthy Women, Healthy Economies initiative strives to unleash the economic power of women by bringing governments, employers and other interested stakeholders together to help improve women's health so women and by extension their families can join, thrive, rise in their communities and live better lives [31]. With this initiative we can seek for gender and professional equality.

It still remains harder, I will give an example by Katherine Zaleski, CoFounder and President of PowerToFly, who was on a final pitch to investor while she was pregnant, and some venture capital asked how she was going to run the business if she had family with kids. In the other hand nobody asks men how they are going to take care of their kids [2]. It is terrible how we have this "motherhood penalty" nowadays.

8. ECONOMIC OUTCOMES

Regarding leadership activities over the years, male participation remains somewhat constant with no relative change, furthermore women had increased their participation in Mexico and Latin America. You can see objectively how it this engagement has evolved, men seem to be linear, women are notoriously are becoming more engaged - leading to an improved economic condition in Mexico and Latin America [15].

There is an epidemiological transition that will create long-term need for providers, primarily driven by the rapid growth in chronic health conditions. Yet despite this, women physicians find themselves at a disadvantage despite this projected trend across the entire health-care system. As mentioned before, women experience lower salaries, and this

The Benefits of Inclusive Leadership among Healthcare ...   87

may vary because it depends where they work or how many hours they work, if they have work benefits or not. According to these studies, women are not reaching the total value of their contributions, they represent a 4.8% total Mexican gross domestic product (GDP) which was 3.8 trillion dollars in 2015, 51% remunerated - implying 49% was not remunerated - almost three times the Mexican economy. For our country we can see that for Mexico GDP percentage, the estimated value of contributions remunerated and not remunerated from women to the health care system remain above Peru but below Spain and Canada. Obviously, this varies because salary structures are different in every country and depends if they are in a developed or undeveloped country [15, 27]. In Mexico depending on the various models, the ratio ranges from 1.6 to 2.2 GDP [15, 27].

Doing a more detailed analysis we can see that the situation between men and women is a crossroad talking about world equality, women represent 2.2% GDP and men 1.1%. What is different? Well, women have more unremunerated contributions, because they do more than men, working much more - such as doing activities that could prevent illness in poor areas. They do more household chores having a great outcome in health. During a week there are a total of 168 hours. There is the question of how much is allocated for rest and sleep if you compare men and women? There was survey that showed men and women older than 20 years and the results were that men rest 73 hours a week, while women have 40 hours to dedicate themselves, meaning less than 6 hours a day, and that included time for sleep - less than the suggested 8 hours a day that is generally recommended. All of this is because it has been shown that most of the women divide their duties almost equally, job, rest, care at home and domestic work meanwhile men invest less time doing care at home and domestic work rather women [15, 27].

The participation of women as health-care providers represents a total of 62%, where most of them are nurses while few of them are doctors. When examining the list of other health-care professions, included on the list are technicians or other professional or skilled-labor titles [15, 27].

Julio Frenk and colleagues conducted a study of employment and unemployment women who graduated medical school. This transition showed a timeline from 1990´s to 2014 where unemployment decreased considerably from 68% to 43%, respectively and employment increased by 25% since then. There is still a lot to do, because there are still few women who are Deans or decision-makers in the health area compared with men who are still occupying most of these positions. Another topic is the difference in women's salaries that are a 30% less than men which could only be partially related to work hours gap [15, 27].

This economic gap will remain until we "Prioritize diversity, because other priorities had eclipsed it," as Nancy Lee said [2].

9. LEADERSHIP EDUCATION FOR MEDICAL STUDENTS

When we decided to study medicine, we may not have known that we will have to lead teams, regardless of whether we choose a clinical, surgical, research, education or administrative role. For example, while we are in an emergency department, we have to give some orders to the emergency crew, indicating to administrate certain medications, intubate or doing a specific study. If we were on an operating room, the decision about making an incision, requesting for a scalpel, Mayo or a Kelly also reflects leadership.

Leadership means inspiring new leaders, and you know you are doing right when they remember you because of the positive things you did while you were leading. It may not be easy at the beginning but once you overcome every obstacle it seems to be easier. What I have learned is that you have to be inclusive, the best way to start it is when you delegate certain activities to your team, listen to them, get new ideas and work as a team.

For example, in Mexico there is a leadership program called Alpha at Anahuac University that has encouraged medical students from the beginning of their career to develop and refine their leadership skills. They are seeking to transform our society into a positive medicine and society. These students have some subjects and clerkships such as decision making, debate, oratory, creativity and solution making, negotiation, social responsibility, team work, entrepreneurship, strategic planning, vocation and emotional intelligence. Usually some of the students participate in national or international seminars where they have the opportunity to visit and interact with lvy-league college students who have similar programs at their campuses. The members also organize medical brigades in poor areas of the country or worldwide, making a positive social impact on this population [32].

There is some data published by Harvard Business Review called *Why Doctors Need Leadership Training,* where we can see that medicine involves leadership as a competency and skill that is not usually taught or reinforced among medical institutions. Those leadership skills have influenced on patient, health-care system, and financially. It has been shown that hospitals with highly rated directors result in higher quality care and also less mortality [33].

If this leadership results to be effective tends to create a better environment associated with less burnout and satisfaction. The benefit of this ability is coordinating teams and giving feedback [33].

Physicians need to understand the business of health-care organization, in order to understand insurances structures. Implementation of leadership training should be formally integrated into medical and residency training programs; it will make an important difference for health-care outcomes and financial sustainability alike [33].

Mexico needs more schools with programs where the young generations can improve their skills and can develop a culture of leadership [33].

CONCLUSION

Both in Mexico and across the world, we must implement and observe a culture of respect, empowerment, inclusiveness and tolerance. There is a lot of talent among our young people, but they need to be guided by a mentor to develop their full potential. But, what do we need to accomplish this noble goal? The answer lies in our understanding of individual determination the motivation to achieve. Moreover, it is critical to educate and sensitize future generations about the importance of inclusiveness in leadership. Doing so will benefit our society, strengthen our economy, improve health and foster harmony. We must stop making excuses for bad behavior - or ignoring it - because the change begins within ourselves.

REFERENCES

[1] Cabot R. C., Women in Medicine. *The Journal of the American Medical Association.* Sept. 11, 1915, Vol 65 pp. 947-948.

[2] Chang E., *Brotopia: Breaking Up the Boys' Club of Silicon Valley.* Portfolio/Penguin, 2018, 320 p.

[3] Wallis C. J. et al., Comparison of postoperative outcomes among patients treated by male and female surgeons: A population based matched cohort study. *BMJ* (Online). 359 (2017), doi:10.1136/bmj.j4366.

[4] Tsugawa et al., Comparison of Hospital Mortality and Readmission Rates for Medicare Patients Treated by Male vs Female Physicians. *JAMA Intern Med.* 2017; 177(2):206–213. doi:10.1001/jamaintern med.2016.7875.

[5] Wittenberg-Cox A., The Saatchi Ouster Shows Leaders Need to Be Gender Smart, Not Gender Blind. *Harvard Business Review.* August 03, 2016.

[6] Koven S., Letter to a Young Female Physician. *N Engl J Med.* 2017; 376:1907-1909 DOI: 10.1056/NEJMp1702010.

[7] Rabinowitz L. G., Recognizing Blind Spots. A Remedy for Gender Bias in Medicine? *N Engl J Med* 2018; 378:2253-2255 DOI: 10.1056/NEJMp1802228.

[8] Anson, Jack (1991). Baird's Manual of American College Fraternities (20th Edition). Bairds Manual Foundation. p. III-32. ISBN 0963715909.

[9] Sandberg S., *TED Talk: Why we have to few women leaders* [web streaming video]. (USA): TED; 2010 [cited 2018 Oct 24]. Available

from: https://www.ted.com/talks/sheryl_sandberg_why_we_have_ too_few_women_leaders?utm_campaign=tedspread&utm_medium=r eferral&utm_source=tedcomshare.

[10] Kimmel M., *TED Talk: Why gender equality is good for everyone, men included* [web streaming video]. (USA): TED; 2015 [cited 2018 Oct 29]. Available from: https://www.ted.com/talks/michael_ kimmel_why_gender_equality_is_good_for_everyone_men_included ?utm_campaign=tedspread&utm_medium=referral&utm_source=tedc omshare.

[11] Lautenberger D. M. et al., The State of Women in Academic Medicine. The Pipeline and Pathways to Leadership. *Association of American Medical Colleges.* 2014.

[12] Instituto Nacional de Estadística y Geografía [Internet]. INEGI: Estadísticas a propósito del día del médico [INEGI: Statistics on the day of the doctor]; 2014 [updated 2014 October; cited 2018 October 24]. Available from: http:// www.beta.inegi.org.mx/ contenidos/ saladeprensa/aproposito/2014/medico0.pdf.

[13] World Economic Forum [Internet]. *WEF: The Global Gender Gap*; 2016 [updated 2016; cited 2018 October 27]. Available from: http://www3.weforum.org/docs/GGGR16/WEF_Global_Gender_Gap _Report_2016.pdf.

[14] Meave A. Gender gap in emerging healthcare systems. *Lecture presented at 66th Annual Scientific Session & Expo*; 2017; Washington, DC.

[15] Knaul F. M. *Valuando lo invaluable: Las contribuciones de las mujeres a la salud y a la economía de México [Valuing the inestimable: The contributions of women in the health and economy of Mexico].* [streaming video] Simposium Mujeres en Medicina. Instituto Nacional de Cardiología "Ignacio Chávez"; 2018 [cited 2018 October 13].

[16] Academia Nacional de Medicina de México [Internet]. *ANMM: Mesa Directiva;* 2017 [ANMM: Board of Directors]. [updated 2017; cited 2018 October 7]. Available from: https://www.anmm.org.mx/acerca- de/mesa-directiva.

[17] Líderes mexicanos [Internet]. *Análisis Los 300 líderes más influyentes de 2018* [*Analysis The 300 most influential leaders of 2018*]; 2018 [updated 2018 July; cited 2018 October 7]. Available from: https://lideresmexicanos.com/ noticias/ analisis- los- 300- lideres- mas-influyentes-de-2018/

[18] Eventbrite [Internet]. *Mujeres en Medicina* [Women in Medicine]; 2018 [updated 2018 september 13; cited 2018 October 24]. Available from: https://www. eventbrite.es/ e/ entradas-simposium-mujeres-en-medicina-50239300 099#.

[19] Detsky A. S. and Baerlocher M. O. Academic Mentoring. How to Give It and How to Get It. *JAMA*. 2007 May 16; 297(19): 2134–2136. doi: 10.1001/jama.297.19.2134.

[20] Chopra V., Arora VM., Saint S., Will You Be My Mentor? —Four Archetypes to Help Mentees Succeed in Academic Medicine. *JAMA Intern Med.* 2018;178(2):175–176. doi:10.1001/jamainternmed.2017.6537.

[21] Sambunjak D., Straus S.E., Marušić A., Mentoring in Academic Medicine: A Systematic Review. *JAMA*. 2006;296(9):1103–1115. doi:10.1001/jama.296.9.1103.

[22] Vaughn V., Saint S., Chopra V., Mentee Missteps: Tales from the Academic Trenches. *JAMA*. 2017;317(5):475–476. doi:10.1001/jama.2016.12384.

[23] The Vernā Myers Company [Internet]. *About Vernā;* [updated 2018; cited 2018 October 26]. Available from: https://vernamyers.com/)

[24] Myers V., *TED Talk: How to overcome our biases? Walk boldly toward them* [web streaming video]. (USA): TED; 2014 [cited 2018 Oct 24]. Available from: https://www.ted.com/talks/verna_myers_how_to_overcome_our_biases_walk_boldly_toward_them?utm_campaign=tedspread&utm_medium=referral&utm_source=tedcomshare.

[25] Proceedings of Aristotelian Society. *Oxford Journals on behalf of the Aristotelian Society.* 1887-2012 (Vol. 1, No. 1 - Vol. 112)

[26] Alexanderson E. and Gamba G., Fisiología cardiovascular, renal y respiratoria [Cardiovascular, renal and respiratory physiology]. *Manual Moderno.* 1ª Edición. 2014.

The Benefits of Inclusive Leadership among Healthcare ... 93

[27] Langer et al., Women and Health: The key for sustainable development. *The Lancet*. 386(2015), pp. 1165–1210.

[28] Harvard T. H. Chan. *School of Public Health* [Internet]. Faculty and Researcher Directory; 2018 [updated 2018 May 23, cited October 26]. Available from: https://www.hsph.harvard.edu/ana-langer/

[29] University of Pennsylvania School of Nursing [Internet]. *About Afaf I. Meleis*; 2018 [updated 2018 May 24, cited October 26]. Available from: https://www.nursing.upenn.edu/live/profiles/69-afaf-i-meleis.

[30] Pan American Health Organization [Internet]. PAHO. *Julio Frenk: Universal health coverage is a global imperative;* 2013 [updated 2013 September 30; cited 2018 October 26]. Available from: https://www.paho.org/blogs/dc-52/?p=446.

[31] Merck KGaA [Internet]. Our vision: 2018 [updated 2018; cited 2018 October 26]. Available from: https:// www.emdgroup.com/ en/ company/ responsibility/ our-strategy/ health/ hwhe.html? global_redirect=1.

[32] Anahuac [Internet]. Alpha. *Programa de Liderazgo en Medicina;* 2018 [*Leadership in Medicine Program*]. [updated 2018; cited 2018 October 24]. Available from: http://ww2.anahuac.mx/alpha/

[33] Rotenstein L. S., Sadun R., and Jena A. B., Why Doctors Need Leadership Training. *Harvard Business Review*. October 17, 2018.

In: Fundamentals of Leadership …
Editors: S. P. A. Stawicki et al.
ISBN: 978-1-53615-729-1
© 2019 Nova Science Publishers, Inc.

Chapter 4

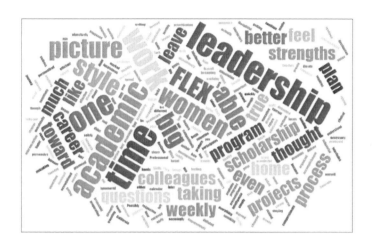

REFLECTIONS ON FLEX: A PROFESSIONAL DEVELOPMENT PROGRAM FOR WOMEN FACULTY OF THE SCHOOL OF MEDICINE AT CASE WESTERN RESERVE UNIVERSITY (CWRU-SOM)

Elizabeth Fine Smilovich[1], MD,
Phyllis A. Nsiah-Kumi[1], MD MPH
and Marion J. Skalweit[1,2], MD PhD

[1]Department of Medicine, Louis Stokes Cleveland Department
of Veterans Affairs Medical Center, Northeast Ohio VA Healthcare

System and Case Western Reserve University School of Medicine, Cleveland, Ohio, US
[2]Department of Biochemistry, Case Western Reserve University School of Medicine, Cleveland, Ohio, US

ABSTRACT

Professional development for women leaders in healthcare is becoming recognized as an important talent retention tool. Case Western Reserve University School of Medicine (CWRU-SOM), through the Office of the Dean and the Women Faculty of the SOM offers a unique program in the form of FLEX, a professional development program for its women faculty. Three recent participants who are practicing physician leaders within the Northeast Ohio VA Healthcare System share their impressions of FLEX and its impact on their leadership. Their reflections show that leadership skills can be learned, honed and must evolve and change with changes in the healthcare field.

Keywords: academic leadership, academic medicine, clinical leadership, leadership, women in medicine

1. INTRODUCTION

During the 2017-2018 academic year, the authors participated in "FLEX", A Professional Development Program for Women Faculty of the School of Medicine at Case Western Reserve University" [1, 2]. The authors were competitively selected for admission to a year-long program sponsored by the Office of the Dean for women faculty in, or destined for leadership roles. The program is the brainchild of executive director, Sumitra Khatri MD, a practicing leader and pulmonologist at the Cleveland Clinic Foundation in Cleveland, Ohio and a faculty member of CWRU Cleveland Clinic Lerner College of Medicine. The program, now in its seventh year, was also generously supported by the Office of Dean (Pamela Davis MD PhD). FLEX is a series of six full-day workshops encompassing diverse topics such as executive presence, public speaking, communication and leadership styles, time management, leading and managing people. Each participant also receives a Korn-Ferry 360 Emotional Social Competency Inventory™.

Each of the authors practices in the Northeast Ohio VA Medical System, an affiliate of CWRU SOM and participates in the rich academic and research life of these institutions. Each author has a different leadership style and goals for her respective sections, but all unanimously agree that programs like FLEX are necessary to develop the current and future women leaders in healthcare. In this series of essays by these three internal medicine subspecialists who each lead specialty care clinics and also provide primary care, unique visions for leadership in clinical medicine are explored.

2. "THE ROADMAP" BY ELIZABETH FINE SMILOVICH, MD

At some point, I began to wonder if slapping the leadership title "medical director" (as in nursing facility or primary care clinic) on a needed, work-intensive position really made it a leadership opportunity. I questioned how can one dedicate the requisite time to deliver excellent primary care and also have time enough to take a birds-eye view on clinic process and implement quality initiatives. I wondered how wonderful same-year colleagues were able to produce enough scholarship that they received career awards that allowed more time for scholarship and were promoted to associate professor so quickly. How can one build diversity and intellectual stimulation into the workday with current demands on productivity? How can one be home for dinner and spend quality time with family on a regular basis? These are questions I am sure I share with my female (and some of my male) colleagues. Overall, these questions left me overwhelmed, stagnant and steadily heading toward burnout. I didn't pursue a career in medicine solely to deliver individual care - I wanted to improve population health in my chosen field (geriatrics), teach and yes, lead.

Even though I had always thought of myself as having "good leadership qualities": fairly confident, assertive, projectable voice (not entirely accurate insights into what makes a good leader, but this was before my time in FLEX), I had the good sense to know that I lacked some of the skills to lead effectively. These are not skills traditionally taught in medical school, despite the implied expectation that physicians should lead. I did make attempts to enhance my career - applying for career awards, writing small grants, but even after reading "Lean In", I wasn't sure how to advance my career in the direction I had envisioned when I applied to medical school.

Knowing I wanted to gain leadership experience, I didn't have to think too much when my boss asked me, after much consideration, would I like to take over as the director of the geriatric medical home or in VA-speak ("geriPACT or geriatric Patient Aligned Care Team). As with many women physicians (anecdotally proven true by raised hands when our FLEX instructors asked, "how many of you discovered yourself in leadership positions because your boss said 'hey, you should do this!' "), I found myself thrust into a leadership role and once there, trying to navigate. I realized I needed, beyond discrete skills, a roadmap for successful leadership.

It's easy to cry "lack of skills" because skills can be taught, and how wonderful to gain a skill set that can change your life trajectory! However, it is the impetus to use skills that drives change. I won't say how many times I applied to career enhancing opportunities. What evaluators certainly recognized was that I didn't have a clear career objective. Possibly after writing several applications, being tapped for more service-related leadership positions and realizing my love for teaching, I began to develop my true career objective in addition to better running the geriatric clinic: expand geriatric knowledge, team communication and yes, leadership/resiliency skills to early health professional students within an inter-professional setting so that they can one day effectively lead…teams, clinics and more.

With this career objective I was admitted to the 6th class of FLEX and despite some initial setbacks in decorum - I couldn't stop laughing during my videotaped exploration into demonstrative gestures during public speaking - I began to see my strengths as a leader. Skills, I thought out of reach or not relevant, became available for use: persuasive, organized presentations; influential (rather than dominant) leadership style, prioritization, and self-care. I had understood even prior to FLEX that I had a high emotional intelligence, though I hadn't always thought of this as a strength, feeling that too much sensitivity and being seen as supportive led me to be overlooked for leadership opportunities. During our 360 Emotional Social Competency Inventory surveys, I found that my supportive nature was very well-received by those with whom I work and lead.

Another misconception that I debunked during FLEX was that I would either leave work terribly late or not be able to complete necessary clinical responsibilities if I took time out of my day to plan or devote time to big picture projects. I promised myself I would work on these things "later" when everything was done or at home. This never happened. I found that, by taking even just an hour once weekly to work on some of my academic priorities or simply plan, I was better able to focus and be efficient. I felt a sense of accomplishment and vigor, actually.

Over the course of the year I learned that, like anything else, effective leadership is a personalized process, one that for me requires interludes of thoughtful preparation (every Tuesday from 9-10:30 is marked on my calendar as "planning meeting" and devoted to organization and big picture projects), risk-taking ("yes" to speaking engagements and chapter writing requests) and caring for oneself, team-members and patients to avoid getting lost in the quagmire of daily, seemingly endless, responsibilities that leave one so deflated. So, did I find my roadmap? Possibly, I've gotten to Colorado on my journey from California to New York, but I remind myself to return to the basic tenets of staying true to my academic objectives, relying on my strengths, taking time out from the weekly grind for organization and big picture planning and to be compassionate to myself and those with and for whom I work. I feel I'm early in the process yet and maybe, objectively, my leadership style hasn't changed all that much, but I feel better which means I can continue traveling toward my academic destination.

3. "Taking My Seat, Overcoming Fear and Using My Voice at the Table to Achieve Results" by Phyllis A. Nsiah-Kumi MD MPH

Leadership is an area where I have always sought to grow and develop. While I have known people that seemed naturally gifted in this area, I also knew that there were genuine principles to learn and skills that successful leaders possess. Excellent leaders push themselves to gain new skills.

I personally have excelled in several leadership roles in both personal and professional endeavors. I knew that in many ways I was shining. But I was very aware that being a strong servant leader is hard. I had reached a plateau in my leadership—a place where I could go no further without some sort of formal leadership training or coaching. I needed something to get me to the next level.

When I became the Medical Director of Women's Health Services for our VA facility (14 locations over 10,000 square miles in Northeast Ohio) in 2013, I was excited for the opportunity to do work on a larger scale than I had in the past. I quickly realized the task I had undertaken was quite sizeable. It gave me opportunities to make a tremendous difference for female Veterans in our large service area. However, it also was tremendously stretching to me. I applied to the FLEX program early in my time as the Medical Director, but at that time I had not been on the Case Western Reserve University School of Medicine faculty for 2 years, and I was not eligible to participate. I was rather discouraged as I had been in many leadership roles for multiple years, and I felt that I could benefit from the training that FLEX had to offer.

Three years later, I was promoted to Women's Health Section Chief. As I faced new challenges in this role, I was reminded again that I needed additional skills. I knew I needed an honest community to get those skills— a safe place to get objective feedback and take a hard look at areas that held me back. I applied to then FLEX program again and was thrilled to be accepted to the sixth class of this important, training program. The FLEX curriculum was excellent, and it pushed me to grow. It wasn't simply about acquiring knowledge, it was about learning and employing practical skills, which did not always come naturally. When I applied, I was a bit apprehensive as I knew there was a chance I would embarrass myself a lot in the learning; I had to be vulnerable and humble there. While it was hard and terrifying, it was freeing. I learned many lessons about overcoming fear, communicating effectively, and using my voice at the table.

As a leader, I knew I was a bridge between the patients I serve, the staff I need, and the senior leadership of our facility. Rodney Sisco, a mentor from my undergraduate days, taught me early that a bridge gets walked on by the people going both directions. A bridge has to be strong and withstand the weight, and sometimes leadership certainly felt like a weight to me. The day I truly realized that tension was inherent in my leadership position, it became much easier to not take things so personally but to try to see what the people from both sides really meant—to listen to what they were not saying directly or to clarify what I was missing.

I learned I needed to pause before giving emotional responses. The pause was a very powerful tool. It allowed me to collect myself. It allowed me to step away from responding to triggers that would make the rest of an interaction ineffective. I was reminded to truly clarify what people meant and not assume that I knew what they meant based on my own perspective. I also learned to clarify what I meant instead of being frustrated by not being understood. Quite often, the disconnect was that we were not truly understanding each other.

A well-known book on negotiation skills for women written by Linda Babcock states it simply: "Women Don't Ask" [3]. That was true for me. Well, I would ask to a point and usually for low-hanging fruit. I realized that I asked for what I thought I could get without too much tension and often not for what I truly needed. Or I would ask for one thing and hope that someone would just offer more. Somehow, I still always came up short. I realized that some of my unmet requests were actually requests that I had not verbalized, and I also became aware that if no one was ever saying "no" to me, I was probably not asking for enough.

I went into FLEX feeling that I could advocate fairly well for patients and for my staff, but I truly struggled with advocating for myself. This contributed to being overextended, and ultimately to overextending my staff. Our program was growing tremendously, and we had many tremendous outcomes to show how effectively we were serving our rapidly growing population. To some degree, I was frustrated that some resources were not as quick to come as I would like. However, on reflection throughout the course of FLEX, I often was not asking often enough, directly enough or to the right people. And to do that, I needed to let go of fear.

I have always been a little afraid of myself. I know that sounds strange. It is not the sound of my voice. Or the force with which I speak. It is the power on the inside. And there is the art of balancing it. I did not want to be perceived as weak, but I did not want to be "too much" for the people around me. I am a passionate, high-energy leader. I am enthusiastic about the endeavors I participate in, and I get excited and often speak quickly. I have long worried about overwhelming those around me. It seemed so hard to be strong and talented and firm while being kind and compassionate and approachable.

As I progressed in my career and accomplished more, each step along the way, I feel like perhaps I gave up a little of my voice. Not in a way that compromises what I believe, but in a way that had me holding my tongue. I did not want to overwhelm or scare anyone off—giving up my priceless seat at the table. However, I realized that in all that silence, I was often rendering my seat as ineffective as an empty one. I was relinquishing the power and opportunity that I had to lead.

Marianne Williamson writes: "Our deepest fear is not that we are inadequate. Our deepest fear is that we are powerful beyond measure. It is our light, not our darkness that most frightens us. We ask ourselves, 'Who am I to be brilliant, gorgeous, talented, fabulous?' Actually, who are you *not* to be? You are a child of God. Your playing small does not serve the world. There is nothing enlightened about shrinking so that other people won't feel insecure around you. We are all meant to shine, as children do. We were born to make manifest the glory of God that is within us. It's not just in some of us; it's in everyone. And as we let our own light shine, we unconsciously give other people permission to do the same. As we are liberated from our own fear, our presence automatically liberates others" [4]. I was always waiting for the right time or the right way to say something, and while appropriate timing and well-articulated messages are key, I was suffering from perfectionism paralysis. Instead of making an attempt to communicate and engage, I often stayed silent, "perfecting" whatever it was that I needed to say. It was like not writing a draft of a paper because the first pass would not be publication worthy. I was so afraid of being misunderstood that I said nothing and left many meetings frustrated. However, I realized that progressions of thought that were obvious to me based on my daily experience were not equally transparent to those around me who spent most of their time in other contexts. I needed to learn to more clearly articulate my experience, the identified needs, the resources needed to address them, and the expected outcomes.

Initially, I was a bit afraid to take a seat at the table, and when I got there, I was often quiet if not addressed directly. I was usually taking it all in, composing my thoughts. Once I finally got my thoughts together (if I did so during the initial meeting), it was hard to get a word in edgewise. So often business meetings felt like jumping Double Dutch to me. You had to jump in at just the right minute while two quickly moving ropes were swinging in opposite directions. I also learned that if I was not able to clearly articulate everything during the initial meeting, the opportunity was not completely passed. A follow-up email or meeting was a reasonable and appropriate way to continue an important conversation.

I was reminded in FLEX that I absolutely needed to be at the table. I deserved to be there. It was not some magnanimous privilege of which I was unworthy. It was the starting point. A late mentor told me often, that "if you aren't at the table, you are on the menu." During FLEX, I learned to advocate more effectively for the resources I needed to serve women Veterans in Northeast Ohio. And I learned how to reframe my requests in a way that was more direct and specific.

I learned to plan requests with the specific audience in mind; to know exactly what I was asking for and why; and to ask for enough. I learned to provide data to support my request. I learned to ask boldly and specifically with intended outcomes included, and watch things happen. The role-playing exercises and practice presentations we gave were actually a powerful tool for me. During the FLEX course, I used a program vision I had had for several years for the Women's Health Program for my practice exercises. I built my argument, presentation of need, business case, and expected outcomes, using the tools we learned. I made my request to our senior leadership. Using a modified version of my FLEX presentation, I effectively advocated a $2 million initiative to bring mobile screening services (3-D mammography, bone density, and ultrasound) to female Veterans throughout our large service area.

Through FLEX, I learned that sometimes you dovetail your message into an ongoing discussion or take the opportunity to add it to the agenda of an existing meeting, but sometimes, you have to call the meeting. Sometimes, *you* must make the opportunity and take the floor.

As I am writing this reflection, I am facing some fairly large decisions about the future of my program. I have made asks and faced some obstacles in getting my program to the next level. I was initially very frustrated, seeing my situation as a possible dead end. THEN, I remembered the new skills in my expanded tool box. I decided to create an opportunity to speak with a key leader in our organization about these issues. I sent an email politely requesting to meet with this individual for some input on my situation. I have prepared a clear, concise discussion that articulates my challenges (supported by data), my proposed solution, including specific requests for this leader and the benefits to female

Veterans and our health care system. I will close reiterating my passion for what we do, the need, the benefits, and the specific requests.

Through my work with women Veterans, I am able to see their needs, understand them and advocate effectively for them. I can be at the table and be a knowledgeable and bold voice for them. In fact, it is my responsibility and honor to be at the table and be a knowledgeable and bold for them because *this* is how I serve them.

I am grateful to the FLEX program for helping me to shine more effectively and encourage others to do the same. The tools from the FLEX program have helped me to develop on my leadership journey. The journey of this servant-leader continues. I am absolutely a stronger leader than I was one year ago. I still have to work to change the behaviors that come naturally, but I feel more equipped to lead and to advocate for my patients, my staff, and myself. Pausing before reacting gives me a greater chance to use more effective techniques to build bridges, lead people and make a difference. I am more effectively taking my seat, overcoming fear and using my voice at the table to achieve results. The best is yet to come, and I cannot wait to see what lies ahead.

4. "Physician, Know Thyself!"
by Marion J. Skalweit MD PhD

As an MD PhD, I entered the Department of Veterans Affairs Career Development program immediately after infectious diseases fellowship and was fortunate to maintain continuous federal, industry and foundation basic research funding for 14 years. In addition to a successful basic science career, I spent approximately 3 months annually on the inpatient wards performing infectious disease consults and practicing general internal medicine. I also was in charge of our local home intravenous antibiotic program. I taught undergraduates, medical students, residents, and infectious disease fellows in a variety of settings, from classroom to bench to bedside. In other words, I was the proverbial "triple threat" that each of my wonderful physician scientist mentors had been.

When our outpatient infectious diseases clinic director left Cleveland to pursue other career options in Boston, I volunteered to "temporarily" take over the management of our outpatient clinical practice until a full time HIV trained replacement could be recruited. In the 7 years that followed, sweeping changes occurred at the VA in encounter documentation, ICD-10 happened, our HIV clinic formally assumed the role as primary care clinic for these veterans, and we ushered in the era of telehealth and electronic consultation. And I remained at the helm, a victim of my success at managing these changes, and budget restrictions that prevented us from hiring additional faculty to take over the clinic leadership. Somewhere along the way, I began to realize that the leadership skills involved in running a productive research program were not quite the same skills needed to run a clinic and manage health care providers. I was clearly at a transition point in my career. How could I continue to do my best in these two competing worlds?

When the FLEX leadership training opportunity came along, I was a mid-career former physician scientist now medical director of outpatient ID services at the third largest VA hospital in the country. I was burned out managing the minutiae of outpatient ID medicine, especially the increasing primary care aspects of HIV care and supervising a staff of 2 nurses, 2 providers, 2 pharmacists, 3 ID fellows and a rotating array of medical residents. In addition, numerous changes in reporting requirements both state and federal had increased the administrative burden of this position to the point that I could not compete effectively for sufficient amounts of research funding. Eking out an existence with small yearlong grants and keeping the lab up and running was becoming a struggle that kept me awake many nights, thinking about the people who depended on me for their livelihood. I had to learn to manage better--time, people, tasks—if I was to be an effective leader. The FLEX program made me realize that a lot of what I was doing was good—I was hardworking and fair minded about allocating tasks to my team, the model of a servant leader—but it was clear to my team, that I wasn't happy in this role. A lot of this was of

Reflections on FLEX 107

my own making in the sense that when I asked for help and didn't get it from my team, I grumpily did the tasks myself and stopped asking. I also had a difficult time communicating to my widely varying team why certain tasks were important, when I myself felt a great deal of resentment at having to do them e.g., coding encounters. In addition, my communication style—direct, firm, but not unkind I thought—was not always appreciated by staff. Different people needed different things, and I wasn't able to understand that at first. Finally, I missed research. Over time, it became harder and harder to make myself focus on keeping up on scientific literature, hypothesis generating and grant writing. Small clinical projects were not the same as basic bench research. There was always some clinical fire to put out anyway, that prevented focused concentration.

One of the most important aspects of the FLEX program to me was an exploration of personality types and how a leader can adapt their own traits to the work and communication styles of those who report to the leader. For example, in the DISC™ personality assessment (a behavior assessment tool utilizing the theory of psychologist William Moulton Marston regarding four different personality traits Dominance (D), Influence (I), Steadiness (S), and Conscientiousness (C)) [5]. I learned that my natural style was to be a dominant (D) leader and my compensatory style, as in when I couldn't get my folks to complete their encounters, was to be conscientious (C) and focus on completing the minutiae of process when others wouldn't….not surprising given what I knew about myself already! I also determined that many of the people I was leading were of different types, such as introverted types ("S's") who liked getting tasks assigned well in advance so that they could spend time processing, or the extroverted "I" types, dreamers, visionaries, influencers but lacking in the ability to really operationalize their ideas. Within the FLEX workshops, we were paired with others who had "opposite" personality types and we practiced different communication styles with one another. As part of FLEX, we also underwent a Korn-Ferry 360™ evaluation of emotional intelligence. I was grateful that my colleagues were able to speak candidly about my burnout, and how it was affecting my leadership effectiveness. It was a painful but ultimately essential part of reimagining what was needed in the clinic director role.

The training I received at FLEX should have been part of my education so much earlier. As physicians, we are all taught that we are leaders, but we aren't taught HOW to lead effectively. For those who are not natural leaders, many of the necessary skills can be learned and must be practiced consistently until they become second nature. The FLEX leadership program has helped me to find my voice to better advocate for my team and myself, to understand the underlying reasons for my positive and negative behaviors as a leader, to better understand the people I lead and serve, to better understand the people that lead ME and to rebalance my leadership goals.

Being a leader within a large healthcare organization involves taking risks, and navigating and advocating for change. It also means knowing when to step away and allow others to have a chance to lead and articulate a new vision for the organization. Since graduating from the FLEX program, I have transitioned a junior colleague into the clinic director position. I remain in this clinical setting to mentor her as she implements her vision and leadership goals to improve our clinical efficiency, improve quality of care and retention in care for our HIV positive veteran population. Our new leader has a wonderful balance of the DISC traits, and possesses a high degree of emotional intelligence. She is what we need at this time. I have also encouraged her to explore FLEX and programs like it, early in her leadership, in order to avoid feeling overwhelmed.

I too am leading again as a physician scientist. My first major research proposal in 3 years was submitted recently, I am a local site investigator for a national VA randomized controlled trial, and I am working with medical and undergraduate students again, honing their research skills. Sometimes being an effective leader means walking away from one leadership role, in order to find one's natural place as a leader.

CONCLUSION

1. Healthcare leaders need to be developed and given opportunities to practice effective leadership skills, in order to succeed. All leaders can benefit from learning new skills and honing old skills. Leadership programs should be offered as part of medical training as early as possible for those seeking leadership positions in the future.
2. Personal fulfillment and satisfaction in one's work is a key to successful leadership, and that means continuing to be an agent for change and improvement in one's organization.
3. Successful leadership requires a "pay it forward" attitude in order for health care organizations to continue to thrive, and to develop the next generation of leaders.

REFERENCES

[1] Khatri SB, Mencini L. What Type of Leader Do I Wish to Be? *New England Journal of Medicine Catalyst.* 2017. Epub August 7, 2017.

[2] Khatri SB, Mencini L, Paynick L, Dickson L, Kyriakides B, Freimark S, et al. *FLEX Professional Development Program for Women Faculty at CWRU individualizes success to create a culture of inclusion and empowerment.* American Association of Medical Colleges Annual Meeting 2015.

[3] Babcock L, Laschever S. *Women Don't Ask: Negotiation and the Gender Divide:* Princeton University Press; 2003.

[4] Williamson M. *A Return to Love: Reflections on the Principles of A Course in Miracles:* HarperCollins; 1992.

[5] Marston WM. *Emotions of Normal People:* Trench, Trubner & Co. Ltd.; 1928.

ABOUT THE AUTHORS

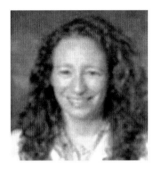

Elizabeth Fine Smilovich, MD is an Assistant Professor of Medicine at Case Western Reserve University School of Medicine and Director of the GeriPACT clinic at the Northeast Ohio VA Healthcare System. Her clinical and research interests are in geriatric medicine and in inter-professional clinical education.

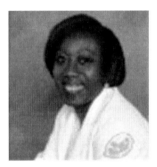

Phyllis A. Nsiah-Kumi, MD, MPH is an Assistant Professor of Medicine at Case Western Reserve University School of Medicine and Section Chief, Women's Health at the Northeast Ohio VA Healthcare System. Her clinical and research interests are in women's health, health disparities and health services research.

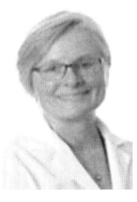

Marion J. Skalweit, MD, PhD is an Associate Professor of Medicine and Biochemistry at Case Western Reserve University School of Medicine and a staff physician in Internal Medicine and Infectious Diseases in the Northeast Ohio VA Healthcare System. Her clinical and research interests are in antibiotic resistance mechanisms of bacteria, diabetic foot infections, and electronic ID consultation.

In: Fundamentals of Leadership ...
Editors: S. P. A. Stawicki et al.

ISBN: 978-1-53615-729-1
© 2019 Nova Science Publishers, Inc.

Chapter 5

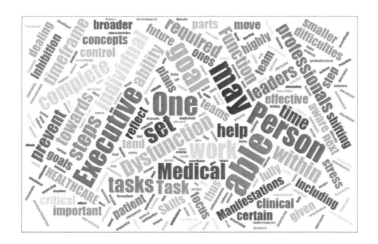

MEDICAL LEADERSHIP SKILLS: EXPLORING THE EXECUTIVE FUNCTION-DYSFUNCTION SPECTRUM

CJ Maron, Alfred DiGregorio
and Stanislaw P. A. Stawicki[*]
Department of Research & Innovation,
St. Luke's University Health Network, Bethlehem, Pennsylvania, US

---

[*] Stanislaw P. Stawicki, MD, MBA, FACS, FAIM; Chair & Network Medical Director of Department of Research & Innovation, St. Luke's University Hospital Campus, Bethlehem, Pennsylvania; E-mail: stanislaw.stawicki@sluhn.org; stawicki.ace@gmail.com.

ABSTRACT

Effectiveness of individual leaders depends heavily on their ability to communicate, coordinate, learn, apply knowledge, implement plans, execute decisions, reflect, and engage in self-improvement – all in exceedingly flexible and seamless fashion. By proxy, teams and team cultures also tend to mirror their leader's characteristics. Thus, the presence of highly effective leaders both directly and indirectly translates into more effective teams, better task execution, and ultimately the attainment of stated goals/objectives. This chapter reviews key components of the conceptual construct of executive function (and dysfunction) and the corresponding manifestations and correlates at both the individual and team levels. Focus is on health-care applications of these important concepts.

Keywords: executive dysfunction, executive functions, leadership skills, objective assessment, professionalism, team design

1. INTRODUCTION

Executive functions can be defined as a set of high-level abilities, such as inhibition, pacing, self-monitoring and emotional control, that contribute to the capacity to live a productive life, both at personal and professional levels [1, 2]. In brief, executive functioning (EF) involves the individual being able to monitor and change behavior, to meaningfully plan for the future, to readily recognize social cues, and adequately/competently interact with others in productive and non-threatening fashion [1]. Summary of EF sub-domains is provided in **Table 1**.

From biological and neuroscience perspective, the frontal lobes of the brain, and in particular the prefrontal cortex, are largely responsible for the control and coordination of EF [3, 4]. People who experience challenges with EF may exhibit difficulties socializing, dealing with stress, shifting between tasks/functions, updating and monitoring of information/working memory, engaging in internally generated "acts of control", and with anticipating and planning for unexpected outcomes [1, 4]. The importance of the above abilities is critical, and individuals who struggle in these domains may at times be considered to have the so-called executive dysfunction complex (EDC) [**Figure 1 & Figure 2**] [2].

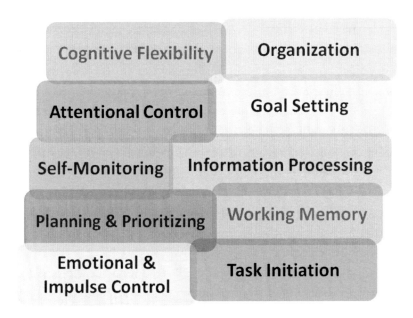

Figure 1. Simplified representation of key components of executive function.

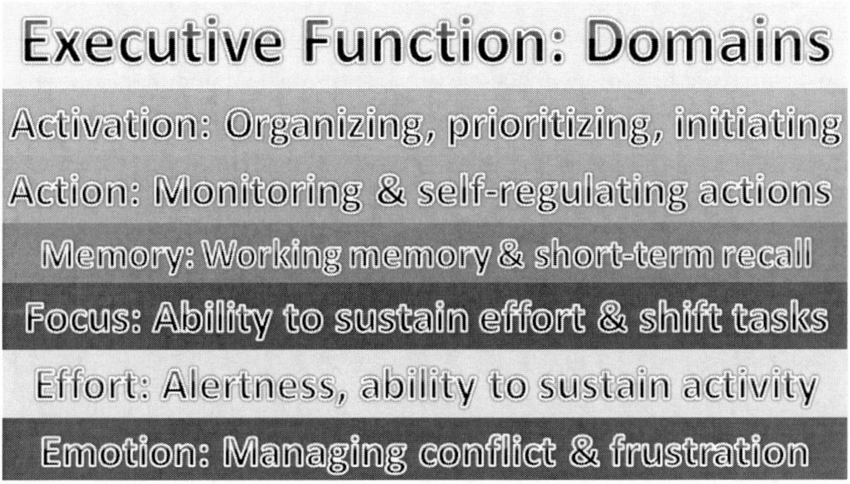

Figure 2. Key concepts pertinent to practical application of executive functioning.

To gain a better understanding of EDF, one can examine specific EFs (**Figure 1**) in isolation to identify with more granularity problems that may arise when corresponding cognitive mechanisms are not operating optimally. For instance, if an individual lacks the ability to inhibit certain undesirable responses, he or she may become more distractible or impulsive in their decisions and/or communication style [2]. Difficulties involving self-pacing and self-monitoring can lead to the affected person being unable to finish their work on time or not checking that each step of a process is fully complete before attempting to move on [2], potentially resulting in suboptimal quality of finished product (or process). As previously mentioned, problems involving emotional control may result in inability to react appropriately to certain situations that may arise during interpersonal or professional interactions. However, it is important to understand that although isolated observations may offer some insight into the underlying pattern of EDF, not every person will exhibit specific characteristics or behaviors [2].

In a health-care setting, high level of EF among medical professionals is necessary to ensure that optimal individual and team functioning is maintained, and that the best patient outcomes can be achieved. Consequently, organizations that foster high level of EF tend to be recognized as having better reputation and are more likely to be known for reliability, safety and quality of care [5, 6]. Within the broader leadership context, one's ability to "withstand" stress and remain calm under pressure is necessary', yet the attainment of the latter may be challenging to health-care providers performing delicate, high-risk procedures or otherwise complex cases [7, 8]. Additionally, medical professionals are required to be aware of, and plan for, any risks that might be present throughout the course of clinical patient management. Finally, strong communication skills have been shown to help improve patient safety, clinical outcomes, as well as hospital and physician ratings [9, 10]. Consequently, one can easily appreciate the critical importance of EF (and the potentially deleterious effects of EDF) on health-care provider's ability to effectively treat patients and conduct meaningful team interactions.

2. EXECUTIVE FUNCTIONS: AN OVERVIEW

The concept of EF was first introduced in the mid-1970's as part of the overall proposed paradigm of a "central executive" [11]. Broadly speaking, EF can be described as the "controller" of our "working memory" and thus a mechanism that allows us to conduct our high level day-to-day problem solving [12, 13]. Since its introduction, it became apparent that the general area of EF is quite heterogeneous, with significant variability across different research schools. Yet, despite these observed differences there appears to be a conceptual "core" that is common across the majority of schools of thought on the topic [11]. Among those "core" concepts is the determination that the frontal lobe of the brain seems to be critical to EF, and that EFs specifically allow us to shift our focus between topics and tasks and adapt to the shifting reality [11]. Finally, while there is no truly comprehensive or universal list of various EF subcomponents (or subsets), the broad concepts of attentional control (mindfulness), planning, set-shifting, and verbal fluency seem to be among the most often recognized themes [4, 14, 15].

Attentional control (mindfulness) is an important component of executive function that encompasses various smaller subcomponents such as attention, initiation, prioritization and – often considered the most important of the set – inhibition [2, 11, 16]. This details a person's ability to not only start a task (initiation) and to be able to select what is important to concentrate on, but then to proceed according to a pre-determined plan (attention and prioritization) [17, 18]. Moreover, mindfulness helps with the maintenance of the focus required to inhibit any distractions and to curb one's impulsive behaviors in the greater context of accomplishing a goal [2, 19]. Developmentally, attentional control tends to appear in infants at around 12 months of age, but is not fully formed until around 12 years of age [11]. Individuals who struggle within this particular skillset are often found to be easily distracted and may have difficulties initiating tasks. Even if able to initiate a task, they may be more likely to fail to maintain their task-specific attention [20, 21]. Also, those who have poor inhibition skills may come off as very impulsive, be overly forthright, and pick relatively smaller, short-term gratification over accomplishing a larger, more ambitious (and often more complex) long-term goal [2, 22].

Table 1. Detailed listing of primary executive functions and signs of executive dysfunction

Executive Functioning Domain	Primary Functional Attribution	Potential Manifestations of Dysfunction
Goal setting	Person is able to identify/set a goal that he or she subsequently works towards	Inability to set goals to work towards; Lack of future orientation
Planning	Person is able to build towards a goal through a series of steps within a set timeframe	Inability to complete tasks or goals within the stated time limit; Starting a task without appropriate preparation
Sequencing	One is able to appropriately space out tasks and ensure that they occur in the correct order	Skipping steps; Difficulty when dealing with (sequential) chronological events
Prioritizing	Person is able to determine the most necessary/important tasks for a given procedural step/time	One may become focused on smaller parts of a project while neglecting the "big picture"
Organizing	One is able to obtain and maintain the tools/resources required to complete a sequence and achieve a goal	One may lose important items, set unrealistic timeframes
Task initiating	Person is able to begin a task within a reasonable timeframe from it being assigned to him or her	The individual may procrastinate or fail to start the required work
Inhibition	Person is able to prevent oneself from being distracted and can selectively prevent actions that may not be most appropriate based on situational awareness	One may become easily distracted, quick to react, sometimes in a way that may be counterproductive in both the short- and long-term
Pacing	One is able to adjust/establish their work speed to meet a specific goal within a given timeframe	The individual frequently runs out of time before he or she is able to finish the required work
Task shifting	Person is able to move from one project to the next within a reasonable timeframe; He or she is able to accept feedback and adjust plans accordingly	One may find it challenging when dealing with unforeseen circumstances; He or she may have difficulties with accepting feedback/criticism
Self-monitoring	Person is aware of their performance (including behaviors and effect on others)	The individual does not check their work before moving on to the next step; He or she may neglect to fully complete certain steps
Emotion control	Person is able to prevent his or her emotions from unduly affecting professional and personal conduct, and is able to choose logical responses over emotional responses	The individual is prone to over-reactions to certain situations, especially when under stress
Task completion	Person is able to finish their goals as assigned/stated	One may not be able to reliably complete tasks; He or she frequently gives up on tasks

The ability to make plans is another key component of one's executive functioning [4, 23]. This domain involves both the act of creating a plan and then the ability to execute it [24, 25]. Being able to set a goal, including the ability to properly sequence, organize, pace and self-monitor are all critical to being a successful planner and an effective leader [2, 26]. The multifaceted skillset associated with effective planning, rational and grounded in reason, begins to emerge around the ages of 7-11, but does not fully develop until the early adulthood [11, 27]. In a more formal setting, individuals with less developed planning skills may come across as somewhat "future-blind", with apparent difficulty in defining what they are ultimately working towards (e.g., goal), forgetting or skipping certain steps in a complicated processes (e.g., sequencing), as well as greater propensity toward impaired task-related organizational skills (e.g., forgetting or not completing tasks) [28, 29]. Moreover, if one lacks requisite pacing and self-monitoring skills, he or she may be more likely to run out of time (e.g., pacing and self-monitoring) or complete a task without ensuring appropriate quality of the process (e.g., insufficient self-monitoring) [2]. When examining these skills further, those who demonstrate difficulties in planning may also exhibit the inability to establish work-life balance, effectively conduct social interactions, or set unrealistic schedules and expectations across various domains of their life [2, 30, 31].

Set-shifting and verbal fluency, while both important facets of executive function, are ultimately less broad than some of the points mentioned above [4]. Set-shifting, also occasionally known as "cognitive fluency" or "cognitive flexibility" [11], is one's ability to move from one task to another [14]. This particular aspect of EF encompasses a general ease of how one can respond to a shifting environment, the introduction of adverse or unexpected circumstances, and how one can adapt and incorporate feedback from others [32, 33]. Those with poorly developed set-shifting ability may experience qualitative differences between various aspects of their life (e.g., one might be excelling in school or work, but their social life may be lacking) [2]. Verbal fluency is important because it is often used in assessing a person's executive ability and is generally viewed as an "overall reflection" of executive functions [34]. This is not surprising because verbal fluency requires significant ability to focus, adherence to time and rule restraints, and inhibition or "filtering" of responses – all extremely important to executive function [34]. In a broader sense, verbal fluency reflects one's ability to "regulate one's thoughts and direct behavior toward a general goal" [34].

3. EXECUTIVE DYSFUNCTION: AN ASSOCIATION WITH BRAIN TRAUMA AND DEPRESSION?

As previously mentioned, EF is intrinsically tied to the frontal lobes of the brain, including the prefrontal/orbitofrontal regions [35, 36]. The orbitofrontal cortex plays an important role in a person's understanding of risks and rewards, and their control over emotions [36, 37]. Physical injury to this region of the brain can cause changes to emotion and behavior which manifest as a lack of social appropriateness and responsibility [37], making it more difficult for patients to detect subtle social signals such as vocal and facial expressions [38]. A famous, while extreme, case of this is that of Phineas Gage, who suffered severe damage to his medial frontal lobes, resulting in profound personality changes [39, 40]. His symptoms, while not explicitly identified as such in empirical observations from the mid-1800's, appear to be those of EDF [39].

Depression is a relatively common disorder, affecting approximately 10 - 15% of the general population [41, 42]. Studies demonstrate that there may be a significant association between depression and executive function [43, 44], including notable changes within the orbitofrontal cortex [43], as well as a degree of prefrontal cortex dysfunction in those with depression [45]. Taken collectively, findings point to a link between depression and EDF, thus highlighting the importance of a comprehensive and highly personalized approach when determining both specific barriers to optimal performance and any assistive steps to help individuals overcome any associated challenges [46-49]. A study among undergraduate students at University College London using the Wisconsin

Card Sorting Test found that those who were considered dysphoric, with a score of ≥11 on the Beck Depression Inventory, were unable to perform tasks as efficiently as the non-dysphoric control group, were more likely to make an error, and had greater difficulty using abstract thinking [50]. In another study from Australia, patients with depression and anxiety were more likely to exhibit symptoms of EDF, with inhibition and volition being most prominently affected [51].

4. BURNOUT AND DEPRESSION AMONG HEALTH-CARE TRAINEES AND PROFESSIONALS

Compared to the general population, burnout and depression among health-care trainees and professionals is disproportionally high [52-55]. These worrisome phenomena begin early in the health education process, as demonstrated in a longitudinal study of depression in students at the University of Massachusetts Medical School [56]. At the beginning of their medical studies, the overall emotional state was comparable between medical students and their peers [56]. However, as their education continued, the students' scores on the Center for Epidemiological Studies Depression scale increased and remained consistently at the elevated level [56]. The link between burnout and depression is well-established [52, 57]. At the same time, these critically important problems continue to be under-reported, under-recognized, and thus relatively neglected.

Although many health-care professionals exhibit symptoms related to depression, majority of them forgo the use of mental health services, often citing concerns about lack of time, lack of confidentiality, and a fear of being stigmatized or misunderstood [53, 58, 59]. When interviewed about their beliefs concerning seeking help from mental health professionals, medical students reported that their future careers may be negatively impacted by using such services [60]. Additionally, many health-care trainees and professionals are unaware that counseling services are available from their employers, thus deciding to seek help and support from friends and family instead [53, 59-61].

A multitude of factors contribute to the high incidence of depression among health-care professionals, including difficulties with balancing personal health/well-being and social life [62, 63], especially in the context of baseline EF and any domains that may affect one's ability to reconcile multiple competing priorities and stressors.

Closely related to depression, burnout, and indirectly to EDF, is the associated decline in empathy and mindfulness [64-66]. During their medical and nursing education, students tend to experience a decline in how much they reflect on their own feelings and how they moderate their behaviors, especially when under significant stress [62, 67]. Another, often neglected, facet of the stress associated with health-care education is the high performance expectation and the associated "test anxiety" [68-70]. For many students, there is a marked disconnect between effort spent in health-care education and the rewards derived from this effort [71]. All too often, students spend disproportionate amount of time (and effort) preparing for an exam, frequently at the expense of their personal well-being. This perpetual cycle only furthers the propensity for depression and anxiety, and consequently EDF [71]. For those who are unable to effectively cope with the stresses and demands of health-care education, the struggle tends to persists well into their careers [72]. Consequently, the connection between EF (or EDF) and personal functioning across various domains of life (e.g., personal and professional) continues to shape one's ability to make a difference and meaningfully contribute to their family and community.

5. IMPLICATIONS FOR HEALTH-CARE TRAINEES AND PROFESSIONALS

Given the propensity toward depression and burnout, coupled with the association between the latter and EF, one can reasonably propose that health-care trainees and professionals may be at a greater risk of experiencing EDF than their professional peers outside of health-care [73-75]. In this context, medical students tend to experience the greatest degree of emotional distress during their third and fourth year clinical rotations [76]. In the face of persistent stress, depression, anxiety, and burnout, those who lack effective coping skills may be at elevated risk of EDF as practicing health-care providers [77-79].

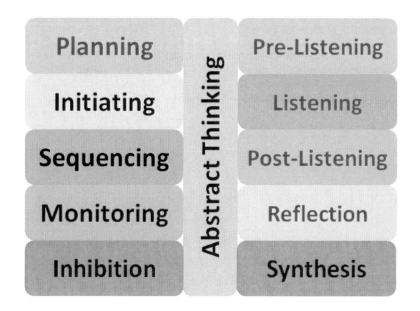

Figure 3. Schematic representation of concepts related to action/implementation and listening/processing, with the abstract thinking ability being at the center of both.

Since EDF can negatively impact a health-care professional's ability across multiple domains, from planning to interpersonal communication [**Figure 3**], individuals with risk factors for EDF (including depression and burnout) are less likely to be effective in relating to, communicating with, and ultimately treating their patients [80-82]. Finally, it is important to remember that EDF may begin to manifest insidiously as a part of cognitive decline related to various pathological states, from mental health issues (including substance abuse) to a plethora of organic disease states (e.g., endocrine dysfunction, malnutrition, neurodegenerative diseases)

[83-85]. The importance of this from leadership perspective is that even subtle deterioration in EF may result in profound consequences when critical organizational functionalities are affected. At the same time, there may be reluctance among peers, co-workers, family members, and other stakeholders to actively point out observations that may potentially be embarrassing or deleterious to the individual in question.

6. THE SYNTHESIS: MOVING FORWARD AND "LESSONS LEARNED"

Executive dysfunction may be more prevalent than previously believed. Given the inherently high risk profile of health-care professionals, EDF appears to affect this population group more frequently, leading to much broader societal implications. Consequently, it is necessary that health-care organizations, from educational institutions to acute care facilities, begin raising awareness and educating personnel about the importance of EF, including manifestations of EDF and effective preventive measures. One important aspect of targeted organizational education should be a focus on self-assessment and self-monitoring, as these skills are crucial to determine a personalized baseline for individual growth and development [86]. It is also very important to ensure the presence of optimal emotional climate for education and awareness of all aspects of EF as well as the non-judgmental approach to addressing EDF at the individual level [87-90]. Formalized organizational programs that foster appropriate coaching and mentoring are critical in this context [90].

Another aspect might be to work on one's communication skills, especially when under stress or out-of-routine situations. In a program described by Ghent University, medical students are evaluated through an objective structured clinical examination, and during the early stage of their education, they are expected to develop high-level communication skills when dealing with an emotional life event [91]. During their advanced curricula, students begin to incorporate medical situations and knowledge into the above skillset, and practice situational scenarios with simulated patients [91]. Students who demonstrated requisite skill fluency were permitted to advance, while those who required additional skill development were given feedback and further education [91].

Similar paradigms may be important in organizational approaches to optimizing employee success and performance. Consequently, individuals with identified EDF may benefit from structured approaches incorporating didactics, coaching, and long-term mentorship. A recently published study suggested that EF can improve markedly when the associated primary stimulus (e.g., depression, medical condition, substance dependence, significant life event) is successfully managed [92]. Additionally, mindfulness-based exercises may help with stress reduction and the reduction in feelings of depression and/or anxiety [93].

CONCLUSION

The presence of adequate EF across all domains is often assumed when evaluating health-care trainees, professionals, and leaders. However, it has become increasingly evident with time that there are many very capable individuals who are able to perform brilliantly in terms of technical skills and competencies, but exhibit various degrees of EDF. The associated lack of requisite social or general life skills may hinder one's ability to perform optimally within increasingly complex organizations and situations, and can become a significant impediment in the personal life domain. In aggregate, this is what makes EDF such a prevalent and high-impact, yet under-recognized and under-appreciated problem.

While it may be relatively easy to see manifestations of EDF in others, a true introspection may be difficult and requires well-developed metacognitive ability. Consequently, organizations need to create an environment of appreciative inquiry and openness regarding EF and associated individual and team dynamics. Most importantly, organizational design should consider team building that focuses on ensuring complementary behavioral skillsets, including supplementing technical talent with EF compatibility, resulting in a well-balanced group-based strategy that helps to prevent the shortcomings of more individualistic, self-reliant approaches. As modern health-care continues to evolve in complexity, multidisciplinary and team approaches are becoming increasingly important. Executive functions are therefore taking on an ever-more-prominent role in the health-care environment of tomorrow.

REFERENCES

[1] Barry, D. Executive Function, in *The Gale Encyclopedia of Mental Health, 3rd Edition*, K. Key, Editor. 2012, Cengage: Boston, MA. p. 592-594.

[2] Packer, LE. *Overview of Executive Dysfunction.* 2017, May 18, 2018]; Available from: https://web.archive.org/web/ 201711060412 55/ www.schoolbehavior.com/ disorders/ executive-dysfunction/ overview-of-executive-dysfunction/.

[3] Zelazo, PD. *Executive function part one: What is executive function?* 2011, December 25, 2017]; Available from: http://www.aboutkids health.ca/ En/ News/ Series/ ExecutiveFunction/ Pages/ Executive-Function-Part-One-What-is-executive-function.aspx.

[4] Miyake, A; et al., The unity and diversity of executive functions and their contributions to complex "frontal lobe" tasks: A latent variable analysis. *Cognitive psychology*, 2000, **41**(1), p. 49-100.

[5] Compton, DS. *High reliability leadership: Developing executive leaders for high reliability organizations.*, 2008, Citeseer.

[6] Barnard, CI; Barnard, CI; Andrews, KR. *The functions of the executive.*, Vol. 11, 1968, Harvard university press.

[7] Clough, P; Strycharczyk, D. *Developing mental toughness: improving performance, wellbeing and positive behaviour in others.*, 2012, Kogan Page Publishers.

[8] Suliman, A; Klaber, RE; Warren, OJ. Exploiting opportunities for leadership development of surgeons within the operating theatre. *International Journal of Surgery*, 2013, **11**(1), p. 6-11.

[9] Quigley, DD; et al., Specialties differ in which aspects of doctor communication predict overall physician ratings. *Journal of general internal medicine*, 2014, **29**(3), p. 447-454.

[10] Green, A; Stawicki, SP; Firstenberg, MS. Introductory Chapter: Medical Error and Associated Harm-The Critical Role of Team Communication and Coordination, in *Vignettes in Patient Safety-*, Volume 3, 2018, IntechOpen.

[11] Jurado, MB; Rosselli, M. The elusive nature of executive functions: a review of our current understanding. *Neuropsychology review*, 2007, **17**(3), p. 213-233.

[12] Coolidge, FL; Wynn, T. Working memory, its executive functions, and the emergence of modern thinking. *Cambridge archaeological journal*, 2005, **15**(1), p. 5-26.

[13] Wynn, T; Coolidge, FL. Did a small but significant enhancement in working memory capacity power the evolution of modern thinking. *Rethinking the human revolution*, 2007, p. 79-90.

[14] Diamond, A. Executive functions. *Annual review of psychology*, 2013, **64**, p. 135-168.

[15] Huizinga, M; Dolan, CV; van der Molen, MW. Age-related change in executive function: Developmental trends and a latent variable analysis. *Neuropsychologia*, 2006, **44**(11), p. 2017-2036.

[16] Teasdale, JD; Segal, Z; Williams, JMG. How does cognitive therapy prevent depressive relapse and why should attentional control (mindfulness) training help? *Behaviour Research and therapy*, 1995, **33**(1), p. 25-39.

[17] Colvin, KW. *Factors that affect task prioritization on the flight deck,* 1999.

[18] Black, P; Wiliam, D. Developing the theory of formative assessment. Educational Assessment, *Evaluation and Accountability (formerly: Journal of Personnel Evaluation in Education)*, 2009, **21**(1), p. 5.

[19] Mann, T; De Ridder, D; Fujita, K. Self-regulation of health behavior: social psychological approaches to goal setting and goal striving. *Health Psychology*, 2013, **32**(5), p. 487.

[20] Miller, EK; Cohen, JD. An integrative theory of prefrontal cortex function. *Annual review of neuroscience*, 2001, **24**(1), p. 167-202.

[21] Sohlberg, MM; Mateer, CA. Improving attention and managing attentional problems. *Annals of the New York Academy of Sciences*, 2001, **931**(1), p. 359-375.

[22] Juchnowski, JA. *Know Yourself, Co-Workers and Your Organization: Get Focused on Personality, Careers and Managing People.*, 2004, iUniverse.

[23] Zelazo, PD; Cunningham, W. *What is executive function?* About Kids Health. Hospital for Sick Children, Toronto. (Part one of a multi-part series). Recuperado el, 2005, **2**.

[24] Georgeff, MP; Lansky, AL. *Reactive reasoning and planning.* in *AAAI.*, 1987.

[25] Ertmer, PA; Newby, TJ. The expert learner: Strategic, self-regulated, and reflective. *Instructional science*, 1996, **24**(1), p. 1-24.

[26] Ley, K; Young, DB. Instructional principles for self-regulation. *Educational Technology Research and Development*, 2001, **49**(2), p. 93-103.

[27] Blakemore, SJ; Choudhury, S. Development of the adolescent brain: implications for executive function and social cognition. *Journal of child psychology and psychiatry*, 2006, **47**(3-4), p. 296-312.

[28] Hughes, C; Graham, A. Measuring executive functions in childhood: Problems and solutions? *Child and adolescent mental health*, 2002, **7**(3), p. 131-142.

[29] Koedinger, KR; Anderson, JR. Abstract planning and perceptual chunks: Elements of expertise in geometry. *Cognitive Science*, 1990, **14**(4), p. 511-550.

[30] Greenhaus, JH; Callanan, GA; Godshalk, VM. *Career management.*, 2010, Sage.

[31] Mowday, RT; Porter, LW; Steers, RM. *Employee—organization linkages: The psychology of commitment, absenteeism, and turnover.*, 2013, Academic press.

[32] Kiesler, S; Sproull, L. Managerial response to changing environments: Perspectives on problem sensing from social cognition. *Administrative Science Quarterly*, 1982, p. 548-570.

[33] Daft, RL; Weick, KE. Toward a model of organizations as interpretation systems. *Academy of management review*, 1984, **9**(2), p. 284-295.

[34] Shao, Z; et al., What do verbal fluency tasks measure? Predictors of verbal fluency performance in older adults. *Frontiers in psychology*, 2014, **5**, p. 772.

[35] Zelazo, PD. *Executive function part one: What is executive function?*, 2011, May 19, 2018], Available from: https://web.archive.org/web/20171108103549/http://www.aboutkidshealth.ca/En/News/Series/ExecutiveFunction/ Pages/ Executive- Function- Part- One- What- is-executive-function.aspx.

[36] Kringelbach, ML; Rolls, ET. The functional neuroanatomy of the human orbitofrontal cortex: evidence from neuroimaging and neuropsychology. *Progress in neurobiology*, 2004, **72**(5), p. 341-372.

[37] Bechara, A. The role of emotion in decision-making: evidence from neurological patients with orbitofrontal damage. *Brain and cognition*, 2004, **55**(1), p. 30-40.

[38] Hornak, J; et al., Changes in emotion after circumscribed surgical lesions of the orbitofrontal and cingulate cortices. *Brain*, 2003, **126**(7), p. 1691-1712.

[39] Van Horn, JD; et al., Mapping connectivity damage in the case of Phineas Gage. *PloS one*, 2012, **7**(5), p. e37454.

[40] Rahman, S; et al., Decision making and neuropsychiatry. *Trends in cognitive sciences*, 2001, **5**(6), p. 271-277.

[41] Ohayon, MM; Schatzberg, AF. Prevalence of depressive episodes with psychotic features in the general population. *American Journal of Psychiatry*, 2002, **159**(11), p. 1855-1861.

[42] Kroenke, K; et al., The PHQ-8 as a measure of current depression in the general population. *Journal of affective disorders*, 2009, **114**(1-3), p. 163-173.

[43] Bremner, JD; et al., Reduced volume of orbitofrontal cortex in major depression. *Biological psychiatry*, 2002, **51**(4), p. 273-279.

[44] Fossati, P; Ergis, A; Allilaire, J. Executive functioning in unipolar depression: a review. *L'encéphale*, 2002, **28**(2), p. 97-107.

[45] George, MS; Ketter, TA; Post, RM. Prefrontal cortex dysfunction in clinical depression. *Depression*, 1994, **2**(2), p. 59-72.

[46] Speller, JL. *Executives in crisis: Recognizing and managing the alcoholic, drug-addicted, or mentally ill executive*, 1989, Jossey-Bass.

[47] Tina Champagne, O; et al., Cognition, cognitive rehabilitation, and occupational performance. *The American Journal of Occupational Therapy*, 2013, **67**(6), p. S9.

[48] Kahn, J; Unterberg, M. *Executive distress: organizational consequences*, in *Mental Health in the Workplace: A Practical Psychiatric Guide.*, 1993, Van Nostrand Reinhold, New York.

[49] Sperry, L; Kahn, JP; Heidel, SH. Workplace mental health consultation: A primer of organizational and occupational psychiatry. *General Hospital Psychiatry*, 1994, **16**(2), p. 103-111.

[50] Channon, S. Executive dysfunction in depression: the Wisconsin card sorting test. *Journal of affective disorders*, 1996, **39**(2), p. 107-114.

[51] Oei, T; Shaw, S; Healy, K. Executive Function Deficits in Psychiatric Outpatients in Australia. *International Journal of Mental Health and Addiction*, 2016, **14**(3), p. 337-349.

[52] Tolentino, JC; et al., What's new in academic medicine: Can we effectively address the burnout epidemic in healthcare? *International Journal of Academic Medicine*, 2017, **3**(3), p. 1.

[53] DeCaporale-Ryan, L; et al., The undiagnosed pandemic: Burnout and depression within the surgical community. *Current problems in surgery*, 2017, **54**(9), p. 453-502.

[54] Dyrbye, LN; Thomas, MR; Shanafelt, TD. Systematic review of depression, anxiety, and other indicators of psychological distress among US and Canadian medical students. *Academic Medicine*, 2006, **81**(4), p. 354-373.

[55] Balch, CM; Freischlag, JA; Shanafelt, TD. Stress and burnout among surgeons: understanding and managing the syndrome and avoiding the adverse consequences. *Archives of surgery*, 2009, **144**(4), p. 371-376.

[56] Rosal, MC; et al., A longitudinal study of students' depression at one medical school. *Academic medicine: journal of the Association of American Medical Colleges*, 1997, **72**(6), p. 542-546.

[57] Stawicki, S. Short timer's syndrome among medical trainees: Beyond burnout. *International Journal of Academic Medicine*, 2017, **3**(3), p. 150-150.

[58] Givens, JL; Tjia, J. Depressed medical students' use of mental health services and barriers to use. *Academic medicine*, 2002, **77**(9), p. 918-921.

[59] Corrigan, PW; Druss, BG; Perlick, DA. The impact of mental illness stigma on seeking and participating in mental health care. *Psychological Science in the Public Interest*, 2014, **15**(2), p. 37-70.

[60] Chew-Graham, CA; Rogers, A; Yassin, N. 'I wouldn't want it on my CV or their records': medical students' experiences of help-seeking for mental health problems. *Medical education*, 2003, **37**(10), p. 873-880.

[61] Subramanian, AP. *Feelin the blues: a survey of depression among medical and dental students at Oregon Health Sciences University.*, 2000.

[62] Stratton, TD; Saunders, JA; Elam, CL. Changes in medical students' emotional intelligence: An exploratory study. *Teaching and learning in medicine*, 2008, **20**(3), p. 279-284.

[63] Uchino, R; et al., Focus on emotional intelligence in medical education: From problem awareness to system-based solutions. *International Journal of Academic Medicine*, 2015, **1**(1), p. 9.

[64] Passalacqua, SA; Segrin, C. The effect of resident physician stress, burnout, and empathy on patient-centered communication during the long-call shift. *Health communication*, 2012, **27**(5), p. 449-456.

[65] Raab, K. Mindfulness, self-compassion, and empathy among health care professionals: a review of the literature. *Journal of health care chaplaincy*, 2014, **20**(3), p. 95-108.

[66] Paro, HB; et al., Empathy among medical students: is there a relation with quality of life and burnout? *PloS one*, 2014, **9**(4), p. e94133.

[67] Beddoe, AE; Murphy, SO. Does mindfulness decrease stress and foster empathy among nursing students? *Journal of Nursing Education*, 2004, **43**(7), p. 305-312.

[68] Peleg, O; Deutch, C; Dan, O. Test anxiety among female college students and its relation to perceived parental academic expectations and differentiation of self. *Learning and Individual Differences*, 2016, **49**, p. 428-436.

[69] Chapell, MS; et al., Test anxiety and academic performance in undergraduate and graduate students. *Journal of educational Psychology*, 2005, **97**(2), p. 268.

[70] Powell, DH. Behavioral treatment of debilitating test anxiety among medical students. *Journal of Clinical Psychology*, 2004, **60**(8), p. 853-865.

[71] Hahn, H; et al., Test anxiety in medical school is unrelated to academic performance but correlates with an effort/reward imbalance. *PloS one*, 2017, **12**(2), p. e0171220.

[72] Barnett, JE; et al., In pursuit of wellness: The self-care imperative. *Professional Psychology: Research and Practice*, 2007, **38**(6), p. 603a.

[73] Quinn, JB; Anderson, P; Finkelstein, S. Managing professional intellect: making the most of the best, in *The strategic Management of Intellectual capital*, 1997, Elsevier. p. 87-98.

[74] Wallace, JE; Lemaire, JB; Ghali, WA. Physician wellness: a missing quality indicator. *The Lancet*, 2009, **374**(9702), p. 1714-1721.

[75] Privitera, MR; et al., Physician burnout and occupational stress: an inconvenient truth with unintended consequences. *Journal of Hospital Administration*, 2014, **4**(1), p. 27.

[76] Rosenthal, JM; Okie, S. White coat, mood indigo—depression in medical school. *New England journal of medicine*, 2005, **353**(11), p. 1085-1088.

[77] Folkman, S. *Stress: appraisal and coping*, in *Encyclopedia of behavioral medicine*, 2013, Springer. p. 1913-1915.

[78] Lloyd, C; King, R; Chenoweth, L. Social work, stress and burnout: A review. *Journal of mental health*, 2002, **11**(3), p. 255-265.

[79] Felton, J. Burnout as a clinical entity—its importance in health care workers. *Occupational medicine*, 1998, **48**(4), p. 237-250.

[80] Ha, JF; Longnecker, N. Doctor-patient communication: a review. *The Ochsner Journal*, 2010, **10**(1), p. 38-43.

[81] Halbesleben, JR; Rathert, C. Linking physician burnout and patient outcomes: exploring the dyadic relationship between physicians and patients. *Health care management review*, 2008, **33**(1), p. 29-39.

[82] Travado, L; et al., Physician-patient communication among Southern European cancer physicians: The influence of psychosocial orientation and burnout. *Psycho-Oncology*, 2005, **14**(8), p. 661-670.

[83] Sher, L. Neurobiology of Suicidal Behavior in Alcohol Use Disorders. *Research on the Neurobiology of Alcohol Use Disorders*, 2008, p. 125.

[84] Schultz, IZ; Sepehry, AA; Greer, SC. Impact of Common Mental Health Disorders on Cognition: Depression and Posttraumatic Stress Disorder in Forensic Neuropsychology Context. *Psychological Injury and Law*, 2018, p. 1-14.

[85] Pandey, VP; Singh, T; Singh, S. Thyroid Hypo-function: Neuropsychological issues. *Indian Journal of Health & Wellbeing*, 2017, **8**(6).

[86] Epstein, RM; Siegel, DJ; Silberman, J. Self-monitoring in clinical practice: A challenge for medical educators. *Journal of Continuing Education in the Health Professions*, 2008, **28**(1), p. 5-13.

[87] McClintic, C. *12 Brain/mind learning principles in action: Developing executive functions of the human brain.*, 2009, Corwin Press.

[88] Solanto, MV. *Cognitive-behavioral therapy for adult ADHD: Targeting executive dysfunction*, 2011, Guilford Press.

[89] Davalos, DB; Pantlin, L; Crosby, H. Depression and Executive Dysfunction in Young Adults; Implications for Therapy. *Journal of Depression and Therapy*, 2016, **1**(1), p. 18.

[90] Western, S. *Coaching and mentoring: A critical text*, 2012, Sage.

[91] Deveugele, M; et al., Teaching communication skills to medical students, a challenge in the curriculum? *Patient education and counseling*, 2005, **58**(3), p. 265-270.

[92] Biringer, E; et al., Executive function improvement upon remission of recurrent unipolar depression. *European archives of psychiatry and clinical neuroscience*, 2005, **255**(6), p. 373-380.

[93] Shapiro, SL; Schwartz, GE; Bonner, G. Effects of mindfulness-based stress reduction on medical and premedical students. *Journal of behavioral medicine*, 1998, **21**(6), p. 581-599.

In: Fundamentals of Leadership ...
Editors: S. P. A. Stawicki et al.
ISBN: 978-1-53615-729-1
© 2019 Nova Science Publishers, Inc.

Chapter 6

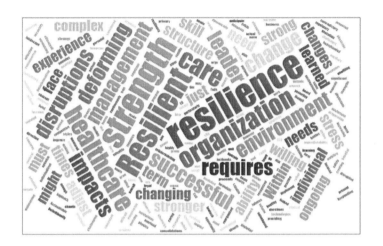

RESILIENCE IN LEADERSHIP

Richard Martin[1], MD FAAEM
and Manish Garg[2], MD FAAEM FAIM

[1]Temple University Hospital Department of Emergency Medicine,
Philadelpha, Pennyslvania, US

[2]Department of Emergency Medicine, Lewis Katz School of Medicine at Temple University, American College of Academic International Medicine, World Academic Council of Emergency Medicine, Philadelphia, Pennyslvania, US

ABSTRACT

The successful organization proceeds with strength, purpose, structure and resource. Resilience is an aspect of strength, particularly valuable in health care enterprises, most of which operate in a highly competitive and dynamically changing environment. In times of unpredictability, there is a need to flexibly adjust and grow when met with surprises, disruptions, and crises—resisting the urge to merely power through. What was successful yesterday may not work tomorrow. The resilient organization requires a resilient leader, willing to learn continuously from experience, listening to the end users from within and attuned to signs of environmental disruptions from the outside. Such qualities are not taught or learned from textbooks or manuals, though they can be modelled and mentored. Fads in management come and go, but resiliency is not formulaic. The resilient group or individual learns by doing, with the ability to adapt and improve with each new experience. In an era of rapid change where disruption is the norm, the capable leader must steer a course between structure and change, cognizant of firm overall direction but willing to make ongoing changes in how and why to proceed. Some are born with intrinsic resilience, able to adjust to misfortune and become stronger. In actual practice, however, resilience is not just a personal trait but a matter of experiential learning in the face of both failures and successes.

Keywords: change management, leadership styles, organizational resilience, resilient leadership, strength, physician wellness

1. LEADERSHIP VIGNETTE #1

The Chief Executive Officer (CEO) of a community hospital sees a bottom line edging into red territory. The hospital has an aging medical staff. The surgeons have comfortable practices, but there has been a loss of operative cases to larger hospitals, offering newer technologies. The obstetrics department has become a loss leader, needing substantial and ongoing subsidies. The primary physician base has been drifting away from the institution, with those who remained referring more patients "out of the system". The emergency department (ED) has seen growing volume, but is operating in a constrained physical space, with long waits and complaints from the community. The Board has become restive, wanting action before the institution reaches the point of bankruptcy. The CEO tries to expand the closed surgical staff and is rebuffed. He attempts to reorganize ambulatory care so that the ED will be under an aggressive administrator, but this is perceived as a heavy-handed initiative and is shouted down. The CEO sees the Chief of Family Medicine, a young and ambitious physician, as a potential ally. Many hours are spent with the Chief of Family Medicine, who enjoys expressing his views and hearing himself speak. Slated to become staff president, this physician instead leaves to become residency director at a university hospital. Continuing to lose business, the hospital is sold to a national for-profit hospital chain. At takeover, the corporation finds the hospital to be poorly run, and the CEO resigns prior to being transitioned out.

This CEO recognized need for change but has not learned how to mobilize alliances, as might have been created between the board and the primary physicians. He has attempted to implement significant changes without adequate preparation and did not anticipate making enemies with heavy-handed decision-making. He has focused on repair rather than innovation. In a city with numerous high-tech institutions, he has not considered capitalizing on the low-tech, caring strengths of his hospital. He has not looked upon disruptions as opportunities, as in the increasing ED volume or an obstetrics unit that might have been re-organized to stress individualized, high-touch care, maximizing the use of ancillary services to optimize stress management and creating niches that promote healthy life styles. He isolated himself with no-win battles, failed to recognize opportunities and was unwilling to risk disruptive innovation.

1.1. Imminent Challenge

The evolving business of health care is one of threats, challenges, competition, and opportunity. The physician leader must navigate out-of-control costs, patient safety concerns, questions of value and efficacy—all in a difficult legal and regulatory environment with rapidly changing technologies and contradictory proposed solutions from lawmakers. Accountable care organizations, the "medical home", value-based care, consolidations, closings, and consumerism present an overload of inflection points. Within this chaotic landscape, there is the day-to-day necessity of providing and maintaining consistent clinical care. Responding to this challenging environment requires complex planning, execution, and on-going crisis management. Such times call for resilient leadership.

1.2. Resiliency

Definitionally, resilience is a simple concept. Resilience, or resilient in physics, is defined as the ability to absorb a deforming impact and then to regain its pre-impact form. A steel plate exhibits strength, but with enough force will bend or shatter. A batted baseball, on the other hand, seen in slow-motion photography, is severely deformed but immediately resumes its spherical shape. Thus, strength is important to the make-up of an individual or organization, but strength needs resilience for the long term [1]. The Maginot line, designed by the French army to resist German invasion during World War II, was strong, but inadequate when the enemy circled and attacked from the flank [2]. All human organizations are complex. In the face of multiple potentially deforming impacts, successful enterprise needs resilience and perseverance [1, 3]. Countless strong businesses – print newspapers, network television, the record industry, manufactures of large automobiles – have been undone by untraditional competitors attacking in untraditional ways [4]. In health care, beset by so many potentially deforming impacts, the skill to lead health care delivery in and around the thickets of disruption requires resilience that not just resists impacts but absorbs them and becomes stronger.

Resilient leadership is not easily described or understood as a skill set. The iconoclast Nassim Taleb, in his book *Antifragile: Things That Gain From Disorder*, drills down into the distinctions between robustness (strength) and antifragility, the latter term meant to describe a person (or organization or civilization) which grows and gains strength from potential setbacks [5]. In this sense the traditional command-and-control organization might be strong, whereas the emergence of the learning organization would, at its best, represent antifragility—resilience. Unlike the "strong", firmly anchored successful corporations of the recent past, success of the learning organization is less predictable. The most spectacularly successful enterprises of this generation are high-tech companies, but many high-tech operations have failed. Doing things differently is certainly no guarantee of success. Resilience implies adaptability and continuous learning, but also navigating risks. Strength implies consistency, planning, anticipation, crisis management and follow-through. One may construct a metaphorical Maginot Line and enjoy a sense of safety behind it, but the attacks and disruptions may come, not from head on assault on the seemingly impregnable defense, but rather from above, below and around. In health care, there is the sense of changes in process and changes to come—but no consensus of the precise nature of the changes. There will be impacts to come, foreseen by no one.

1.3. Inflection Points

Inflection points are disruptors. Andy Grove, who guided Intel to dominance in computer chips, noted that "a strategic inflection point is a time in the life of business when its fundamentals are about to change. That change can mean an opportunity to rise to new heights. But it may just as likely signal the beginning of the end [6]." Health care is not unique in contending with barrages of inflection points, many of which require naturalistic thinking. Naturalistic thinking is non-linear, partially intuitive, and can be crucial when there is not time for meticulous study and planning. In his book *Only the Paranoid Survive*, Grove describes specific inflection points faced by Intel. When there was a flaw in some computer chips, Grove made the expensive and resource-intensive decision to recall and replace all chips immediately. The result was a strengthened company in multiple ways. When Starbucks suffered sudden massive negative publicity after the forced removal of two African-American visitors in a Philadelphia franchise, Howard Schulz responded immediately with new policies and a closure of all Starbucks for a day of diversity training [7].

Such decisions contain real risk, do not guarantee benefit, invite unintended consequence(s) and cannot be made with months of deliberation. Ideally, we should anticipate rather than react. As Grove put it, "You can be the subject of a strategic inflection point but you can also be the cause of one."

1.4. Leadership Styles

Generic leadership characteristics might be considered as valuable to every organization—decisiveness, firmness, flexibility, and planning skills. On a more granular level, varying styles of leadership are recognizable, with differing applicability and importance in different arenas. The "Gamesman", a well-received study written by Michael Maccoby in 1976, identified four such distinctive styles [8]. Maccoby and his staff performed in-depth interviews and psychological testing on CEOs of large corporations to find specific qualities that made it possible for an individual to make it "to the top". The study identified the following styles:

1. The "Craftsman" is the person who succeeds on the basis of focused knowledge, skill and self-reliance. Physicians most often view themselves as this style, but clinical competence does not in itself translate to organizational success. Contemporary high-tech start-ups, usually brought into existence by computer engineers, are in some ways a throwback to this individualistic approach.
2. The second personality type, the "Jungle Fighter", represents the executive who fights to the top, viewing every encounter as win-lose. This type has appeared in literature and drama as thriving on conflict, perhaps visible politically as a Richard Nixon-like figure. The "Jungle Fighter" often is eventually thwarted to succeed by the baggage of too many accumulated enemies.
3. A third type, as opposed to the "Jungle Fighter", is the "Company man", who predicates success on relationships, conformism, "who you know", and on acquiring the right mentor and avoiding overt

conflict. This style was prevalent in the 1950's and 1960's, dramatized in such works as "The Man in the Gray Flannel Suit" and, more recently, "Madmen". This type, though still and always present, is somewhat outmoded, not disposed to the risk-taking required in the rapidly moving current business culture.

4. The final style, the "Gamesman", is suggested by Maccoby to be the successful personality type of the modern CEO. The "Gamesman", considered in this work to be typified by President John F. Kennedy, sees leadership as a grand game, serious but non-linear, involving constant thrust and parry, anticipating and responding with agility to competitors within and without, operating with intelligence but not necessarily with predictability [9]. The "Gamesman" is argued to be the truly successful captain of industry, from high-tech and entertainment, but also in formerly staid businesses that must adapt rapidly to changes in taste, innovation, globalism and culture. The potentially crushing pitfall of the "Gamesman", as the type has evolved since Maccoby's writing, is to focus purely on the game itself, without overarching vision or responsibility. Examples abound, as seen in crash-and-burn game players who led such companies as Enron and Global Crossings into bankruptcy and those financiers who contributed mightily to the credit crisis of 2007. A particular genre of business literature, sometimes referred to as faith-based, as in the writings of Steven R. Covey, counters the excesses of game-playing with emphasis on the moral and ethical imperatives important to successful leadership [10].

The delineation of leadership styles in "The Gamesman" is useful, but simplistic [8]. In the real world, the successful leader of a complex enterprise combines some elements of all four personality styles. The genuine "Gamesman" possesses specialized knowledge as the "Craftsman" but does not micromanage. He or she can jungle-fight but generally chooses fights with great care. He or she is sensitive to political contingencies, and aside from a handful of celebrity CEOs, is adept and polished in personal relationships. In the era of rapidly multiplying inflection points, a significant dose of gamesmanship is called for.

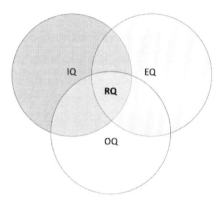

Figure 1. Resilience quotient as an amalgamation of intelligence, emotional, and operational quotients; Legend: RQ = Resilience Quotient; IQ = Intelligence Quotient; EQ = Emotional Quotient; OQ = Operational Quotient.

1.5. Defining Your Resilience Quotient: IQ + EQ + OQ = RQ

How can you define your resilience quotient? Although simplistic, the complexity of such a question may be summarized in a combination of a health care practitioner's "book smarts" or intelligence quotient (IQ); "street smarts" or emotional (intelligence) quotient (EQ); and "situational awareness" or operational quotient (OQ) [11, 12]. The term "adversity quotient" has also been utilized by some authors [13]. A health care practitioner's IQ is the most important leadership predictor according to leadership researchers. In addition to fact retrieval, the benefit of high IQ helps in mental reasoning and making better decisions. As the complexity of tasks increase, having a high IQ will allow for optimal variable analysis, risk mitigation, decisional capacity, and ultimately leadership resilience. EQ is best thought of as an ability to perceive and understand the feelings of others and to manage emotions to predict interpersonal relationships [14]. The leader with high EQ can integrate thoughts and feelings to advance the growth of the collective. This enhances both personal and collective resilience within the organization. A leader's OQ represents real-time information gathering, scene evaluation and cognizance to determine maximal decision-making strategies. It requires perceptual, diagnostic and inferential processing and is enhanced with practice, preparation, and stored algorithms. As resilience is tested with a leader's real time adaptability, having a high OQ will lead to better decision making and ability to withstand stress and complexity. Thus, a health care leader's resilience quotient (RQ) will require versatility and evolution from the intersection of IQ, EQ, and OQ (Figure 1).

1.6. The Learning Organization

Peter Drucker, the godfather of management consulting, was among the first to speak of the learning organization [15]. The learning organization, as Drucker described, is knowledge-based. The popular television show, Undercover Boss, follows disguised CEOs as they claim to be trainees at different points in the ground-level workings of their companies [16]. The humor is in observing them flail away as they try to perform tasks that are routine to their employee (i.e., flipping hamburgers, coordinating retail sales, performing basic plumbing or lawn care labor, etc.). Were the show to feature a hospital CEO, there would be humor as well in watching the CEO try to run a blood count in the lab, take care of an incontinent patient or prepare an intravenous solution. The CEO would and should recognize every worker in the organization as his or her own "Craftsperson", with particular sets of knowledge and skills that the leader does not have. The concept is not new. Napoleon Bonaparte referred to every soldier as carrying a general's baton in his pack [17]. Every corporation is, to an extent, like the military, a command-and-control structure. However, as with the military, where every soldier must be able to think in fluid battle conditions, a competitive company must allow a degree of autonomous thinking on the part of the end user.

1.7. Resilient Leadership: Theory and Practice

Yogi Berra may or may not have actually said, "In theory, there is no difference between theory and practice. In practice, there is" [18]. Resilient leadership is not theory but a way of being, or experiential learning. The naturalistic thinking of the soldier or firefighter is crucial to the modern leader. Preparation is always necessary, but, in the heat of battle, every house in flames or every military skirmish is different. Resilient leadership is in-the-moment decision-making, based on knowledge with adaptability of rigid protocol. The resilient leader cannot function in isolation, as the "Craftsman" of the past; cannot lead by constantly engaging in head-on battles; and cannot get ahead by going along.

The building up of a resilient organization is more of a process, and certainly not a "set formula." The knowledge worker is respected and listened to, but middle management needs people who themselves are resilient. Micromanagement is the ever-present pitfall, a commonly seen self-destructive organizational behavior [19]. In *Memoirs of Hadrian*, the Roman Emperor is said to have proposed, "The mistake most often made is to expect qualities of people that they do not possess, and to fail to cultivate qualities they have" [20]. The resilient organization is organic, not constructed like a building, but rather cultivated like a garden. The resilient leader experiences setbacks and challenges in terms of necessity and opportunity for growth [21].

2. LEADERSHIP VIGNETTE #2

An ED nurse manager retires. The replacement is a younger nurse manager who wants to lead a learning organization. This new nurse manager comes into conflict with an entrenched command-and-control nursing administration. The CEO respects the consistent quality of nursing care overseen by nursing leadership but sees opportunity for a fresh look in the ED, a scene of ongoing problems of crowding, long waits, safety issues and patient complaints. The CEO recognizes the sensitivities of those involved, and she avoids taking sides and invests considerable time in informal discussions with the director of nursing (DON). The CEO studies ED metrics, including patient experience scores, elopement rates, ambulance diversions and throughput times. She joins rounds in the ED, trying to visit at times of peak patient overload. She has non-directed discussions with the physician medical director of the ED, speaking of her vision and how she would go about achieving it. The physician ED director agrees that the ED does need a new set of optics and would like for the new ED nurse manager to re-think processes and re-motivate staff. The CEO also recognizes that the physician ED director is new to the culture of the hospital, does not appreciate how nursing has traditionally been a strength of this hospital and that there will be destructive conflict if the new ED nurse manager is given free reign. She suggests to the DON as part of an ongoing discussion that there is new opportunity to make a notoriously problematic department better and that supporting change might make the DON a star in the eyes of the medical staff and the trustees, whereas insisting on the status quo and resisting necessary change will make everyone look bad. She has a breakfast meeting with the DON, the new ED nurse manager and the physician medical director of the ED, suggesting that the hospital administration needs to get behind a joint effort to improve ED safety and the patient experience. She manages to get all parties committed to pointing the ED on a new course of improvement, with some risk, but with great upside potential for the institution.

CONCLUSION

A complex melding of different qualities, in varying proportions, makes for the effective leader of a successful enterprise. In the context of an ever-changing environment, resiliency is paramount. Resiliency is not a specific skill and cannot be attained through non-experiential learning. It can be described, modelled and perhaps mentored. It is a way of being and interacting, responding to each personal or systemic challenge without rigidity or preconception, and learning from each such encounter. In the real world, the individual or organization suffers hurtful impacts and cannot easily respond with a consistently positive attitude. An organization overall needs structure and confidence, and the leader needs (per Andy Grove) a healthy paranoia and "an acute sense of when to stick to a current course of action or change". Resilience implies an organic type of strength capable of anticipatory learning. The effective leader gains understanding and, with less drama, acts to prevent progressive disruptions from cascading into crisis.

KEY POINTS

- Resilience is not just a personal trait but a matter of experiential learning in the face of both failures and successes.
- Resilient leadership is defined by strength and the ability to grow from adversity.
- Successful leaders possess stylized qualities that combine specialized knowledge, strategic fighting, mastery of personal relationships, and the ability to adapt in real time.
- A leader's resilience quotient is a combination of intelligence, emotional, and operational quotients.
- A learning organization requires each member of the team to contribute specialized knowledge and skill, and the resilient leader must understand, support and cultivate members of the organization.
- The resilient leader experiences setbacks and challenges in terms of necessity and opportunity for growth.

REFERENCES

[1] Maddi, S.R. and D.M. Khoshaba, *Hardiness training for resiliency and leadership.* Promoting capabilities to manage posttraumatic stress, 2003: p. 43-58.

Resilience in Leadership 145

[2] Jackson, J., *The fall of France: The Nazi invasion of 1940*. 2004: Oxford University Press.

[3] Stagman-Tyrer, D., *Resiliency and the nurse leader: The importance of equanimity, optimism, and perseverance*. Nursing management, 2014. **45**(6): p. 46-50.

[4] Christensen, C., *The innovator's dilemma: when new technologies cause great firms to fail*. 2013: Harvard Business Review Press.

[5] Taleb, N.N., *Antifragile: Things that gain from disorder*. Vol. 3. 2012: Random House Incorporated.

[6] Grove, A.S., *Only the paranoid survive: How to exploit the crisis points that challenge every company and career*. 1996: Broadway Business.

[7] Associated_Press. *Starbucks to close 8,000 US stores for racial-bias training*. 2018 January 1, 2019]; Available from: https:// www. theguardian.com/ business/ 2018/ apr/ 17/ starbucks-racism-training-close-stores-may-us.

[8] Maccoby, M., *The Gamesman: The New Corporate Leaders, New York (Simon and Schuster) 1976*. 1976.

[9] O'Connelt, J. and T.E. O'ConneW, *Kenny's Kennedys: A Study in Power*.

[10] Covey, S.R., *The 7 habits of highly effective people*. 1991: Simon & Schuster New York, NY.

[11] Sucaromana, A., Resilience quotient: RQ. *Journal of MCU Peace Studies*, 2016. **4**(1): p. 209-220.

[12] Reivich, K. and A. Shatte, *The resilience factor: 7 keys to finding your inner strength and overcoming life's hurdles*. 2003: Harmony.

[13] Tripathi, S., *Use of Adversity Quotient (AQ) in creating strong business leaders of tomorrow*. 2011, Doctoral thesis, SNDT Women's University). Retrieved from http://shodhganga ....

[14] Mayer, J.D., P. Salovey, and D.R. Caruso, Emotional intelligence: New ability or eclectic traits? *American psychologist*, 2008. **63**(6): p. 503.

[15] Drucker, P., *Innovation and entrepreneurship*. 2014: Routledge.

[16] McGlothlin III, J., In good company: corporate personhood, labor, and the management of affect in "Undercover Boss". *Biography,* 2014: p. 124-144.

[17] Chandler, D.G., N. Bonaparte, and D.G. Chandler, *The Military Maxims of Napoleon*. 2016: Skyhorse Publishing, Inc.

[18] Fullan, M., *Change leader: Learning to do what matters most*. 2011: John Wiley & Sons.

[19] Eiring, H.L., Dynamic office politics: Powering up for program success! *Information Management,* 1999. **33**(1): p. 17.

[20] Yourcenar, M. and G. Frick, *Memoirs of Hadrian*. 2005: Macmillan.

[21] King, G.A. and M.G. Rothstein, *Resilience and leadership: The self-management of failure*, in *Self-management and leadership development*. 2010, Edward Elgar Publishing.

Chapter 7

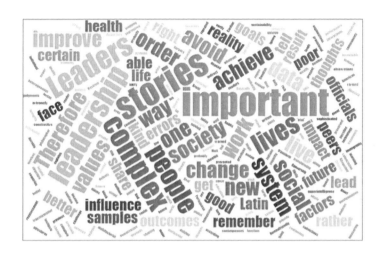

LEADERSHIP IN COMPLEX MEDICAL SYSTEMS WITH LIMITED RESOURCES: SOCIAL AND ECONOMIC CONSIDERATIONS

*Rodolfo A. Neirotti[1], Luiz F. Caneo[2]
and Aida L. Ribeiro Turquetto[2]*

[1]Clinical Professor of Surgery and Pediatrics,
Emeritus Michigan State University, East Lansing, Michigan, US
[2]Heart Institute, University of Sao Paulo, Medical School,
Sao Paulo, Brazil

"A leader is best when people barely know he exists. Not so good when people obey and acclaim him. Worse when they despise him. But a good leader who talks little, when his work is done and his aim fulfilled, they will say: We did it ourselves".

Lao-Tzu, the 6th Century B.C. Chinese Philosopher

ABSTRACT

This chapter is about leadership in complex medical systems with limited resources—a mix of connected topics. A lot has been written about leadership, but not enough on the kind of leaders needed for the challenges we face today, especially in societieis with limited financial resources and access to advanced technology. Real leaders are those that get people to confront reality and influence their life by showing them the way to change values, habits and practices to deal with the threats they face. Conversely, indirect leaders do not defy authority, but have a constructive impact on those around them through the life they live, their work and their capacity to transform their defeats in opportunities. Leaders play an important role in handling knowledge workers— whose main capital is to think for a living— by understanding them and providing the conditions and autonomy to innovate, try new things, generate strategies and growth by helping people to comprehend the convoluted nature of complex systems that are made up of individuals, activities, connections, and pathways.

Keywords: complexity, leadership, limited resources, outcomes, system

1. INTRODUCTION

Hopefully, the readers can find in this chapter a series of concepts with potential applications to their daily practice— some of them borrowed from previous work in this area by the Authors, and some from selected books and publications, both with the proper citations and quotation marks— in an attempt to expand the horizon of my knowledge and the message. Returning to some of these subjects after presenting and writing on them, as well as adding new ones, is not just to offer new information but more importantly to propose some provocative viewpoints and theories. The purpose of combining a mix of ideas, and perspectives on leadership, complex medical systems and limited resources, intended to avoid a piece structured around narrow fields of views [1].

In recent visits to some leading centers, it was encouraging to observe that they are already applying many of the concepts that will be discussed in the different sections. However, the readers should be warned that most likely, several of the thoughts outlined in this manuscript might change in the future as a result of the impact of sophisticated technology— according to Nick Bostrom a Swedish philosopher known for his work on existential risk. He stated "Basically we should assume that a 'super-intelligence' would be able to achieve whatever goals it has. Therefore, it is extremely important that the goals we endow it with, and its entire motivation system, is human-friendly" [2]. Technological systems with goals that are not identical to or very closely aligned with human ethics are intrinsically dangerous unless extreme measures are taken to ensure the safety of humanity.

The Latin American context— our example of a framework with limited resources and one the most unequal part of the world despite of its great natural resources— is a difficult setting to lead, and keep a complex system running because of its low social and human capital, poor social bonds, and high level of corruption.

History and the colonial processes shaped today's Latin America. Spanish extractive colonization divided their settlements into separated communities, each with its own "expat community," that eventually became a collection of very different and even rival's sovereign states. Although, the Portuguese colonization of Brazil preserved the integrity of the territory, it did not do a good job with the amalgamation of the mixed population, where black slaves and Indians were segregated, and the poor low class white immigrants were prevented from moving up – all with limited socio-economic resources and opportunities. Altogether, it is a complex social structure with wide disparities in income, wealth, education and economic opportunities.

By the time the colonies gained their independence, each had become an independent socio-economic society, with its own economy, social structure and moral belief that fragmented into so many different countries— with great parts of their population in extreme poverty and underdeveloped stages. As a result, people there have the notion that "the game" can be played by its own rules and code of conduct— rather than by those of the rest of the world, a mix of ignorance and arrogance that preclude them to be a part of a collective project. The teenager's attitude in which it is fine to break rules you do not like, thinking that you will get away with it is common and viewed as acceptable. If not, it is because the world is against you. The laws are for other people, not for you [3]. Moreover, it is important to remember that worldwide, government officials are samples of the society that share their values with their peers.

This heterogeneous framework, explains why Latin American countries continue to have poor quality of governments as well as why has this rich region not been able to develop mature and durable democracies.

1.1. Why is Latin America Facing Frequent Government Crises?

The answer to this question is most likely multifactorial. Perhaps the explanation is that contrary to the United States and English-speaking countries that adopted England's basic model of law, Latin America opted for laws based on Roman law— the system of jurisprudence elaborated by the ancient Romans, that had a strong influence on the legal systems of many countries. This could be a root cause for the Latin America's bad governance because it inherently leads to a dysfunctional and disrespected weak judiciary that does not function effectively or efficiently, and to excessive and inefficient bureaucracies that delay decisions.

As always, the counterexamples abound, what about prosperous, functional Japan, Germany, and France— the latter pioneered the notion of lots of nit-picking laws?

2. HISTORY IS WHERE FUTURE BEGINS

Although "the future" almost never had "enough voters" because those interested in present gain almost always win out, we should hope for a future that most likely will be quite different from the recent past [4].

Because we live in a transforming world, we cannot ignore the present forces shaping our realm and what these transformative changes will bring to the way we live, work, and invest, by their influence on the global economy and societies. A future that will challenge the reader in the belief that a continuous reassessment of our thoughts and convictions by defying reality can be helpful to verify the sustainability of previous judgments. "By studying how new observations led to the revision of important theories, one can see that science is not about immutable laws but provisional explanations that get revised when a better one comes along. The repeated `trial` of a certain event is precisely what leads to new understandings— which in turn can instigate even newer understandings" [5].

3. COMPLEXITY

The American Heritage Dictionary defines complex and complicated as "things whose parts are so interconnected or interwoven as to make the whole perplexing". If we add rarity and small numbers to complexity, the results is a distinctiveness that explains many aspects of our profession and specialty such as variability with institutional differences in outcomes; inconsistency of results in treating rare diseases and uncertainty on any inference about results of complex rare lesions [6].

4. COMPLEX SYSTEMS

A system is a group of mutually supporting elements that are working together with a common objective. They are made up of individuals, activities, connections, and pathways. Ideally, in complex systems, all members contribute to the quality of outcomes through an integrated manner in which, communication, organization, interdependence and reciprocal supervision are crucial. Still, like in an orchestra, a conductor is needed because complexity demands rehearsal [7].

Complex systems generate complex products or provide complex services and their performance and outcomes depend on complex individual and organizational factors and their interactions [8]. In developed countries, high velocity organizations set themselves apart in how they address the problems of unpredictable systems and how they deal with the unexpected problems of complex systems [9].

5. HOW COMPLEX SYSTEMS FAIL

Regardless of the effort to design the "system of work", it is impossible to do it perfectly and to predict behavior under the circumstances in which they must perform. In those that fail, their parts come together through hard work, goodwill, and improvisation, without a diagnostic work to determining the principal challenge. Their components are managed and operated independently when in fact they are quite interdependent [9].

6. COMPLEX MEDICAL SYSTEMS: THE INFINITE QUEST

At the "atomic" level, medical organizations consist of individuals, activities, connections, and pathways with the following characteristics, qualities or peculiarities of other complex systems:

- Heterogeneity of the parties (diverse nature and multiple);
- Cause-and-effect relationships may be nonlinear and obvious only in retrospect;

Leadership in Complex Medical Systems with Limited Resources 153

- Richness of interaction between them— including their contradictory character;
- Multidimensional and multi-referential;
- Many variables commonly present;
- Provide information that by itself reveals the extent of its complexity; Under an apparent simplicity, they often hide the true dynamics of these processes and interactions between its parts;
- Vulnerability— are influenced by factors and surprising circumstances that may affect, cause, or facilitate a change in behavior and expected results, altering all or changed significantly.

Altogether, they are rich in a diverse interdependent events that frequently manifest unforeseen consequences that are nonlinear and often asymmetric— often called "black swans" [10].

All of the above, explain the increasing percentage of workers time consumed to avoid the organization from collapsing under the weight of its own complexity— a bureaucracy that is difficult to dismantle [11]. Because cardiac surgery was my specialty— 1964-2005— it is used as an example of a complex medical system in this essay The field of cardiac surgery has become so sophisticated and the technology so advanced that those patients that would have died years ago can now be safely treated.

Cardiac surgery involves a large number of components, in which human errors are possible and can carry major consequences. It has much in common with other complex structures in which their function depends on technical and organizational factors. A system, a whole, which would not be strong and complete should one of its modules fails [7].

7. Demanding Medical Excellence

We have often taken quality for granted, assuming that if people have access and there are enough resources, quality will be sufficient. In many instances, access to poor quality care will do more harm than good. Given that for many years physicians and surgeons have been able to implement new treatments with minimal oversight— safety and quality are today an understandable concern— in an era in which society is demanding medical excellence and is more critical of the actions of the medical profession.

Quality is complex as the following equation shows:

Quality = $\sum$ Technical Quality + Service Quality + Ethical commitment + Social accountability

Moreover, "as the public becomes better informed about the work inside the hospitals and the medical care, their doctors have come under more scrutiny and monitoring than before, pushing medical errors into the public spotlight" [12]. Subsequently, the learning curve has changed, standards are stricter and the measuring stick more exact, hence, doing the right thing and doing it right the first time, both throughout the process, is important to avoid errors, improve outcomes, saving lives, and cutting costs.

7.1. Issues around and Outside the Operating Room

In addition to our clinical and technical work, there is a need to search outside for collaboration and for lessons from other complex systems that have identified solutions for similar problems, indicating that the general theory is independent of any industry or activity.

Thinking of the big picture matters because the health care is multidimensional and therefore it is affected by the economy, social issues and politics, particularly in the developing world. As J. Matloff put it, "The future of medicine would evolve almost entirely as a function of leadership and management capabilities. Beyond whether this evolution could happen, concern was expressed having to do with where that leadership would emerge from government, business, or **medicine**" [13].

Therefore, it is important that physicians and health professionals take an active role in the political, economic, and social aspects of society— social cure— in order to defend the interests of those suffering. Folks

Leadership in Complex Medical Systems with Limited Resources 155

involved have to increase their participation in finding potential answers to improve their institutions and as a result the existing troubled health care system. Additionally, getting people to understand what they are doing and developing co-workers relationships by encouraging communications among them, helps to increase efficiency, solve disputes more quickly, and improve general satisfaction.

7.2. Calls to Action

The time has come when those involved have to decide if they will continue to be a part of the problem, or whether they will be part of the solution. It is not just making progress against the problems facing our profession, but to move forward to position it in the right place. Then, how about evaluating what we're doing right now and say, in a constructive way? 'It's not good enough until we conquer the current limitations. Ask what you can do and imagine what we can do together!

7.3. Mission Possible

Reevaluating outdated models with critical thinking is essential to understand the limitations of archaic models, to address creatively, and effectively the needs of the patients with a modern approach. There will be barriers & external influences that are the limitations that block people reasoning, such as:

- Psychological state: arrogance, ignorance, and low inventive capacities.
- Group culture: is acceptable or unacceptable due to social barriers.
- Context in which the problem occurs.

However, barriers also include those people or groups who are supportive of the current order and those who might feel threatened by creative work. Therefore, we should look for a model that is more open, more balanced, more equitable and beneficial to all [14].

In general, people with the ideas do not have the power to implement them, whereas the people with the power are so embedded in the system that they are unlikely to come up with new thoughts. In addition, it is important to bear in mind the policy/implementation principle gap— an important barrier to modernization nicely explained by the public choice theory— developed by James Buchanan and Gordon Tullok to try to explain how public decisions are made— which results in fewer implementations of good ideas. Often, people tend to agree when principles and policies are discussed, but their support diminishes when those bearing the costs— interest groups, more influential than those who would benefit from action— have rational incentives to do precisely what they are doing [15].

8. MANAGING COMPLEXITY

Steven Spear aptly describes the problem and manner of managing complexity: "There are high velocity organizations— whom everyone chases but never catches— that manage to stay ahead because of their endurance, responsiveness, and an exceptionally high velocity in self correction. They see and seize opportunities and, by the time rivals responded, the leaders have raced on to further opportunities— these systems pose both the capacity to retain their viability and the capacity to evolve" [9].

"These organizations—complex adaptive, self-improvement systems— face a common problem and have identified a common solution, which keeps them performing way ahead of the pack and always getting better— the two go together. The solution has been used successfully by a wide variety of organizations indicating that the general theory is independent of any particular industry or activity" [9].

"This leads to collaborative rationality, of getting better together, which is a different way of knowing and generating, of making and

Leadership in Complex Medical Systems with Limited Resources 157

justifying decisions based on *diversity, interdependence and authentic dialogue*— not always accepted by the chain of command despite of the limitations of acting unilaterally." The agents interact dynamically, exchanging information and the effects of these connections flow through the system. There are many direct and indirect feedback loops; the overall system is open. "The behavior of the system is determined by these interactions, not the components; and… it cannot be understood by looking only at the components" [16].

8.1. Diversity

"Diversity implies that a collaboratively rational process must include not only agents who have power but also those who have needed information or could be affected by outcomes of the process". As in direct democracy, their success depends on the amount and quality of the information available to those involved in the decision making process [16].

8.2. Interdependence

"Agents must depend to a significant degree on other agents, considering that each stakeholder has something that the others want. This condition ensures that participants maintain a level of interest and energy required to engaging each other and pushing for consensus— such interdependence means that players cannot achieve their interests on their own" [16].

8.3. Authentic Dialogue

"Deliberations must be characterized by direct engagement so that the parties can test to be sure that claims are accurate, comprehensible, and sincere. Deliberations cannot be dominated by those with power outside the process, and everyone involved must have equal access to all the relevant information and an equal ability to speak and be listened to. In authentic dialogue— nothing is off the table" [16].

9. THE IMPORTANCE OF DEFINITION

As Lord Kelvin— an Irish mathematical physicist and engineer, 1824-1907— rightly put it: "What is not defined cannot be measured. What is not measured cannot be improved. What is not improved always deteriorates."

10. THE CHALLENGE OF DEFINING WHAT IS POSSIBLE

Like in the universe, in the world of cardiac surgery there are visible galaxies emitting light and five times as much dark matter. The purpose of introducing theories and ideas from other disciplines attempts to lighting up— if that is the appropriate word— the dark matter of our specialty and if possible contribute to diminish its size.

How do we generate the necessary cohesion to implement reforms? First, we have to preserve the leadership, patience, perseverance, dedication, the capacity to adapt, and the creativity that comes with having to work under adverse circumstances, that were the keys to success. At that point, we need to transform exogenous ideas into endogenous dreams through leadership, persuasion, and empowerment. By breaking down complexity into individuals, activities, connections, and pathways, it should be possible to act on the different levels, particularly on individuals to build the system of work required in complex successful organizations [1]. In addition, it is essential to identify what should be improved, what must be transformed, by whom, and how to engender a better future for the incoming generations. Then, in order to address these issues is crucial to avoid complacency— that is feeling satisfied with your own abilities or situation and believing that there is no need to try harder.

11. UPWARD COMPARISON: THE MORAL POWER OF RAISING THE BAR

Since we tend to overestimate where we stand in contrast to others, comparing our self to others it is not bad if fraud and Pseudo-Mathematics are avoided— a twisting strategy to fix and improve data— [17]. Upward comparison, can diminish our success— we are not the best anymore — but also encourage us to learn. Although looking around us can be punishing, it is better to watch good players and improve your performance, than bad ones and feel superior [18].

12. BUSINESS INTELLIGENCE

In order to compare, it is important to know how we are doing. Due to the current demand for excellence and transparency, institutions should start collecting and analyzing data remembering what Leonardo Da Vinci suggested: "No human investigation can claim to be scientific if it doesn't pass the test of mathematical proof". Therefore, it is imperative to define the situation or problems to avoid confounding and to facilitate the application of methods and strategies for improvement and meaningful comparison.

The systematic use of information requires good data and commitment of executives to fact-based and analytical decision-making as a way to learn rather that doing it out of gut feeling or intuition— cognitive illusions, and misconception of validity. Gathering solid data, working analytically, and leaving emotions aside, help those on the top to reflect critically on their own behavior, and then change how they act to make better decisions.

The people who construct statistics are often not the same kind of people needed to publicize them. Therefore, an effective leader should be able to comprehend number-laden reports, evaluate the information provided to him, and draw conclusions from data, rather than be dependent on others to interpret for him [10].

Analytic capabilities can be improved through adding *estimative intelligence* to gauge uncertainty and make assumptions about different scenarios, to anticipate the consequences and probabilities [10].

13. LEADERSHIP: WHAT IS A LEADER?

"It is hard to define, but you know it when you see one" [19].

"A leader is an individual who significantly affects others—their beliefs, feelings, and behaviors." [20]. Leaders achieve their mission in two ways, they tell stories and they lead certain kind of lives—leading by example. Stories feature characters who are trying to achieve things. Leaders tell stories with the hope that they affect what people do. In addition to their stories, it is important to pay attention to the kinds of lives they lead. If their lives rebuff their stories, they are hypocrites. In this case, their stories do not last long. Furthermore, the stories have to be related to the circumstances and not too distant in the past in order to avoid been unnoticed [20].

14. PROFESSIONALIZING LEADERSHIP

Barbara Kellerman, an expert on leadership has recently critiqued leadership and the leadership industry. In her new book she claims that leadership is treated as an occupation rather than a profession. Leadership has no commonly recognized body of knowledge, and no curriculum or expertise considered indispensable. In addition, unlike the professions, there are no clear standards for qualification, no metric and no license requirement. As a result, it is difficult to identify those who are trained to lead. Therefore, is the time to start thinking that as a career requires adequate training, particularly because if your leadership skills slip you are out [21].

15. REAL LEADERSHIP

As Dean Williams properly put it, is the kind of leadership that helps organizations, communities, and nations face their challenges with the best probabilities of success and is now a day missing in the world. Most of what we see today are people after a frontrunner and buying into his plan. Basically, real leadership get people to challenge reality and change values, habits, practices and urgencies in order to deal with the real threat they face [14].

Again, the time has come when we physicians have to decide whether we will continue to be a part of the problem, or whether we will be part of the solution. "If we, who have the talent and knowledge, don't look after the problems ourselves, then others who are less talented and more ignorant of those problems will certainly do it for us," stated Professor Francis Fontan in his presidential address read in Vienna in 1987, at the 1st Annual Meeting of the European Association for Cardio-Thoracic Surgery. A feasible task if one follows Vision → Skills → Incentives → Resources → Action Plan → Change as the road map to accomplish it.

We need people who can provide leadership in multiples and diverse contexts to solve problems and generate progress. Real leaders can help societies by diagnosing their critical defies and designing and recommending solutions [14]. An effective leader is a person who does the following:

1. Creates an inspiring vision of the future by teaching, and persuading;
2. Motivates people to engage with that vision;
3. Manages delivery of the vision;

4. Coaches and builds a team, so that it is more effective at achieving the vision, and brings together the skills needed to do these things;
5. Negotiate to satisfy the interests of the persons they lead.

Transcendent transformative leaders — exceed usual limits— help organizations, people, and cultures experience deep, lasting meaning and purpose from the work and outcomes they produce. They foster a culture that nurtures in people the ability to feel they are contributing to making a real difference in the world. For them, leadership has nothing to do with *formal* authority; it has to do with *moral* authority [22].

After making a difference in many lives by performing thousands of cardiac operations on children in different countries, it is obvious that my help reached only a minority of those in need. It is then important that physicians take an active role in the political, economic, and social aspects of the society in order to defend the interests of those suffering [23]. Leading is hard work and success depends on people and if leadership is an activity. To emphasize this, others prefer to use *leading* instead of *leadership*— a verb instead of a noun, it does something— a process rather than a position.

"The kind of continuous innovation alone... it comes from human creativity and commitment, from employees giving their best at all level of the organization. In short, success depends on people— and in order to achieve success, people depend on leaders" [24].

16. LEADERS AND FOLLOWERS: AN INDIVISIBLE UNITY

Leaders have people following them, and managers have people working for them— an important difference. Countries are not great for their military might or wealth, but for the quality and moral values of their leaders, followers and institutions— their society.

Aristotle once noted that "all great leaders must first learn to follow" [25]. Since leadership is about results, leaders and followers are equally important for organizational success and development. Leadership and

Leadership in Complex Medical Systems with Limited Resources 163

followership represent two sides of one dynamic relationship; without followers, there can be no leaders. This means that followers' behaviors are a vital component of the leadership process, and that leadership cannot be fully understood without a proper understanding of followership— therefore, it is essential to educate individuals to become effective followers [26].

16.1. Partners for Growth

There are three key things companies want to know when they are thinking about where to invest: speed, risk, and cost [27].

Therefore, leaders-followers public-private partnerships working on projects such as industries, including energy, automotive, aerospace, financial services, biotechnology, and information technology— focused on areas where those industries together can create new opportunities to drive social and economic development.

Although it is accepted wisdom that there is no leadership without followers, yet followers are very often left out of the leadership research equation— with very few training sessions and courses offered on cultivating follower's skills. Fortunately this problem is being addressed in recent research, with more attention being paid to the role of followership in the leadership process [28].

"Today's followers are influenced by a range of cultural and technological changes that have affected what they want and how they view and communicate with their leaders. Followers are different from one another. Using the level of engagement with a leader or group as a defining factor…. Barbara Kellerman segments followers into five types:

Isolates are completely detached; they passively support the status quo with their inaction.

Bystanders are free riders who are somewhat detached, depending on their self-interests.

Participants are engaged enough to invest some of their own time and money to make an impact.

Activists are very much engaged, heavily invested in people and process, and eager to demonstrate their support or opposition. And

Diehards are so engaged they're willing to go down with the ship— or throw the captain overboard" [29].

17. RELEVANT FACTORS FOR THE LEADERSHIP-FOLLOWERSHIP DYNAMIC RELATIONSHIP AND EVENTUALLY FOR THE QUALITY OF FOLLOWERS

Knowledge is power. The greater quantity and quality of skilled knowledge workers— know how— in rich countries suggest that human capital is vital for social and economic development. Better education = better Income— the famous simple equation that dates back to 1597 when Sir Francis Bacon published the maxim in his book, *"Meditationes Sacrae and Human Philosophy"*.

17.1. Human Capital

The knowledge and expertise embodied in a workforce acquired through education and training, used to produce goods, services or ideas [30].

17.2. Social Capital & Social Bonds

The levels of trust, tolerance, cooperation and reciprocity among individuals in a particular social environment— the base for team work and social cure. Bad things happen when good people do nothing.

17.3. Physical Capital

The general belief that buildings— physical capital— are important has resulted in new facilities spread around in many towns, schools, universities, hospitals, research centers and even convention centers without realizing that the quality of the crew— less visible— is the real determining factor for progress. The view that increasing buildings and machinery is the fundamental determinant of growth, called "capital fundamentalism" by the economists is another panacea that has not met expectations, unless it is combined with human capital. Societies can grow rapidly by relying on a well-trained, educated, hardworking and conscientious labor force that makes good use of modern technologies [8].

17.4. Motivation

The desire to do things and the reason for people's actions, desires, and needs. Self-motivation, the ability to do what needs to be done, without the influence from other people or situations. Instilling motivation is not easy, but it's essential if you want your employees to grow and stay satisfied with their jobs. Unfortunately we cannot teach motivation or incentive [31].

17.5. Attitude

The tendency to respond positively or negatively towards work, ideas, objects, persons, or situations. Attitude influences an individual's choice of action, and responses to challenges, incentives, and rewards. A positive attitude helps people to cope with the daily activities of life, brings optimism, and makes it easier to avoid negative thinking. The right combination of attitude, culture fit, motivation and skills are difficult to find in one person. Skills can be taught, but attitude is forever.

18. Leading Knowledge Workers

Coined by management expert Peter Drucker in 1959, the term knowledge workers refers to people whose main capital is to think for a living. They have high degrees of expertise, education or experience and rely on their brains! This classic quote from Steve Jobs describe them, *"It doesn't make sense to hire smart people and tell them what to do; we hire smart people so they can tell us what to do."* Their jobs involve the creation, distribution and application of their knowledge that needs to be constantly updated.

They are willing to try new things, and are responsible for the organizations' innovations, strategies and growth, thus the importance of their production.

They are different from other workers in their motivations, attitudes, need for autonomy, and require an unconventional management to be more productive [32].

How do you manage highly paid, independent thinkers who like to control the process of their own work and don't like to be managed, and who own their organization's means of innovating, developing, and producing? By treating them as valued human being. We should give those more to say in how they do their jobs, opportunities to learn and grow, and adequate compensation. In addition, it can be a smart way of increasing the number of qualified followers. As leaders, hiring competent people can be the most difficult aspect of our jobs.

19. Leadership in Medicine

In addition to our clinical practice, our commitments as physicians also carry other implications. We have a social responsibility to speak out on health issues, their practices, their communities, their professional associations— in ways that can influence public policy and putting us in a position of leadership not only on direct health issues but also on determinants of health.

"Good medical leadership is vital in delivering high-quality healthcare, and yet medical career progression has traditionally seen leadership lack credence in comparison with technical and academic ability" [31]. Interestingly, the Canadian Medical Association asked its members for their views on leadership, and whether there was a need to develop leaders in medicine. Physicians responded that there is both a need and a void. They recognized the need for physicians to assume leadership roles, but did not feel prepared to do it in the current health care environment.

With the exception of public health and epidemiology, medicine focuses on issues related to the physician-patient relationship. Doctors mentioned the different reasons for becoming involved in leadership roles— but for most of them it was not their choice.

"Given such a context… what kind of support can professional associations, provide to doctors who want to develop these non-clinical aspects of their careers"? It is our professional responsibility to ensure that our core values are represented in all important leadership issues. How do we prepare ourselves? [31].

Oliver J. Warren, and Ruth Carnall, provides an excellent description about the leadership attributes and training required for doctors and methods available to develop medical leadership. Among them, schemes courses, mentoring, coaching, action learning, networking, peer networking, networking with senior leaders, and experiential learning that can be useful for the readers in their article "Medical leadership: why it's important, what is required, and how we develop it" [33].

20. LEADERSHIP AND CULTURE

It is important to understand medicine, health care, illness and disease from a socio-cultural perspective. What is medically obvious in one culture might be incomprehensible in another. What is possible in a rich country might be almost impossible in the developing world - regardless of authority, leadership and technical competence.

Having worked in South America, Europe, and most recently in the United States, differences in culture, resources and technology had a significant impact in my practice and interactions with colleagues, patients and the public. The link between leadership and culture is complex. It is not easy to appreciate or comprehend what people do, mean, and say because of the variations from one culture to the next. Therefore, it is almost impossible to lead without understanding the local culture. A leadership style that would be effective in one culture may be dysfunctional in another. We all have seen very bright people making mistakes because they didn't recognize the cultural differences of the environment in which they were working. In complex cross-boundary interactions, it is hard to assess risks and make decisions requiring the calculation of the probability of outcomes and the prediction of people's behavior. Summarizing, it is difficult to judge anything at all without walking a few miles in the other person's boots.

My leadership challenges in my home country and abroad, resulted in a mix of successes, some failures and like everybody some mistakes, related at time, to insufficient resources, my personality, my emotional intelligence, the feasibility of the task, the limitations in my authority, and occasionally not enough knowledge of the local cultural narrative. However, when something did not go well, a critical analysis was helpful to learn from it and leveraged strengths before blaming anyone else. Effective leadership from the middle is possible but can be extremely difficult and even unmanageable when those holding the platforms of power at the top are not receptive [34].

21. ADAPTIVE LEADERSHIP

Flexibility and a diagnostic approach allow leaders to adapt, react and operate according to the needs of different contexts. The capacity to adapt enables both individual and business needs to be met through making changes to the time (when), location (where), and manner (how) in which people work [34].

22. LIMITED RESOURCES

The scarcity of the human capital— knowledge, skills, and expertise and economic support to get the daily work done. The social and business environment that has to deal with a scarcity situation involving limited resources has a negative impact on individuals and institutional quality.

23. LEADERSHIP UNDER LIMITED RESOURCE CONDITIONS: MAKING THE IMPOSSIBLE POSSIBLE

The most conspicuous advantage of the human mind is its remarkable ability to simplify complex tasks, but due to the limitations of simplification it is both a strength and a weakness. The escalating costs and the lack of money required to simplify the surgical process led those affected to adopt an ingenious multi-principle adaptive work— the KISS (Keep It Simple and Safe) approach— in order to help more patients with the available funds, equipment and manpower.

However, the risk of oversimplification of the complex process of policy formulation is substantial, particularly when complexity requires complexity!

Solutions often reside not only in the executive suite but also in the collective intelligence of people at all levels, who need to use each other's resources and learn their way to those solutions [35].

24. LEADING UNDER ADVERSITY: A WORD OF CAUTION

"There is always a risk of being satisfied with delivering substandard care in resource-limited settings, assuming that offering some care is better than no care, or that reaching a larger number of people with sub-optimal care is preferable to reaching fewer people with more sophisticated –and therefore more expensive —care" [36].

25. RESISTANCE TO CHANGE: AN OBSTACLE TO PROGRESS

What is it about how our brains are wired that resists change so tenaciously? Why do we fight even what we know to be in our own vital interests? Resistance of people to change and human nature's tendency to apply the "minimal risk" and "least effort" strategies that result in incomplete adaptive work allowing subsistence but no optimal result, explain the frequency and persistence of maladaptive practices. Unfortunately, maladaptive practices eventually become permanent adaptive challenges that do not subside with the application of technical skills provided by a profession because people are unwilling to probing their values, habits, practices and priorities [14].

Often people prefer to look outside their organization for the cause of what is flawed. Yet, answers often reside not in the executive suite but in the collective intelligence of workers at all levels, who require to use one another's resources, and learn their way to those solutions. The response is leadership, an important piece of the leadership/management philosophy that nurtures transformation by encouraging creative thinking, challenging the status quo, removing obstacles and promoting "bottom up" changes. To think creatively means to think "outside the box." That kind of thinking needs role models that can bring us new visions and possibilities. Sometimes, we need to speak the truth to power, and challenge conservative wisdom, orthodoxies, powerful institutions, and people, rather than to be part of the chorus. Sucking up to power, which is not always effective, let others think that the status quo is good enough. Therefore, sometime it is necessary to push audiences to the very limits of what they could understand or accept– and far beyond even if it sounds dissonant and very little immediate tradition lies behind it. Although in their own way, some may hear it and become a factor of change altering the course of the events [37].

"In a crisis we tend to look for the wrong kind of leadership. We call for someone with answers, decision, power, and a map of the future, someone who knows where we ought to be going— someone who can make hard problems simple. Rather than looking for saviors, we need a leader that will challenge us to face difficulties for which there are no simple solutions, requiring us to learn new ways. Making progress on these problems demands not someone who provides answers from on high but changes in our attitudes, behavior, and values— with a viable strategy" [14].

26. NEEDING HELP? ARE CONSULTANTS USEFUL?

Yes, when they are familiar with the context and they participate in the implementation of their recommendations. Despite of the extensive use of foreign advisors in emergent countries, there has been little examination of their roles. They work by different set of rules than nationals, their roles differ from those of the host country and the context determines how outsiders acquire influence and to whom are they accountable. Although they exercise vast influence with limited accountability, and without organizational authority, they have the responsibility to consider the feasibility of their recommendations [27].

26.1. Useful Rules for Wise Advisors

What every professional should know about consulting and counseling. Giving advice is an essential task in all professions. "The ability of…. a consultant to help another person with a problem depends as much on the command of the process of giving advice as on an understanding of their situation" [38].

- Encourage your advisee to tell their stories to understand the problems faced by locals. First listening, then letting them tell you why they need your help, and then ask what help they feel they need.
- Do not talk too soon. Self-control is crucial, avoiding to prove your value by offering advice before you know the problem fully. This ability, provides the basis for mental flexibility, social skills and discipline [39].
- Avoid early judgment. If the advisee senses that you are judgmental, he/she will probably become defensive and guarded. An open-minded understanding helps to gain trust and cooperation [38].
- "To observe without evaluating is the highest form of intelligence" [40].

27. Be Cautious about Models that Work in Other Contexts

Why, models with proven effectiveness in other settings, fail to take hold in in different contexts even despite having enough support? The name for the practice behind the problem is *isomorphic mimicry*. This happens when consultants and public officials drop a replica of a verified model into an old-fashioned system with unaccounted conditions [41].

28. Limited Resources Affect Sustainability

Why some developed nations are rich and others are poor and volatile? Critical thinking is essential to answer this question, to understand the limitations of obsolete models in order to address creatively and effectively their needs with a long term objective. Therefore, it is the time to accept that old ideas and norms which were well-understood and governed behaviors in the past may no longer be effective in our time. New good ideas by themselves, have no power if they are not implemented.

Thus a reassessment of our thoughts and beliefs requires persuasion that by inviting reasoning, logic, and challenge, can be helpful to verify the sustainability of our judgements [42]. Countries with a long history of incentivizing the growth of strong political institutions— constitutions, regulatory authority, legal systems, and distribution of power— are more likely to succeed. They are an example of the importance of the rule of law and institutional quality.

In contrast, those that fail to develop— often afflicted by corruption, inequality, and dysfunction— have weak institutions where the government violates property rights and concentrates wealth and power in a class of elites at the cost of the majority [43].

Cardiac surgery has been available for many years in several developing countries, thanks to the creativity and hard work of individuals who were able to produce good work in spite of the limited resources. Leadership, patience, perseverance, dedication, and the capacity to adapt to adversity have been the keys to success. Limited resources were a constant problem forcing us to focus on short-term creativity about tomorrow's needs. While, a great deal of energy in the form of leadership and negotiations was used to convince people to continue to work hard for low pay, our efficiency was suboptimal.

Under those circumstances, it would be wise to induce change from the top, by influence or persuasion, commitment to education, and encouraging bottom-up grassroots involvement and cooperation— an important component of the W. Edwards Deming's principles of total quality management. Both the top-down and the bottom-up approaches are not mutually exclusive but rather complementary.

29. THE CULTURE FACTOR

Strategy and culture are the primary levers at leaders' disposal in their quest to maintain organizational viability and effectiveness. *Strategy* offers a formal logic for the goals and orients people around them. *Culture* expresses goals through values and beliefs and guides activity through shared assumptions and group norms [44].

30. CULTURAL STAGNATION: A BARRIER TO DEVELOPMENT

The real problem is bias, based on the sameness of world view caused by social, intellectual, educational, and professional inbreeding. These are people who travel in the same circles, go to the same parties, talk to the same people, compare their ideas to people with the same ideas, and develop a standard view on issues that make any deviation from them seem somehow marginal, or even weird. There is no diversity of thoughts!

Opposite poles have always more to say to each other than people who share exactly the same views.

31. NON-TECHNICAL SKILLS

In complex systems, technical skills are necessary but not sufficient. Paying attention to interpersonal non-technical/non-cognitive skills, such as decision making, team working, leadership, situation familiarity, and communications, increase the probability of a good performance. "People get a job because of their technical skills but non-technical skills help them to keep their jobs by showing that they fit in organizational culture" [45].

32. ORGANIZATIONAL FACTORS: TEAM WORK IS A NON-TECHNICAL SKILL

Can anyone recall watching migrating geese would discover that they fly in diagonal lines, or "V" formations, to save energy and allow them to

Leadership in Complex Medical Systems with Limited Resources   175

fly longer distances? Most importantly, the leader rotates— and we often do not, attempting to solve the puzzle with a personal effort rather than a collective one. Collectively intelligence—the ability of individuals to solve problems well in a group—has emerged as an important interdisciplinary area of study with applications in understanding and supporting the performance of groups and teams [46].

Team work improve collaboration among disciplines by removing barriers to produce complex outputs by the exchange of knowledge, and promoting bottom-up participation to find solutions in the collective intelligence of people at all levels. Connected entities centered on getting better together, generate, make and justify decisions based on diversity, interdependence, and dialogue. Those having a vested interest in one another's success, facing a common problem, interact sharing information in an open system, to identify a common solution for the benefit of all, avoiding the limitations of acting unilaterally [16]. Ask what you can do. Imagine what we can do together!

33. COMMUNICATIONS, INTERACTIONS, NEGOTIATIONS, COMPROMISE

33.1. Communications and Interactions

When a physician, collaborates to manage a patient, the relationship with others requires respect and cooperation, without patient ownership. If the conversation starts with someone saying: this is my patient! It is a bad start.

33.2. Negotiations

In these discussions keep a few rules in mind: *First*, there are certain basic principles of care that should not be compromised. *Second*, both parties can learn from the interaction. *Third*, there is much in medicine that can be approached in more than one-way.

33.3. Compromise

Ultimately, the best plan results from honest open communication between physicians and the adoption of the best option.

It is difficult to have a team unless every member has respect for people who have different skills.

34. TEAMWORK IN LATIN AMERICAN CARDIAC CENTERS: WHEN IT WORKS

Collaboration at work is generally seen as a good think. In an orchestra, an example of team work, a conductor is needed— the chief cardiac surgeon in most centers— to address the problems collectively, with the individual orchestra members, promoting cooperation by building a group based on addition not subtraction, multiplication, not division. Latin American Cardiac centers have "conductors and musicians", but do they have an orchestra? The answer is obvious— if the readers remember our previous description enumerated in the introduction about the dominant cultural trait in that part of the word.

The leader should keep in mind those issues around and outside the operating room since we are constantly watching much of the world around us but sometimes failing to notice things right in front of our eyes. Altogether, too many variables for the surgeon to understand in depth and deal with them. This scenario should encourage us to ask the following question— can a truly sustainable organization afford to depend on one leader?

Perhaps, the current model should evolve into a collaborative problem-solving approach that is working in the United States in which the co-directors from cardiology, intensive care, cardiac surgeon and a business person — with a common objective are leading together [47]. However, this approach can creates doubts about who is in control, complicating the decision making process, and defers solutions— when in the end someone has to make a decision.

Although, modern communication methods encouraging collaboration by keeping people constantly in touch, its impact on performance is not clear. Previous research has shown that when people interact and influence each other while solving complex problems, the average problem-solving performance of the group increases, but the best solution of the group actually decreases in quality [48]. What's more, in their paper *"How intermittent breaks in interaction improve collective intelligence"* Bernstein et al. advocate intermittent collaboration as an alternative option for group activities, to avoid delays and improve performance [49]. Summarizing, collaboration might be a valuable tool that has to be adapted to the context because it does not always work.

34.1. Turning Doctors into Leaders

In addition to our clinical and technical work, there is a need to search *outside* for collaboration, ideas and lessons from other complex systems that has identified solutions for similar problems, indicating that the general theory is independent of any industry or activity.

Altogether, this essay reflects an array of personal views in an era with a tendency to rewards those who can accrue technical knowledge, a skill that is only marginally related to the ability of being sensitive to context and it is not linked at all to skills like empathy— an immeasurable variable of human capital. Sometimes diplomacy is necessary to pass the borders of ignorance, culture and geography.

34.2. Point of View

Often, people consider my articles "philosophical". If we accept that philosophy— the base of critical thinking— is "The critical analysis of fundamental assumptions or beliefs"; "A set of ideas or beliefs relating to a particular field or activity" or "A system of values by which one lives", they could be rightly regarded as philosophical [50].

35. INFERENCES

Some important take-home messages and inferences for the reader:

- Talking directly about problems is risky because most people do not like it.
- Enumerating the problems may be easy, finding the solution is proving increasingly difficult in settings without political stability and sustainable economic growth.
- To-date, in developing countries we have been unable to secure support from governments, professional organizations, philanthropists, patients, or peers for our practice.
- We need to improve the quality of the decisions we make. How we decide often determines what we decide. Ask yourselves, what strategies and processes would you advise to overcome these problems, and what parts of society and other professionals would you want to engage to aid the courses of action?
- It is important to determine what should be preserved, what needs improvement, how it can be done, by whom, and what we must transform.
- Which problems might be encountered in implementing the recommended strategies?
- Complex systems are not immune to the waves of innovations— Kondratieff waves— sweeping the world at large over the past fifty years starting with disruptive new technologies that have

Leadership in Complex Medical Systems with Limited Resources 179

transformed industries, societies and economies beyond recognition.

- We should be prepared for changes in the patient population requiring surgery because of the unilateral decision making process for surgical indications. Conventional surgical procedures are expected to diminish. Hybrid procedures requiring special facilities and team work with the participation of people with different skills will be more often adopted.
- Many obstacles remain, but physicians and professional societies can and must play an important role in overcoming them.
- Ask what you can do. Imagine what we can do together. Say yes to the future!

ACKNOWLEDGMENTS

The authors are grateful to Marcelo Cardarelli, MD for his valuable suggestions in preparing this manuscript.

REFERENCES

[1] Neirotti, RA. Cardiac surgery: the infinite quest. *Rev Bras Cir Cardiovasc.*, 2012, 27(4), 614-20.

[2] Bostrom, N. Superintelligence Paths, Dangers, *Strategies*, 2016.

[3] Suarez, L. Argentina's debt stand-off reflects a teenage attitude that rules are there to be broken. *The Economist.*, 2014.

[4] Faust, D. History is Where the Future Begins. *Harvard Magazine.*, 2012, 63.

[5] Willingham, DT. Trust me, I'm a scientist. *Sci Am.*, 2011, 304(5), 12.

[6] EH, B. *The challenge of rare diseases*. Joint Meeting of the Congenital Heart Surgeons Society and the European Congenital Heart Surgeons Association, 2004.

[7]   de Leval, MR; Carthey, J; Wright, DJ; Farewell, VT; Reason, JT. Human factors and cardiac surgery: a multicenter study. *J Thorac Cardiovasc Surg.*, 2000, 119(4 Pt 1), 661-72.

[8]   Neirotti, RA. Cardiac surgery: complex individual and organizational factors and their interactions. Concepts and practices. *Rev Bras Cir Cardiovasc.*, 2010, 25(1), VI-VII.

[9]   Spear, SJ. *Chasing the Rabbit: How Marked Leaders Outdistance the Competition and How Great Companies can Catch U and Win.* McGraw Hill, 2009.

[10]   Neirotti, RA. Cardiac surgery: the infinite quest. Part II. *Rev Bras Cir Cardiovasc.*, 2013, 28(1), 129-36.

[11]   Hamel, G; Zanini, M. Assessment: Do you know how bureaucratic your organization is? *Harvard Business Review.*, 2017.

[12]   Gaynor, JW; Pasquali, SK; Ohye, RG; Spray, TL. Potential benefits and consequences of public reporting of pediatric cardiac surgery outcomes. *J Thorac Cardiovasc Surg.*, 2017, 153(4), 904-7.

[13]   Matloff, JM. The practice of medicine in the year 2010. *Ann Thorac Surg.*, 1993, 55(5), 1311-25.

[14]   Deam, W. *Real Leadrship Helping People and Organizations Face Their Toughest Challenges*, 2005.

[15]   Buchanan, JM; Tollison, RD. *The Theory of Public Choice - II*2009.

[16]   Innes, JE; Booher, DE. *Planning With Complexity: An Introduction to Collaborative Rationality for Public Pollicy*, 2010.

[17]   Foley, S. When you of pseudo maths adds up to fraud. *Financial Times.*, 2014.

[18]   Tugend, A. Shortcuts. *The New York Times.*, 2011.

[19]   Bennis, W. *The leadership advantage*, Leader to Leader Institute, 1999.

[20]   Gardner, H. K12 - *Education. Perspectives on the Future.* The Van Andel Education Institute.

[21]   Kellerman, B. *Professionalizing Leadership*, 2018.

[22]   Caprino, K. How To Stop Being A Boss And Become A Trnascendent Leader. *Forbes*, 2018 [Available from: https://www.

forbes.com/ sites/ kathycaprino/ 2018/ 05/ 01/ how-to-stop-being-a-boss-and-become-a-transcendent-leader/ - 21099fdd24e4.

[23] Neirotti, R. *Cultural narrative. Leadership course: A Cross-Cultural and International Perspective.* Harvard's Kennedy School of Government, 2006.

[24] Rosen, RH; Brown, PB. *Leading People.* 1th Edition ed 1996.

[25] Goffee, R; Jones, G. The art of followership. *European Business Forum.*, 2006, 25, 5.

[26] Cruickshank, V. Followership in the School Context. *Open Journal of Leadership.*, 2017, 6, 9.

[27] O'Neill, R. Partners for Growth: Andrew Deye MC/MPC 2015 is working to bring jobs back to Ohio. *Harvard Kennedy School Magazine.*, 2018.

[28] Uhl-Bien, M; Riggio, RE; Lowe, KB; Carsten, MK. Followership theory: A review and research agenda. *The Leadership Quarterly.*, 2014, 25, 21.

[29] Kellerman, B. What every leader needs to know about followers. *Harv Bus Rev.*, 2007, 85(12), 84-91, 145.

[30] Jones, BF. The Human Capital Stock: A Generalized Approach. *American Economic Review.*, 2014, 4, 25.

[31] Collins-Nakai, R. Leadership in medicine. *Mcgill J Med.*, 2006, 9(1), 68-73.

[32] Davenport, T. *Thinking for a living.* Harvard Business School Press, 2005.

[33] Warren, OJ; Carnall, R. Medical leadership: why it's important, what is required, and how we develop it. *Posgraduate Medical Journal.*, 2010, 87, 6.

[34] Heifetz, RA; Linsky, M; Grashow, A. *The practice of adaptive leadership: Tools and tactisfor changing your organization and the world.* First eBook edition ed: Harvard Business School Publishing, 2009.

[35] Neirotti, R. Paediatric cardiac surgery in less privileged parts of the world. *Cardiol Young.*, 2004, 14(3), 341-6.

[36] Delauney, S. *Medicins sans Frontieres* 2012 [Available from: http:// www.princeton.edu/ news-and-events/ news/ item/ sophie-delaunay-doctors- without- bordersm% C3% A9decins- sans-fronti% C3% A8res-msf.

[37] Burton-Hill, C. *Stravinsky's ballet: 100 years on BBC Culture*, 2013 [Available from: http:// www.bbc.com/ culture/ story/ 20130529-i-predict-a-riot].

[38] Salacuse, JW. *The Wise Advisor: What Every Professional Should Know About Consulting and Counseling*. First ed: Praeger, 2000.

[39] Kureishi, H. The Art of Distraction. *The New York Times*, 2012.

[40] *The Philosophy of Jiddu Krishnamurti - Indian philosopher* [Available from: https://www.jkrishnamurti.org/about_landing.

[41] Andrews, M; Pritchett, L; Woolcock, M. *Building State Copability: Evidence, Analysis, Action*. Oxford Scholarship Online, 2017.

[42] *Social Norms Stanford Encyclopedia of Philosophy*, 2018 [Second: [Available from: https://plato.stanford.edu/entries/social-norms/.

[43] Accmoglu, D; Robinson, JA. *Why Nations Fail. The Origins of Power, Prosperity, and Poverty*, 2012.

[44] Scimeca, V; Dunne, A. *The Culture Factor - Strategic Insights.*, 2018.

[45] Levin, H. *Teachers College*, 2011 [Available from: https://www.tc. columbia.edu/bigthinkers/segments/henry-levin-/.

[46] Woolley, AW; Chabris, CF; Pentland, A; Hashmi, N; Malone, TW. Evidence for a collective intelligence factor in the performance of human groups. *Science.*, 2010, 330(6004), 686-8.

[47] Cardarelli M, Vaikunth S, Mills K, DiSessa T, Molloy F, Sauter E, Bowtell K, Rivera R, Shin AY, Novick W. Cost-effectiveness of humanitarian pediatric cardiac surgery programs in low-and middle-income countries. *JAMA network open*. 2018 Nov 2;1(7):e184707.

[48] Lorenz, J; Rauhut, H; Schweitzer, F; Helbing, D. How social influence can undermine the wisdom of crowd effect. *Procceedings of Natural Academy of Sciences of United States of America.*, 2011, 108, 6.

[49] Bernstein, E; Shore, J; Lazer, D. How intermittent breaks in interaction improve collective intelligence. *Proc Natl Acad Sci U S A.*, 2018, 115, 6.

[50] Neirotti, RA. Cardiac surgery: the infinite quest. Part III--pediatric cardiac surgery: a discipline on its own. *Rev Bras Cir Cardiovasc.*, 2013, 28(2), 248-55.

In: Fundamentals of Leadership … ISBN: 978-1-53615-729-1
Editors: S. P. A. Stawicki et al. © 2019 Nova Science Publishers, Inc.

Chapter 8

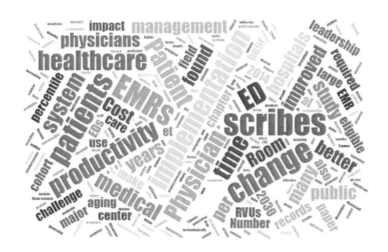

MANAGING CHANGE IN HEALTHCARE: THE RISE OF ELECTRONIC MEDICAL RECORDS

Veronica Sikka[1,2], MD, PhD, MHA, MPH, FACEP, FAAEM,
Raaj Popli[2,3], MD and Naazli Shaikh[1,2,4], MD

[1]Orlando VA Medical Center, Orlando, Florida, US
[2]University of Central Florida College of Medicine, Orlando, Florida, US
[3]Digestive Disease Consultants, Altamonte Springs, Florida, US
[4]Florida State University College of Medicine, Tallahassee, Florida, US

ABSTRACT

This chapter addresses a common theme in healthcare management - managing change. The U.S. healthcare system has gone through rapid change over the past several years and none has been more drastic than the implementation of EMRs. The benefits of EMRs are many but the impact on productivity has been questionable. EMRs have affected every type of healthcare organization from large hospitals to smaller group practices. In an effort to make the implementation of EMRs more palatable to physicians who have been resistant to change, this chapter discusses a case study of a Level 1 Trauma Center that also used scribes to make the transition from paper to electronic both seamless and actually satisfying to physicians. The stages of change are also discussed as the Kubler Ross Model for Change and the role for managers in managing the change so that something as daunting as EMR implementation is actually pleasant and organizationally unifying.

Keywords: clinical productivity, electronic health record, electronic medical record, health information management, physician satisfaction, system implementation

1. INTRODUCTION: CHANGING HEALTHCARE LANDSCAPE

Few sectors of the United States economy undergo as dramatic and as frequent a change as the health care system. From the evolution in patient management to the varied regulatory requirements of delivering care, changes within the healthcare system can be dramatic and rapid. In particular, economic realities of healthcare spending loom large in many of these changes.

One of the key concerns in health care management is management of change. Healthcare professionals are obligated both to acquire and to maintain the expertise needed to perform their professional duties and associated tasks, and outside of emergency/life-saving situations are obligated to undertake only those tasks that are within their competence. Managing change is about handling the complexity of the process. It is about evaluating, planning and implementing operations, tactics and strategies and making sure that the change is worthwhile and relevant. Managing change is a complex, dynamic, and challenging process. It is never a choice between technology or people-oriented solutions but a combination of all.

One of the challenges in healthcare is managing change in an environment where spending is on the rise. Health care spending in the United States is greater than in any other country in the world. Spending on health care reached $2.9 trillion in 2014, amounting to more than 17% of the US economy and more than $9,110 per person. Between 2013 and 2014 alone, spending on health care increased 5.3%. Spending on diabetes, ischemic heart disease, and low back and neck pain accounted for the highest amounts of spending by disease category [1].

Widening economic inequality in the USA has been accompanied by increasing disparities in healthcare outcomes. The life expectancy of the wealthiest Americans now exceeds that of the poorest by 10–15 years. Poor Americans have worse access to care than do wealthy Americans, partly because many remain uninsured despite coverage expansions since 2010 due to the Affordable Care Act. Medicaid has helped some in narrowing the gap between adults with Medicaid versus those with private insurance. According to the 2014 Commonwealth Fund Biennial Health Insurance Survey, adults with Medicaid coverage were better protected from the cost of illness than uninsured and even private coverage adults [2].

For individuals with private insurance, rising premiums and cost sharing have undermined wage gains and driven many households into debt and even bankruptcy [3]. The reforms resulting from the Affordable Care Act (ACA) over the past 6 years have led to increases in health care coverage. There is broad consensus that an estimated 20 million to 22 million individuals have obtained health care insurance since 2010 primarily through the expansion of Medicaid, coverage through parents' policies for young adults until age 26 years, and the health care exchanges. But that leaves more than 25 million US residents without health insurance [4].

A major public policy concern in the long-term care field is the potential burden an aging society will place on the care-giving system and public finances. The "2030 problem" involves the challenge of assuring that sufficient resources and an effective service system are available in thirty years, when the elderly population is twice what it is today. Much of this growth will be prompted by the aging of the Baby Boomers, who in 2030 will be aged 66 to 84. Various aspects of economic burden are associated with an aging population: social security payments, medical care insurance costs, the burden associated with uncovered medical expenses such as pharmaceuticals, and long-term care costs. Every elder has to prepare for four key "aging shocks": uncovered costs of prescription drugs, the costs of medical care that are not paid by Medicare or private insurance, the actual costs of private insurance that partially fills in the gaps left by Medicare, and the uncovered costs of long-term care. If the lifetime costs of each of these "aging shocks" are calculated, the typical 65-year-old faces present value lifetime costs for uncovered long-term care of $44,000 [5].

2. LEADERSHIP VIGNETTE: IMPLEMENTATION OF EMRS

Application of leadership theory to change management is evident in the implementation of electronic medical records (EMRs). This has been a challenge that many organizations, small and large, have faced over the years. As part of the American Recovery and Reinvestment Act, all public and private healthcare providers were required to adopt and demonstrate "meaningful use" of EMRs by January 1, 2014 in order to maintain their existing Medicaid and Medicare reimbursement levels. The Medicare and Medicaid EMR Incentive Programs provided incentive payments to eligible professionals, eligible hospitals and critical access hospitals (CAHs) as they adopted, implemented, upgraded or demonstrated meaningful use of certified EMR technology. Eligible professionals could receive up to $44,000 through the Medicare EMR Incentive Program and up to $63,750 through the Medicaid EMR Incentive Program [6].

Given that the implementation of EMRs involves a significant cash outlay, loss of productivity during implementation, and an organizational culture change, there can be much resistance when implemented in any institution. Studies have shown that EMR implementation has obvious decreases both during and after complete implementation. Practice reimbursements increase but the overall productivity decreases for providers [7-9].

This is an opportunity for leadership to make the EMR transition as seamless and cost effective as possible. The vignette presented in this chapter discusses the challenges and leadership solutions involved with the implementation of EMRs in an inner-city Level 1 Trauma Center ED with an annual volume of 100,000.

Implementation of EMRs in a busy ED where documentation went from written T-sheets to electronic medical records was not well received by providers who were accustomed to a written documentation system and others who were not as technologically proficient. This required the ED leadership to be proactive in convincing providers the value of this major healthcare process change and breaking the hopeless-helpless cycle. The biggest hurdle was the documentation in EMRs which was more tedious than simple pen and paper. This beget the proposal of having scribes in the ED and convincing higher management that scribes were cost neutral if not profitable.

A common solution that many EDs across the country have found to deal with increasing lengths of stay and stalled throughput is scribes. This results in better documentation, better coding and better capture of RVUs [10]. Scribes are often students working while in school toward an eventual career in the field of medicine. Scribes assist physicians with the clerical aspects of patient care with the intent of improving physician productivity. Their roles are diverse, but may include recording patient histories, documenting details of the physical examination, documenting procedures, following up on lab reports, and assisting with discharges. The significant impact of scribes in EDs has been proven in multiple studies. The pivotal study amongst the literature on this topic was by Arya et al. (2010) [11]. He found that in 243 clinical shifts over an 18-month period in an academic medical center the use of scribes was associated with improved overall productivity as measured by patients treated per hour (Pt / hr) and RVUs generated per hour by physician. Another study by Bastani et al. (2014) [12] compared patient data from a total of 11,729 patients in the before cohort to 12,609 patients in the after cohort. They found that the implementation of scribes improved the overall door-to-doc time by 13 minutes. Furthermore, patient and physician satisfaction was improved from the 58th and 62nd percentile to 75th and 92nd percentile, respectively.

Table 1. Project goals and milestones or key events

August - September 30, 201X	October 1, 201X – October 31, 201X+1	Sustainment Plan
1. Submit bid for contracting agencies for scribes 2. Collect pre implementation data with analysis	1. Implementation of 4 scribes to work with providers 10 hours a day on the weekdays (total of 40 scribe hours a day; 200 scribe hours a week) 2. Collection of post implementation data with analysis	Fully operational, scribe program integrated into the operation of the ED

It was anticipated that the volume of patients who would be affected would be over 100,000 patients [13]. The anticipated challenges were the scribes learning the new EMR. Table 1 presents a detailed plan for project implementation, with a target timeline for when the project will be fully operational.

By having a scribe assist with documentation and facilitating consults, more patients will be seen per hour which will help with lower wait times, lower number of patients leaving before being evaluated, and higher satisfaction. The core measures that would be used to determine the impact of this project include:

- Number of patients impacted
- Median time from ED arrival to ED departure for admitted and discharged ED patients (further stratified by medical and mental health patients)
- Waiting room times
- Door to room time
- Room to physician time
- Physician to disposition time
- Number of patients who are left without being seen
- Patient satisfaction
- Cost of scribes versus productivity gained (benefit of RVU and productivity per scribe)
- Cost to benefit ratio

Table 2. Project Specific Evaluation Measures

Measures (Quality, Access)	Anticipated Outcomes
Median time from ED arrival to ED departure for admitted and discharged ED patients (further stratified by medical and mental health patients)	⇓
Waiting room times	⇓
Door to room time	⇓
Room to physician time	⇓
Physician to disposition time	⇓
Number of patients who are left without being seen	⇓
Patient satisfaction	⇑

Table 2 specifies the evaluation measures that will be tracked and the anticipated outcomes.

2.1. Operational Feasibility

Scribe agencies across the country are very experienced in working in different EDs and do all of the training. The average hourly rate for a scribe is $20/hour which includes computer training which the agency facilitates. The question is often also raised by what is the difference between scribes and voice recognition programs such as Dragon which is a dictation system via a handheld device. Table 3 below lists the significant differences between these modalities.

Table 3. Scribes versus voice recognition modalities

Service	Voice Recognition Software	Scribes
Real-time, parallel documentation of all elements of the medical record		√
Real-time ED course updates	√	√
Tracking and prompting of result status		√
Assisting with consultant paging		√
Preparing aftercare instructions / discharge planning		√
Capturing procedures and ancillary interpretations		√
Ongoing quality assessment and performance feedback		√
Coding of exam and procedures		√
Editing notes	√	√

2.2. Customer Satisfaction

Leadership had to convince providers who were hesitant to adopt EMRs that scribes would provide both qualitative and financial benefits. Among the qualitative benefits, scribes will help improve physician satisfaction and physician recruitment and retention. Instead of clerical work, providers will be able to focus on the clinical tasks that allow them operate at the top of their clinical license. Scribes will allow providers to end their shifts on-time and "note-free". Also, scribes will allow providers to focus on the patient, by removing the technology and EMR from the patient-provider relationship. The provider can deliver better care to the patient, because they will no longer be burdened by the heavy clerical requirements of documenting and clicking in the EMR [14].

Because scribes will remove the burden of documentation, they will inherently make the provider more efficient during their shift. In fact the data suggests that the average emergency providers spend 44% of their clinical shift entering data into the EMR. Moreover, they will assist in coding with a focus on capturing workload and productivity. By outsourcing that task to the scribe, providers will have the capacity to treat more patients in the same clinical shift, thus expanding patient access and throughput in the ED. Scribes will also improve the accuracy, completeness, and timeliness of physician notes, which can result in better communication with other clinicians who read the patients' notes. Timeliness of notes will also help in ensuring that if the patient immediately follows up for care elsewhere after their ED visit, the ED note will be updated and complete.

Patients will also be more likely to be satisfied if they are able to be seen by a provider and experience lower wait times and quicker dispositions. Also, by providers not having to jot down notes for their documentation during the patient encounter, the provider will be more engaged with the patient.

3. DISCUSSION

The above vignette illustrates how leaders can manage change in a cost-cutting healthcare environment while also garnering provider buy-in who are resistant to change. EMRs was a given reality for implementation and convincing the team to use scribes allowed for the transition to be seamless and cost-neutral and even, profitable. The biggest factor in an organization resistant to change are individuals. Any healthcare change in an organization goes through several stages, like individuals.

A common organizational model that has significant parallels to individuals in the organization is the Kubler-Ross Change Curve (Figure 1).

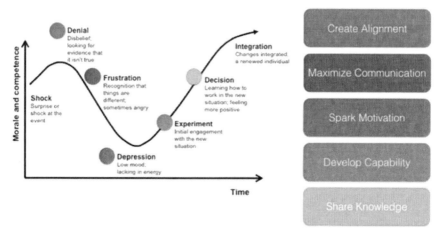

Figure 1. Kubler Ross Change Curve.

The stages of change in an organization progress over time (x-axis) with an increase in morale and competence (y-axis). As with the implementation of EMRs, it is important to *create alignment* by ensuring the individuals in an organization feel vested in the change. *Maximizing communication* with such a large change is critical with emails, newsletters, and meetings that can never be too frequent as an organization undergoes a major change. Also, when individuals are frustrated, they need to be listened to. As part of this, it is important to understand what is holding people back from trying new practices. Seeking what motivates different members and capitalizing on unique strengths *sparks motivation*. It is important to then *develop capability* by getting the appropriate training for EMRs and implementation of scribes in the ED workflow. Finally, it is important to encourage team members to share knowledge. With a new system like EMR, everyone learns new nuances that they should share and integrate into their workflow. When it is evident that everyone is trying to develop capability and integrate EMRs into their workflow, acceptance is achieved.

CONCLUSION

Every organization needs to support the individuals in the process of making transitions or changes. These individual transformations can be traumatic and may involve a lot of power loss and prestige issues, especially among veteran physicians who have always been practicing healthcare a certain way for years. The easier it is for the physicians to move along on their journey, the easier will it be for the organization to move towards success. Thus, this impacts the success rate and overall profits experienced by the company. The Kubler Ross Change Curve in healthcare is thus a powerful model that can help one understand and deal with changes and personal transitions. It helps managers to fathom how one will react to change and how to provide support during the process of change.

REFERENCES

[1]   Dielman JL, Baral R, Birger M. (2016). US spending on personal healthcare and public health, 1996-2013. *JAMA.* 316(24): 2627-2646.

[2]   Commonwealth Fund Biennial Health Insurance Survey. (2014). *Does Medicaid Make a Difference?* URL: http:// www. commonwealthfund.org/ publications/ issue-briefs/ 2015/ jun/ does-medicaid-make-a-difference. Accessed: 5/25/18.

[3]   Dickman SL, Himmelstein DU, Woolhandler S. (2017). Inequality and the healthcare system in the USA. *Lancet.* 389(10077): 1431-1441.

[4]   Bauchner H. (2017). Healthcare in the United States: A right or privilege. *JAMA.* 317(1): 29.

[5] Knickman JR & Snell EK. (2002). The 2030 problem: Caring for aging baby boomers. *Health Services Research.* 37(4): 849-884.

[6] Assistant Secretary for Public Affairs (2017). *About the Affordable Care Act.* URL: https:// www.hhs.gov/ healthcare/ about-the-aca/ index.html. Accessed: March 10, 2018.

[7] Howley MJ, Chou EY, Hansen N, and Dalrymple PW. (2015). The long-term financial impact of electronic health record implementation. *Journal of the American Medical Informatics Association, 22(2): 443-452.*

[8] Health Data Management. (2011). *Survey: EHRs often don't increase doc productivity. URL:* https:// www. health data management.com/ news/ survey- ehrs- often- dont- increase- doc-productivity, *Accessed: March 10, 2018.*

[9] Healthcare IT News. (2011). *HITECH drives docs to EHRs, but cost, productivity issues remain. URL:* http:// www.healthcareitnews.com/ news/ hitech- drives- docs- ehrs- cost- productivity- issues- remain. *Accessed March 11, 2018.*

[10] Schultz CG and Holmstrom HL. (2015). The use of medical scribes in health care settings: a systematic review and future directions. *Journal of the American Board of Family Medicine,* 28(3): 371-381.

[11] Arya R, Salovich DM, Ohman-Strickland P, and Merlin MA. (2010). Impact of scribes on performance indicators in the emergency department. *Academic Emergency Medicine,* 17: 490-494.

[12] Bastani A, Shaqiri B, Palomba K, et al. (2014). An ED scribe program is able to improve throughput time and patient satisfaction. *American Journal of Emergency Medicine,* 32: 399-402.

[13] Hess JJ, Wallenstein J, Ackerman JD et al. (2015). Scribe impacts on provider experience, operations, and teaching in an academic emergency medicine practice. *Western Journal of Emergency Medicine,* 16(5): 602-610.

[14] Hess JJ, Wallenstein J, Ackerman JD et al. (2015). Scribe impacts on provider experience, operations, and teaching in an academic emergency medicine practice. *Western Journal of Emergency Medicine,* 16(5): 602-610.

Chapter 9

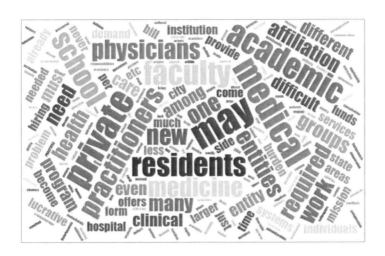

PITFALLS OF ACADEMIC AFFILIATIONS: HEALTH CENTER AT A CROSSROAD

Thomas J. Papadimos[1,*], James P. Hofmann[2], Steven J. Margolis[1] and Andrew B. Casabianca[2]

[1]The Department of Anesthesiology,
The Ohio State University Wexner Medical Center,
Columbus, Ohio, US
[2]The Department of Anesthesiology,
The University of Toledo College of Medicine and Life Sciences,
Toledo, Ohio, US

---

[*] Corresponding Author's E-mail: Thomas.Papadimos@osumc.edu.

ABSTRACT

The health and practice of academic medicine/academic medical centers is changing. In its attempt to preserve itself financially and to provide training sites for increasing class sizes and the addition of new medical schools, the academic health enterprise has been engaging in affiliations with non-governmental private health systems in order to acquire needed training venues and funds for their training and educational coffers. In so doing, academic health centers and their schools of medicine should not negotiate from a position of fear, but of knowledge and astute situational awareness. They should understand their own strengths and weakness and those of their potential partners with whom they are negotiating, and they should never give up their independence, or their oversight of the educational mission. Here we will address pitfalls related to affiliations, who is responsible for the educational mission, the blending of medical practices, conflict, billing and liability, inequality of compensation, concerns about the Accreditation Council for Graduate Medical Education requirements, and long- and short-term agreements between academic medical centers and private health systems.

Keywords: academic affiliations, academic health center, academic practice, hybrid model, medical education, private practic

1. INTRODUCTION

The landscape for healthcare, generally, and academic medical centers specifically, has changed significantly over the last 30 years [1-3]. This has led to partnerships that at one time would have been thought to be impossible. Though mergers are well accepted in the business community this concept for academic medical centers had been uncharted territory the last several decades [4-12]. Mergers and acquisitions have been replaced with terms such as affiliations, integrations, collaborations, alliances and just working together. Several changes in healthcare were cited as contributing factors:

1. there was a transition to more managed care and the reluctance of health plans to enter into contracts with academic medical centers because of their higher costs generally attributed to their teaching function [13];
2. congressional legislation to reduce Medicare payments to support graduate medical education [14]; and
3. consolidation of healthcare delivery at larger centers have negatively impacted teaching opportunities for medical students and residents, especially smaller academic medical centers [15].

Academic medicine and academic medical centers are concerned with their future [16, 17]. Such changes may jeopardize the academic mission to care for vulnerable patient populations, conduct ground breaking research and teach and train the healthcare providers of the future [18]. Decisions to affiliate or merge are made despite the knowledge that the challenges are enormous and they have a low probability of success [19]. Throughout it all there have emerged several common themes, critical for the successful organizational transformation of the academic medical center. There are also several key factors that were identified as reasons for those that ultimately failed. We will explore the pitfalls of academic affiliations, the challenges and what can be done to improve the chance of success.

2. AFFILIATION VERSUS MERGER

An academic affiliation is not a merger [20]. The merging of two organizations, especially in the same geographic or catchment area, may encounter problems from the Federal Trade Commission (FTC) in that in a merger between two or more organizations combines assets and the two entities become one [21]. If the combined entity would capture a majority of the market share, or if the move could limit competition (by elimination of one of the few independent entities in that particular catchment area) the FTC may scrutinize the effort, and even possibly step in to prevent or reverse the merger. Lessons can be learned from academic-industrial relationships regarding pitfalls to success [22-24].

In an affiliation, a hospital system may offer its facilities, services, and/or assets (including monetary inducements) to an academic organization, such as medical school, to not only assist the school, but also to further their own goals [25]. This frequently occurs because the medical school has a facility (university medical center) that does not provide enough patient volume for the students and residents, or the medical school needs income (from the affiliate) in order to insure the medical center's financial viability, or possibly the medical school lacks an adequate faculty to resident ratio [26, 27]. In other words, the university medical center may not, itself, be viable and may have to reinvent itself [28].

In some instances, an affiliation will cause the "teaching hospital" to cease being the primary academic center, and the private hospital system (non-governmental) will become the sole site for the provision of medical training. One of the goals of a hospital system housing the medical school's trainees and faculty is an effort to control costs through the use of cheaper help, i.e., trading nurse practitioners, physician assistants, and private physicians for medical students, residents, and faculty. The most interesting and curious aspect to an affiliation is that both entities remain competitors while housed under the same roof. More precisely, students, residents, and faculty from a school of medicine which no longer has a viable academic health center, will now be housed and operating in a facility under total control of a competitor; placing both residents and faculty in direct competition with the non-university personnel.

In some cases, the university medical center may cease to exist completely. If a perception exists that the elimination of competition was a major incentive for the health system to engage in the merger, the FTC may become interested in the action as it would in a merger. Excessive fear of this situation may produce difficulties in successful integration of programs. Actual plans or motives may be withheld from the chairman, program directors, faculty, and even hospital administrations; exchange of necessary information may be prohibited; and the future requirements for personnel (although known at some high level of administration) may be withheld from those responsible for actually hiring and assigning those people.

Although the reassignment of learners, and a change in the practice of a university medical center may be the most obvious outward signs of an affiliation, these may not be the only motives behind an affiliation. On the part of the medical school, one of the most common motives is future viability. In an era of increasing costs, reduced financial support from the state, and mandates at the state level that tuitions not be raised; many state sponsored medical schools have legitimate fears for their continued existence. This has driven a large number of schools in the recent past and the present to seek out partners with "deep pockets" to support their ongoing efforts. It will drive many more in this direction in the near future.

On the part of the private health care system, perception of reduced costs is only one of the major driving forces to align with medical schools and train students and residents. Many large health care systems own or act as health care insurers. In the absence of an academic medical center of their own, they are forced to send complex patients out of their network. By affiliating with a medical school, they are able to boast of a major academic medical center within their network. Thereby increasing their prestige in order to attract more patients. This allows not only retention within the system of fees for complex care, but also prevents the loss of those patients sent out of network to another entity for follow-up and ongoing future care and testing.

Perhaps the largest incentive for a private system to affiliate with a medical school is for recruitment [29]. As health care systems become larger and enter into more markets they are in constant need for new physicians to expand services, provide service in less desirable areas (rural, inner city, etc.), and to replace attrition due to age, or more lucrative offers from other large entities. One answer to this problem, other than increasingly more lucrative (costly) offers, is to develop your own physicians [30, 31]. By affiliation with a medical school many offers and inducements can be made at all steps along the training path. As an example, scholarships can be given to promising students in return for a commitment to practice at the entity for a specified number of years [32].

This is, of course, a win-win for both entities in the affiliation. The health care system insures a crop of needed physicians without having to enter into a bidding war with other systems. At the same time the medical school is able to continue to collect tuitions, and also demonstrate to the LCME that they are engaging in practices to help limit student debt. Nonetheless, there are academic centers who have affiliated with private entities and then cut ties for their own welfare [33].

3. WHO IS IN CHARGE?

In an affiliation, in which the private entity now houses medical school operations, the question is raised as to who is in control of the mission? While it can be argued that the school of medicine should direct any medical educational activities [34, 35], this may not become the reality. Private practitioners will loathe to give up control of the direction of their hospital practices. Of particular note is that by agreeing on an affiliation the controlling management of both institutions or parties must be sure that everyone below the top management level is willing to teach, support research efforts, and give up some clinical control to academicians. And what will it take to keep the current academicians from leaving [36, 37]?

When a private group and academic group are thrust into each other's arms the question will arise as to whether there are enough qualified teachers (or those willing to teach) [27]. If more are needed to be hired, who shall pay the costs? Many private entities may wish to burden the school of medicine with hiring the required faculty because hiring faculty that do not themselves bring in as many new patients (because of teaching and research requirements) requires an outlay of cash. If a school of medicine is already lacking in funds, how can there be an insistence, or directive, that the school of medicine should hire any new faculty that are required? When you add students and other learners (residents) to a hospital system you will likely need more faculty, not less. Oversight responsibilities for trainees can be extensive and expensive. How do you engage private physicians or other health care providers who never "signed up for this?" It will be difficult to demand such cooperation. It is difficult to blame anybody outside of the school of medicine for having a lack of academic motivation, for such motivation may never have been present.

This may be compounded by the private physicians practicing in a manner in which they have become accustomed, i.e., as they have practiced for many years (and successfully), but not necessarily using current evidence-based medicine. For instance, the use of renal dose dopamine, intraoperative paralysis of all patients with open abdomens, or using intermittent hemodialysis for all patients and ignoring the use of continuous renal replacement therapy.

Furthermore, who will appoint department chairs and program directors? While it seems simple to answer that those on the academic side will do so, this is not such an easy tasking. For example, a department chair of surgery will have particular aims and desires for the faculty and trainees. However, he or she will not necessarily have control of who is faculty, who gets hired, and requiring scholarly work from all participants. An academic chair will have faculty under his or her control, but by the nature of the affiliation, or more specifically, the need for it, chairs will not be able to dictate the course of their department as would be done at a university-run medical center [38]. In effect, private practitioners can hold the academic side of the house hostage. While the administration of the private health system may give public support to affiliation efforts, they will have difficulty demanding the cooperation of private physicians in these efforts. These administrations will have contracts for which they are beholden, and they cannot suffer the loss of institution profit by causing rebellion among their private physicians, whether hospital-based or otherwise.

An additional stumbling block will be that as the initial university chairs or program directors leave (resign or retire), will the private institution support true academic outsiders for positions as leaders or will they try to influence or demand that one of their private physicians take over an academic chair position [39]? They could also attempt to require that appointed academic chairs must report to, or seek permission of, a clinical chair or administrator appointed by the hospital. Ultimately, how much influence should a private, non-academic entity have in the appointment of a Dean of a school of medicine?

4. THE BLENDING OF PRIVATE AND ACADEMIC PRACTICES

The blending of practices presents inherent problems [40]. The actual blending of practices, or mixing/creating a group of private and university physicians may create a problem with the FTC. So, instead these two groups may work side by side in competition with each other. A two-pronged problem occurs immediately. Where are the origins of your patient base and what are, or will be, the referral patterns?

If a university practice moves over to a private institution because of a lack of patients or funds that signals that there was an inadequate base of patients and remuneration to support the university group [41]. In the new environment how will they create a patient base? Will they take patients from the private practitioners and who will refer to them? How will they grow their base of patients? Will private practitioners stop referring to their colleagues of many years? This is highly unlikely. Additionally, if one examines electronic medical records for consultation forms and referrals it is evident that there are choices to be made by the practitioner needing the consult. For instance, one does not just have the choice of a university group or "the" private group, the referral list will have all practitioners within 25-50 miles, including *other* university and private groups. Some of these practitioners may even be located in a different city or state.

To create additional difficulties for the university groups, their clinics, at least initially, will be near their original university medical location (for the most part), not at the new institution. Space will have to be made for them if they are to be competitive. Will such space be made available, and at what price, and of what size, and in what proximity? In the end, some of these some of these collaborations fail and some succeed [42-45].

5. CONFLICT MANAGEMENT

Conflict may be the result of cultural differences, which can be detrimental to an affiliation [10, 46]. Culture dictates how physicians approach their work, how they interact among other colleagues, and how they respond to administrations [47]. Culture can also take the form of intangible nuances. Likely, the two institutions have intangible nuances that will create friction and eventual conflict. Reconciling these cultural differences will lead to an improvement in communication, satisfaction and overall productivity. However, this will be a monumental task.

Resolution of conflict will be extremely important. Conflicts between individuals, between the practices, and between the administrative bodies of both organizations will need to be approached equitably [48, 49]. Protocols and provisions for conflict need to be addressed and put into place. However, the leaders of the academic effort will be in a disadvantageous position as it relates to conflict resolution. The academic organization has made the move to the private entity because of a need for patients and funds [50]. While it is true that the private entity may have motives for the affiliation including, a less expensive employee pool to assist in curbing costs, an expanded patient base, and a source for future physicians; it is the academic center that is in the needier position. For the private party the affiliation is a means to an end: lower costs, more profit, expansion, and the like [51]. For the medical school the overwhelming need for the affiliation is almost always a matter of survival. Why else would they decide to make their living in another's house? A private entity may be tempted to rule in a manner that will preserve its economic viability at the expense of the learner, wherein there must be a close understanding and working relationship between the two organizations. Also, as mentioned above, conflicts may arise over time as to how the academic mission will be organized, and who will be its leaders, and what research will be pursued.

Furthermore, if an academic institution receives advances of millions of dollars per annum that extend over a decade or more, in exchange for medical students and residents and program support (not for faculty salaries or research support, which is the usual case) there is a heavy burden of obligation placed on the medical school to comply and perform their tasks, or they may have to forfeit funds they have already received from the private entity. Unfortunately, there may be pressured entreaties from higher administration to avoid conflicts between those working in the educational and research missions and those in the clinical areas.

6. ADDRESSING BILLING AND LIABILITY

The manner of remuneration and the ability to bill for a particular individual's clinical work is very important [52]. In some instances, the health system will rent or lease the university physicians for a specified dollar per hour amount, while taking over the billing for the practice(s). This may or may not be to the advantage of the university physician group [53]. Additionally, if the health system owns or operates an insurance plan it can control the reimbursement for services and it may or may not proffer an advantage to physicians they directly employ over other private physicians, vis-a-vis the university/school of medicine. The health system might also be the billing service, or provide the billing service, for all or some of the clinical principals involved. Academic institutions should take steps to ensure equitability among all those involved. An additional complication arises in cross-coverage involving physicians of both groups for those services for which a single fee is usually remitted, such as surgery and post-operative care, and intraoperative anesthesia. This opens up questions of who will bill, and who will be paid, and how much.

Similarly, protection from liability is required of all practitioners. In many cases the practitioners from the separate entities will be covered by different malpractice insurers. One or the other of the entities may have chosen to self-insure their respective employees. While a liability claim involving a single practitioner may remain straight-forward, the same would not be true of one involving practitioners from both. Not only may both institutions be judged liable as well as the individuals, but different rules may apply to each. Some states provide a degree of protection for faculty members from malpractice claims as long as their clinical practice furthers the educational mission of the institution, e.g., by the teaching of medical students, or residents. Such protections may come in the form or limitation of venue to a state court, or hearing by a judge rather than a jury, caps on dollar amount for non-financial loss like pain and suffering, and even the provision of defense by the state's office of the attorney general without compensation. These protections from liability may not extend to the private practitioners, even if they are working with medical students and residents. This may dampen their enthusiasm for teaching or taking the risk of allowing trainees to participate in procedures or complex diagnostic work-ups. Nonetheless, regardless of the liability coverage (academic vs. private practice faculty) close supervision of residents is important because in leads to better outcomes [54]. Therefore, those private physicians in an affiliation will have to keep high supervisions standards, regardless of how they feel about the affiliation.

7. INEQUALITY OF COMPENSATION

Compensation of clinicians from an academic vs. a private practice is considerably different [50, 55]. When an affiliation is put together there is usually an expectation that clinical work will be equally shared among the two groups, even though they are competitors. While some expect that academic clinicians engage in more research and therefore are deserving of less clinical compensation, there is a fallacy in that thought process [56]. In today's academic environment faculty are expected to produce their share of relative value units or weighted relative value units. Some faculty members, in fact, compete well with those in private practice. However, the per hour compensation for clinical work between the two groups will vary, with the private practitioners earning more.

Such an inequality of compensation will lead to morale problems among faculty [57]. This is particularly true if academic titles are bestowed upon those private practice physicians who work with the learners, without at the same time giving them any requirement for further academic accomplishment. Giving those physicians some financial stipend to accompany their title will promote more rapid decay of faculty morale, no matter how token in value the stipend. There will be faculty who will leave the institution to go to a more traditional setting (a university that owns its own hospital/health system for instance), where the concept of the "team" and the compensation formula is consistent and equitable for all members. Also, the private hospital may attempt to "poach" faculty members from the academic side so as to incorporate those perceived as the best economic producers and the best teachers. Curiously enough, even though they may recruit those who they see as most valuable of the faculty for their employees, they may seek to increase their clinical activities and downplay their academics, in direct conflict with the stated goals of the affiliation. Eventually the faculty side may become depleted, especially if they are required to cover the new private entity and a potentially failing university entity (an academic medical center in financial trouble) at the same time.

Many times, as mentioned above, when there is a need for more academic faculty the private entity may insist that the university hire any new faculty required for the teaching mission. This is difficult because it is very challenging to recruit faculty to work side by side with private practitioners for less money while at the same time not having the required funding (on the university side) to hire the needed personnel [58]. Also, the space needed for faculty members at the new entity may be severely limited. Such space is needed, not only for administration, but for day to day medical student and resident interactions [59]. Solving this conundrum requires a resolve on the part of the private entity to support the academic mission which may be sorely lacking at some levels of the administration and clinical workforce.

This ultimately ends with the private entity and the university trying to hire hybrid personnel that can both teach and work and perform and administrate as if in private practice [60]. Many private entities (community hospitals) have residency training programs, but their ability to provide cutting edge state of the art care and scholarly activity of a premier university academic center is limited or hindered, both by the type of personnel and the attitude of their administrators and private practitioners.

8. ACCREDITATION COUNCIL FOR GRADUATE MEDICAL EDUCATION: THE STUMBLING BLOCKS

The Accreditation Council for Graduate Medical Education (ACGME) has mandatory requirements for residency programs to follow to retain their certification [61]. Failure to follow these requirements may result in sanctions including probationary status and even withdrawal of certification. Some requirements (the Core Program Requirements) are universal throughout all residency programs. These requirements address such things as maximum work hours per week, interventions for the mental of health of residents and faculty, and mandatory time off, to name a few. Each specialty program also has requirements that are specific to residency programs training in that specialty. These requirements may demand such things as a particular caseload, appropriate supervision ratios, amount of scholarly work required of the faculty and residents, the number and type of rotations the residents must complete and protected nonclinical time for key personnel. Private practice groups need to become well-versed in these requirements and to abide by them, including a review of their performance by the academic faculty and medical students and residents. Again, such requirements and expectations may be difficult for the private practitioners to agree or adhere to, as well as health system administrators to understand.

A good example would anesthesiology residency training [61]. Adding anesthesiology residents to a private health system may lessen the system's need for certified registered nurse anesthetists (CRNAs). However, residents are not only in the operating room. They have required rotations in pain medicine, critical care medicine, the post anesthesia recovery unit (PACU), and obstetrical anesthesia, all of which take the resident out of the operating room. Furthermore, they can only be supervised by the faculty at most a 1:2 ratio of faculty to residents, and, in some cases, require a ratio of 1:1. In the anesthesia care-team model CRNAs and AAs can be supervised for medical direction at a ratio of 1:4. To make such an integration successful, administrators must be cognizant of the requirements of an academic environment. Another difficulty is with the case assignments. CRNAs may have to be assigned to less complicated cases in order for anesthesiology residents to receive the necessary education. Again, this may be difficult to implement if private anesthesiologists and CRNAs are at odds with this need. Difficulties can be further compounded if a student registered nurse anesthetist (SRNA) program is present. ACGME requirements state that other learners must not compete with the residents for educationally required cases. This may necessitate the reduction or even curtailment of a student CRNA program.

The specialty of anesthesiology is not alone in ACGME requirements affecting the clinical practice. This situation is found for many specialties; however, those formulated for the hospital based specialties may have the greatest impact on the health care system involved in an affiliation. The specialty of emergency medicine requirements [61], for example, limit the faculty's clinical work to no more than 28 hours per week, and no more than 4 patients per hour on average while supervising residents. Numbers which are much smaller than that usually seen in a private practice group, especially one which employs mid-level providers as physician extenders. At the outset, it may seem lucrative to replace physician assistants and nurse practitioners with the lower paid longer working residents; but any anticipated savings may evaporate in the face of reduced supervision ratios, and decreases in allowable clinical physician hours.

9. PROS AND CONS OF LONG-TERM AGREEMENTS

Getting a medical school on sound financial footing and avoiding its closure or probation is of the utmost importance. Completing and implementing agreements between private entities and academic medical centers is difficult, especially if all the residents in training are required to go to the private entity by a certain date. There must be detailed ground work laid, not just among what is brokered by the negotiators at the highest levels, but an acceptance and setting of expectations among and between private physicians, nursing staff, and other allied health professionals. If this groundwork is not done properly, and the allotted time for its completion is not adequate, many difficulties will arise that will compound the concerns expressed in the above sections [62, 63].

A university and a private entity may find it advantageous to pursue a long-term agreement. Short-term agreements to have medical students and residents come to work and observe are less difficult to negotiate than those of longer term. Agreements for the long-term require trust between and should have parsing of as many details as possible. Long-term agreements, especially those that entail the elimination or severe downgrading of an academic medical center's capacity to provide care (or specialty care it had previously been providing), require exquisite attention. When hundreds of millions of dollars, or billions of dollars, are promised for support of a medical school there needs to be agreement at many levels. Such agreements are usually made between small or medium size failing academic medical centers, and the negotiators on the academic side should be cognizant of their disadvantage in the negotiations and hold their impulse to take money at any or all costs. They should realize that the health care system with whom they affiliate is not entering into the agreement altruistically, but for their own benefit and continued health, well-being and expansion. As such they should not negotiate from a position of weakness, but as a potential partner (albeit a lesser one) in a mutually beneficial enterprise [64]. A matter that could be potentially devastating to retention or recruitment of academic faculty is the perception or fact that they personally, and their practices, are not protected from the private sector through some unfair advantage (referrals, consults, remuneration, and even bullying). There must be a way for a university to pull out of an agreement without entailing repayment of untold millions of dollars from a situation that is detrimental to medical education and scholarly activity.

CONCLUSION

In an environment of scarce medical resources, especially in locales where there is stiff competition for a limited amount of compensation, smaller medical schools and their accompanying institutions (academic medical centers and the university, in general) may face incredible stressors to stay financially solvent. Money is needed for new equipment, research endeavors, general repairs, etc. It may come to pass that such institutions will need to form new alliances, sometimes with new partners and sometimes with current competitors who will remain competitors. These endeavors will be riskier to the smaller academic competitor/institution.

Schools of medicine have much to offer in regard to cutting edge technology use, patents, research projects, national reputation, and the provision of cheap labor. Universities must not allow themselves to be taken advantage of and not portray themselves as desperate or inferior to larger hospital systems. Academic medical centers and their academic faculty should always speak truth to power [65]. It is incumbent upon university administrations to provide, not only for protection of the educational experience and the learners, but also for their faculty.

REFERENCES

[1]   Moses, H; 3rd, Matheson, DH; Dorsey, ER; George, BP; Sadoff, D; Yoshimura, S. The anatomy of health care in the United States. *JAMA*, 2013, **310**(18), 1947-1963.

[2]   Wartman, SA. Toward a virtuous cycle: The changing face of academic health centers. *Academic Medicine*, 2003, **83**(9), 797-799.

[3]   Blumenthal, D; Meyer, GS. Academic health centers in a changing environment. *Health Aff (Millwood)*, 1996, **15**(2), 200-215.

[4]   Lowery, K; Shi, L; Weiner, JP; Patow, C. Money, mission, and medicine: an innovative managed care partnership between the

community health centers of Maryland and Johns Hopkins University. *J Ambul Care Manage*, 1999, **22**(4), 13-27.

[5] Longenecker, R. Crafting an affiliation agreement: academic-community collaboration in a rural track family practice residency program. *J Rural Health*, 2000, **16**(3), 237-242.

[6] Leeman, J; Kilpatrick, K. Inter-organizational relationships of seven Veterans Affairs Medical Centers and their affiliated medical schools: results of a multiple-case-study investigation. *Acad Med*, 2000, **75**(10), 1015-1020.

[7] Garcia, FA; Miller, HB; Huggins, GR; Gordon, TA. Effect of academic affiliation and obstetric volume on clinical outcome and cost of childbirth. *Obstet Gynecol*, 2001, **97**(4), 567-576.

[8] Jaklevic, MC. New bedfellows. Baylor medical school switches hospital partners. *Mod Healthc*, 2004, **34**(17), 4.

[9] Lambert, CR; Bunker, S; Garrison, LF; Means, MD; Pepine, CJ; Conti, CR; Dewar, MA; Goldfarb, T. An academic-community cardiovascular service line affiliation: design, implementation, and performance. *Am Heart Hosp J*, 2006, **4**(2), 86-94.

[10] Fleishon, HB: Itri, JN; Boland, GW; Duszak, R. Jr. Academic Medical Centers and Community Hospitals Integration: Trends and Strategies. *J Am Coll Radiol*, 2017, **14**(1), 45-51.

[11] Clancy, GP. Good Neighbors: Shared Challenges and Solutions Toward Increasing Value at Academic Medical Centers and Universities. *Acad Med*, 2015, **90**(12), 1607-1610.

[12] Sussman, AJ; Otten, JR; Goldszer, RC; Hanson, M; Trull, DJ; Paulus, K; Brown, M; Dzau, V; Brennan, TA. Integration of an academic medical center and a community hospital: the Brigham and Women's/Faulkner hospital experience. *Acad Med*, 2005, **80**(3), 253-260.

[13] Zwanziger, JMG. Can Managed Care Plans Control Health Costs. *Health Affairs*, 1996, **15**(2), 185-199.

[14] Iglehart, JK. The uncertain future of Medicare and graduate medical education. *N Engl J Med*, 2011, **365**(14), 1340-1345.

[15] Pizzo, P; Braddock, CH; III. Prober, CG. The Future of Graduate Medical Education: Is There a Path Forward? In: *The Transformation of Academic Health Centers*. Edited by Wartman S. London, U.K.: Academic Press, 2015, 101-110.

[16] Rodriguez, JL; Jacobs, DM; Zera, RT; Van Camp, JM; Muehlstedt, SG; West, MA; Bubrick, MP. Academic practice groups: strategy for survival. *Surgery*, 2000, **128**(4), 505-512.

[17] Balser, JR; Stead, WW. Coordinated Management of Academic Health Centers. *Trans Am Clin Climatol Assoc*, 2017, **128**, 353-362.

[18] Meyer, D; Armstrong-Coben, A; Batista, M. How a community-based organization and an academic health center are creating an effective partnership for training and service. *Acad Med*, 2005, **80**(4), 327-333.

[19] Rice, AM. Successful affiliations: principles and practices. *Front Health Serv Manage*, 2011, **27**(4), 13-18, discussion 39-41.

[20] *From Dave's Desk: Understanding Mergers, Acquisitions, and Affiliations. Health Care Business Solutions*. [https:// www. cookmedical.com/ healthcare- business- solutions/ from- daves-desk-understanding-mergers-acquisitions-and-affiliations/].

[21] *Merger Review* [https://www.ftc.gov/enforcement/merger-review].

[22] Martin, JB. Academic-industrial collaboration: the good, the bad, and the ugly. *Trans Am Clin Climatol Assoc*, 2002, **113**, 227-239, discussion 239-240.

[23] Martin, JB; Reynolds, TP. Academic-industrial relationships: opportunities and pitfalls. *Sci Eng Ethics*, 2002, **8**(3), 443-454.

[24] Pizzo, PA; Lawley, TJ; Rubenstein, AH. Role of Leaders in Fostering Meaningful Collaborations between Academic Medical Centers and Industry While Also Managing Individual and Institutional Conflicts of Interest. *JAMA*, 2017, **317**(17), 1729-1730.

[25] Hegwer, LR. Strengthening an affiliation without a merger. *Healthc Financ Manage*, 2015, **69**(4), 50-57.

[26] *The Rise and Fall of Academic Medicine: AMC Competitivenss in Post-Reform Healthcare*. [http://www.miramedgs.com/web/57-focus/

past-issues/ spring-2017/ 667- the- rise- and- fall- of- academic-medicine-amc-competitiveness-in-post-reform-healthcare].

[27] Porter, S. Just-released clerkship study: growing shortage of clinical training sites challenges medical schools. *Ann Fam Med*, 2014, **12**(5), 484-486.

[28] Kirch, DG; Grigsby, RK; Zolko, WW; Moskowitz, J; Hefner, DS; Souba, WW; Carubia, JM; Baron, SD. Reinventing the academic health center. *Acad Med*, 2005, **80**(11), 980-989.

[29] Kocher, R; Sahni, NR. Hospitals' race to employ physicians--the logic behind a money-losing proposition. *N Engl J Med*, 2011, **364**(19), 1790-1793.

[30] Scott, KW; Orav, EJ; Cutler, DM; Jha, AK. Changes in Hospital-Physician Affiliations in U.S. Hospitals and Their Effect on Quality of Care. *Ann Intern Med*. 2017, **166**(1), 1-8.

[31] Kirch, DG; Salsberg, E; Association of American Medical C: The physician workforce challenge: response of the academic community. *Ann Surg*, 2007, **246**(4), 535-540.

[32] Broderick, PW; Nocella, K. Developing a community-based graduate medical education consortium for residency sponsorship: one community's experience. *Acad Med*, 2012, **87**(8), 1096-1100.

[33] Conn, J. Standing on its own. University hospital cuts ties with two systems. *Mod Healthc*, 2007, **37**(28), 22-23.

[34] D'Aunno, THR; Munson, FC. Decision Making, Goal Consensus, and Effectiveness in University Hospitals. *Hosp Health Serv Admin*, 1991, **36**(4), 505-523.

[35] Lobas, JG. Leadership in academic medicine: capabilities and conditions for organizational success. *Am J Med*, 2006, **119**(7), 617-621.

[36] Kubiak, NT; Guidot, DM; Trimm, RF; Kamen, DL; Roman, J. Recruitment and retention in academic medicine--what junior faculty and trainees want department chairs to know. *Am J Med Sci*, 2012, **344**(1), 24-27.

[37] Ries, A; Wingard, D; Gamst, A; Larsen, C; Farrell, E; Reznik, V. Measuring faculty retention and success in academic medicine. *Acad Med*, 2012, **87**(8), 1046-1051.

[38] Sarfaty, S; Kolb, D; Barnett, R; Szalacha, L; Caswell, C; Inui, T; Carr, PL. Negotiation in academic medicine: a necessary career skill. *J Womens Health (Larchmt)*, 2007, **16**(2), 235-244.

[39] Lieff, S; Banack, JG; Baker, L; Martimianakis, MA; Verma, S; Whiteside, C; Reeves, S. Understanding the needs of department chairs in academic medicine. *Acad Med*, 2013, **88**(7), 960-966.

[40] Macfarlane, B. The Morphing of Academic Practice: Unbundling and the Rise of the Para-academic. *HEQ*, 2010, **65**(1), 59-73.

[41] Gallagher, CEM. (ed.). *Ethical Challenges in Oncology*, 1st edn: Academic Press, London, United Kingdom, 2017.

[42] Mallon, WT. The alchemists: a case study of a failed merger in academic medicine. *Acad Med*, 2003, **78**(11), 1090-1104.

[43] Their, SO; Kelley, WN; Pardes, H; Knight, AW; Wietecha, M. Success factors in merging teaching hospitals. *Acad Med*, 2014, **89**(2), 219-223.

[44] Sidorov, J. Case study of a failed merger of hospital systems. *Manag Care*, 2003, **12**(11), 56-60.

[45] Cohen, MD; Jennings, G. Mergers involving academic medical institutions: impact on academic radiology departments. *J Am Coll Radiol*, 2005, **2**(2), 174-182.

[46] Munich, RL. Transplanting an organization: how does culture matter. *Bull Menninger Clin*, 2011, **75**(2), 126-144.

[47] Ovseiko, PV; Melham, K; Fowler, J; Buchan, AM. Organisational culture and post-merger integration in an academic health centre: a mixed-methods study. *BMC Health Serv Res*, 2015, **15**, 25.

[48] Leape, LL; Shore, MF; Dienstag, JL; Mayer, RJ; Edgman-Levitan, S; Meyer, GS; Healy, GB. Perspective: a culture of respect, part 1: the nature and causes of disrespectful behavior by physicians. *Acad Med*, 2012, **87**(7), 845-852.

[49] Leape, LL; Shore, MF; Dienstag, JL; Mayer, RJ; Edgman-Levitan, S; Meyer, GS; Healy, GB. Perspective: a culture of respect, part 2: creating a culture of respect. *Acad Med*, 2012, **87**(7), 853-858.

[50] Regev, aMA. Integrating Academic and Private Practices. *Anesthesiology Clinics*, 2018, **36**, 321-332.

[51] Adashi, EY. Money and Medicine: Indivisible and Irreconcilable. *AMA J Ethics*, 2015, **17**(8), 780-786.

[52] Tseng, P; Kaplan, RS; Richman, BD; Shah, MA; Schulman, KA. Administrative Costs Associated With Physician Billing and Insurance-Related Activities at an Academic Health Care System. *JAMA*, 2018, **319**(7), 691-697.

[53] Cappell, MS. The art of salary negotiation in academic medicine: lessons from a 32-year career. *Gastrointest Endosc*, 2012, **75**(4), 857-860.

[54] Farnan, JM; Petty, LA; Georgitis, E; Martin, S; Chiu, E; Prochaska, M; Arora, VM. A systematic review: the effect of clinical supervision on patient and residency education outcomes. *Acad Med*, 2012, **87**(4), 428-442.

[55] Wai, PY; Dandar, V; Radosevich, DM; Brubaker, L; Kuo, PC. Engagement, workplace satisfaction, and retention of surgical specialists in academic medicine in the United States. *J Am Coll Surg*, 2014, **219**(1), 31-42.

[56] Balch, CM; Shanafelt, TD; Sloan, JA; Satele, DV; Freischlag, JA. Distress and career satisfaction among 14 surgical specialties, comparing academic and private practice settings. *Ann Surg*, 2011, **254**(4), 558-568.

[57] RJ. Retaining Talent at Academic Medical Centers. *IJAM*, 2016, **2**(1), 46-51.

[58] PF, D. *Management Challenges for the 21st Century*. New York, New York: HarperCollins, 1999.

[59] Pober, JS; Neuhauser, CS; Pober, JM. Obstacles facing translational research in academic medical centers. *FASEB J*, 2001, **15**(13), 2303-2313.

[60] Spyridonidis, D; Hendy, J; Barlow, J. Understanding Hybrid Roles: The Role of Identity Processes Amongst Physicians. *Public Administraiton*, 2014, **93**(2), 395-411.

[61] *ACGME Common Program Requirements* [https://www.acgme.org/Portals/0/PFAssets/ProgramRequirements/CPRs_2017-07-01.pdf].

[62] *The Pros and Cons of Multi-Year Client Contracts* [https://www.continuum.net/blog/pros-and-cons-of-multi-year-client-contracts].

[63] *The Advantages and Disadvantages of Sort- and Long-Term Contracts* [http://www2.westsussex.gov.uk/ds/cttee/ses/ses060711 i6b.pdf].

[64] Angell, M. Is academic medicine for sale? *N Engl J Med*, 2000, **342**(20), 1516-1518.

[65] Papadimos, TJ; Murray, SJ. Foucault's "fearless speech" and the transformation and mentoring of medical students. *Philos Ethics Humanit Med*, 2008, **3**, 12.

In: Fundamentals of Leadership ...
Editors: S. P. A. Stawicki et al.
ISBN: 978-1-53615-729-1
© 2019 Nova Science Publishers, Inc.

Chapter 10

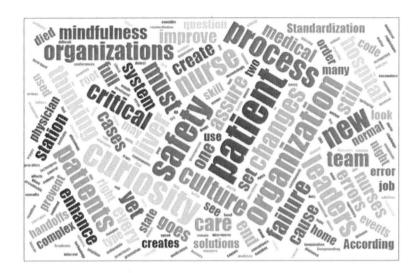

CREATING A CULTURE OF CURIOSITY TO IMPROVE QUALITY AND PATIENT SAFETY

Dianne McCallister, MD, MBA
Chief Medical Officer, The Medical Center of Aurora,
Aurora, Colorado, US

ABSTRACT

In an increasingly complex healthcare system, it is the duty of leaders to continuously improve the safety of the patients we serve. While standardization and process are key components of a Patient Safety Culture, in the end, it is the critical thinking of our teams that prevent many errors from reaching the patient. The development of curiosity as a central skill set to detect aberrances from normal operations or patient physiology can and must be developed, reinforced and recognized to assure patient safety. Methods to enhance this skill set exist, and can be leveraged to improve culture and care.

Keywords: change management, culture of curiosity, medical leadership, patient safety, process

1. INTRODUCTION

Patient Safety is an imperative of healthcare organizations, and yet as leaders, the ability to eliminate harm to patients remains a challenge unmet by all organizations. Solutions and techniques abound in the literature from experts and consultants, yet many leaders remain with the haunting notion that there are pieces missing in the puzzle. We attend and speak at conferences devoted to the topic, yet medical leaders still return to the home organization to battle the root causes of errors that were preventable.

The challenge resides in the complexity of the system in which we care for patients. In an IHI study on infection prevention, it was found that there are a median of 5.5 visits to a patient room per hour. This included nursing staff, visitors (25%), medical staff, nonclinical staff, and other clinical staff [1]. The range of visits per room ranged from 0 to 28 per hour. Correcting out the visitor visits, this is, at median 4.125 visits per hour of hospital/medical staff, or 99 visits per day. Assuming a 3.5 day length of stay, it is 346 visits per patient per stay. Add in the non- visit interactions of remote entry of orders, critical lab result calls/texts, radiology reads, equipment sterilized, pharmacist reviews/verifications, are all adding to the number of "touches" per patient. With these non-contact interventions, the crucial process interactions per patient, easily reach the thousands in a single patient hospitalization.

In addition to patient centered encounters, one should add the processes of hand-offs between shifts, medication reconciliation, home treatments that are or are not available to hospital providers, order strings, allergy histories, physician to physician handoffs and consults, EMR

Creating a Culture of Curiosity ... 221

downtimes, updates to systems that may create new traps, changes in equipment, shortages of drugs and supplies and the resulting complexity of the system staggers the imagination. Compounding this complexity is the fallacy that 100% reliable process is an achievable goal when both technology and humans have fallibility. According to the Academic Medical Center Patient Safety Organization, we must consider that there is always an "inherent error rate" that affects our systems and processes [2].

Policies, rules, regulations and check sheets, regulatory reviews and safety huddles are methods commonly employed to contain and combat the complexity, yet we still find variability and normalized deviance springing up like weeds. In the end, no matter how robust our systems and processes, our dependence on human critical thinking creates the last defense. This is a process that must be triggered, and in the prevention of errors, the trigger is curiosity. We invoke the "5 Whys" in our root cause analyses after events. How do we as leaders create a culture of curiosity – one that questions why something is different, why an alarm is going off again, why the patient is suddenly "difficult", and why intuition is pointing to something "not being right"? Those team members that take the moment to invoke their curiosity are often the ones to whom we give the Great Catch Awards. They have put a plug in the last slice of Swiss cheese. How do we empower all our staff with this gift of curiosity in the midst of complexity?

2. VIGNETTE ONE

A postoperative, full code, tonsillar cancer patient is placed on the Oncology Unit for post-operative care. His night nurse is given hand off from the day shift, including the pain medications and physician's orders from the standardized head and neck oncology order set. The patient is doing well for the first four hours, but then begins with hypoxia and changes in mental status. The night nurse, newly oriented to the organization, and with years of clinical experience in hospice care, assesses the patient, who talks to him and while she is in the room, his oxygen saturations to normal. The nurse returns to the nursing station and is charting when, suddenly, the patient experiences a cardiopulmonary arrest. The nurse goes to the room, but does not begin CPR or call a code. She goes to the nurse's station, where the charge nurse is asked what to do when a patient has died. The charge nurse fails to ask which patient, and answers the question. Several minutes afterward, another nurse returns to the nurse's station and asks why Mr. X's pulse ox is alarming. The nurse replies that the patient has passed away. The second nurse asks what the patient's code status is, since the board indicates full code. It is then that the first nurse realizes that she assumed, on an oncology floor with a number of no code patients, that this patient was a no code. At that point, a Code is called, CPR started. The resuscitation is unsuccessful. The CMO leads the investigation of the incident, which shows normalized deviance in assuming no code status, and a culture that does not verify for "No Code" armbands. Further questioning shows that the nurse had not changed her mindset from hospice work to acute care work. The family is invited to a meeting where there is full disclosure of the mistake. Training, changes in the cohorting of patients and new oversight by the house supervisor and charge nurses is implemented to prevent a recurrence. As a result of the required state reporting of the incident, the nurse, who did not follow policy, or do critical thinking, despite documented and appropriate training, loses her nursing license and hence her job.

2.1. Skill Set

As medical leaders, this scenario plays on our deepest insecurities. How do we assure the safety of our patients in a complex organization over which we have much influence and little control? Our training to be the expert, and give directives, does not assure safety when we are not present, and when others direct and fulfill the process. High Reliability Organizations (HRO) are organizations that create "organizational mindfulness" [2], and a key component of an HRO is the "constant, proactive vigilance by all staff to help identify signals of potential and actual risk" [2].

Creating a Culture of Curiosity ...

According to Simon Walker, curiosity is the attribute everyone, and particularly leaders, must develop to compensate for complexity and uncertainty [3]. He states that "deep, (but narrow) insight becomes obsolete during times of change, where new developments/disruption where "something from left field" can catch us off guard and unprepared. The significance of responding to change is emphasized by an article from the Journal of General Medicine: "This continued proliferation of medical advancements has resulted in an exponential growth of medical knowledge, increased complexity of medical practice, and greater medical specialization" [4]. There is no standardized process that can flex to accommodate every situation. Standardization should be present, and is necessary, to deal in a consistent and predictable way with the 80% of our work that is standard. We are adding artificial intelligence to monitor sets of data to look for the aberrations from the norm. However, in the end, we still rely on the critical thinking and curiosity of the professionals to see the changes, or respond to signals from artificial intelligence and monitoring, to have the curiosity to look for and respond to the unusual and use their curiosity and critical thinking to pursue an answer rather than make an assumption.

Merriam Webster defines curiosity as "interest leading to inquiry" [5]. In the end, curiosity is the crucial element that allows individuals remaining vigilant and able to learn in situations that on the surface appear to be static. In the complex medical world, curiosity is a foundational to the personal attribute to foster in each member of the team to help create safety for the patient. How, as leaders, do we instill curiosity into our culture?

We have guidance from the methods we currently employed in response to mistakes. For example, when performing a Root Cause Analysis, we invoke the process of the "5 Whys" from the IHI [6]. The underlying supposition is that the obvious answer may not be the actual problem. To get to the correct solutions to repair systems, we must be curious enough to look past the obvious. We can take this paradigm, and apply it as a proactive tool used by the team at the bedside by looking to other industries that have successfully implanted curiosity into the fabric of their companies. Drs. Toussant and Ehrlich suggest that this is best modeled into the culture by leaders respecting those that do the work by going to where the work is done and asking them open ended questions and seeking input [7]. With the place of comfort for experts being providing answers, this can be challenging, however, open-ended questions are also the foundation of a good history, and therefore an accessible skill for most clinicians.

According to Simon Walker, the first step is to model curiosity in the way we behave, to recognize and reward curiosity in others, and to expose our teams to new perspectives [3]. Some concrete examples used by organizations are relatively easy to incorporate into leadership styles and vary from the simple change of asking for differing perspectives and insights when rounding and in meetings and challenging our teams to question the status quo to find solutions. We must emphasize having this curiosity in positive situations in order to develop the curiosity that is needed in the moment in a tense or difficult situation. These can be ingrained into the organizational culture using a variety of systems that positively reinforce thinking beyond the obvious.

One positive way of incorporating curiosity into our management paradigm is the technique of Appreciative Inquiry, developed at the Weatherhead School of Business at Case Western Reserve. This is an approach to asking questions, with the assumption that every organization and person has strengths inherent to the way it functions. Appreciative Inquiry "begins by identifying this positive core and connecting to it in ways the heighten energy, sharpen vision, and inspire action for change" [8]. This methodology uses positive questioning to determine and reinforce the positive goals of the individual, the team and the organization. Or, in other words, it takes the training we have in determining the problem, and turns the line of questioning to determine what is going well and how to enhance it. Obviously, there is still need to problem-solve and trouble shoot, yet having a hospital/organization filled with people seeking the positive goal of patient's best interests is a powerful preventive force.

Appreciative Inquiry, "centrally involves the mobilization of inquiry through the crafting of the "unconditional positive question" [9]. One example would be the CEO going to the unit and asking "What is going well today?" Following up with, "how does your team assure that the patients are safe at all times?" Boiled down, the goal is to use positive questions, rather than negative, to inspire the ownership and engagement of each team member. While not a complete answer to patient safety, this approach does lay down a foundation of assuming good intentions that is a foundation to another well documented safety process, Just Culture, which also encourages curiosity as a value.

A Just Culture is a systematic approach to safety in which the organization is constantly seeking to improve to enhance patient safety by encouraging curiosity. It goes beyond identifying problems and solutions to one in which every individual is constantly seeking ways to enhance the safety of the system. This will not happen when the individuals feel "unsafe" and thus there must be an assumption of positive intent and bad process. In other words, it's not about who is wrong, it's about what is wrong, at the fundamental level. It's about a state of mindfulness. According the Dr. Boysen, "mindfulness throughout an organization considers, but moves beyond, events and occurrences. Everyone in the organization is continually learning, adjusting, and redesigning systems for safety and managing behavioral choices" [10]. Thus mindfulness, in this definition, is curiosity in action. It is also curiosity as a general cultural expectation which is embodied in the way each individual performs their work and interacts with the system and one another. Just culture is a topic in and of itself, yet the way we lead can either create a just culture or destroy it, particularly in moments of error. The approach we take as leaders sets the culture. We can have accountability in a way that teases out the real cause of error, and at the same time sets an expectation that each individual will be rewarded for having the curiosity to think beyond the obvious, to deviate from the standardized process when needed to achieve the goal of patient safety. In Just Culture, the response to the error is done in a consistent way that responds to the type of error made. Some errors are intentional, such as falsifying data, and require a disciplinary response. Other errors, are unintentional, and are a product of the system, and so the response is to involve the "2nd victim", i.e., worker involved in the error, to devise a way to prevent similar errors in the future by their engagement in creating a solution. On an organizational level, this is a structure of curiosity that looks into the details of the issue rather than responding to assumptions or appearances.

Another reinforcement of the value of curiosity comes from what the organization is perceived to value. As leaders, we must constantly monitor our public dialogue. Do we recognize those who positively question the status quo to create improved processes? Do we stop to answer questions to assure understanding rather than cutting off conversation to "save time"?

Organizationally, formal recognition is symbolic of values, including the value of curiosity. "Great Catch Awards" publicly celebrate an individual who averted an error by using their curiosity to question a situation that did not appear to be right. Awards for innovation are used by some organizations to recognize curiosity that creates improvements in patient care.

Structurally, curiosity is engendered by exposure to new environments. When there is discord between interdependent teams (OR and ICU, Nursing Unit and Environmental Services) we can send member of the team to job shadow the work on the other unit. It is an experiential method to create knowledge that trumps assumptions. This can be a breakthrough methodology to creativity and has lasting effects to remind the teams that processes are most often the issue, not people and work ethics.

As leaders, we need to feed our own curiosity. Structures such as Community Advisory Boards can help us see our organization from the outside in. Input from other industries can also shatter glass ceilings that are self-imposed. By delegating with confidence, and "having their backs", we can empower those who report to us to innovate.

3. VIGNETTE TWO

A postoperative low risk patient died from a rare type of liver failure seen in patients with exposure to a specific chemicals. The multidisciplinary team, concerned and curious regarding the source of the toxic insult immediately met to brainstorm and identify all of the chemicals used anywhere in the hospital in or near this surgical process. While they could not identify a source, they did institute a new protocol to assure patient safety as they continued research. A few weeks later, they saw LFT changes similar to the sentinel case in another post-operative patient in the same service line. They immediately consulted hepatology and with expert support were able to avert complete liver failure. The coincidence of two cases closely linked in time triggered involvement of hospital administration to mobilize a full investigation comparing every detail of the two cases, including personnel, drug and implant lots, storage of all chemicals in this class throughout the hospital, patient demographic similarities in an attempt to identify any issue that would cause this type of liver failure. While the root cause of the issue was under investigation, the team also initiated a new bloodwork protocol on all post-operative patients with this type of surgery to detect any increase in LFT's. If LFT's were elevated beyond a trigger level, the hepatology team was consulted to assure optimal care. The lead surgeon, still concerned and curious despite no identified cause, contacted acquaintances at the CDC to perspectives from the national experts in this type of liver failure. The case was so unusual that the CDC joined the hospital team in the investigation.

No obvious cause for the cluster of liver failure was identified, however, still determined to protect patients, the team adopted new protocols re: use of implants and cements, and continued surveillance of all patients with liver function monitoring. After changes in process worked out with the CDC, there were no more cases identified of liver failure.

As a result of the relentless curiosity of the entire clinical team, and the processes developed, the team's agility in quick turn-around for process improvements was greatly enhanced as indicated by key quality metrics.

CONCLUDING REMARKS: SUSTAINABILITY OF CULTURE

Any culture is dynamic as new members join the team. The new members bring both important new ideas, as well as "old baggage" that may not support the culture the organization has created. Attention, therefore, must be placed on creating an onboarding process that instills or reinforces, a value for curiosity. The organization must lead with a sense of positive curiosity regarding the new team member. Why did this person choose the job they now have? What are their priorities and motivations? How can we incorporate their goals into the mission of the hospital/clinic/unit?

Values must be consciously reinforced in "how and why" priorities are added and subtracted. As management team members change do we train them to value curiosity in the people for whom they are responsible? Are there feedback mechanisms in our annual evaluations that can foster and sustain the curiosity of the organization? How are skillsets incorporated into the flow of the organization, such as checklists, patient rounding, and meeting constructs? For example, do we ask the patient what their goal for care might be? Do we open meetings by asking what the goals of the group are for the time to be spent? Patient safety and quality are rooted in the soil of the organizational culture, and so as leaders, we must find every opportunity to add the ingredient of curiosity to even the most mundane business aspect of our work.

REFERENCES

[1] Cohen, Bevin; et al., Frequency of Patient Contact with Health Care Personnel and Visitors: Implications for Infection Prevention, *The Joint Commission Journal on Quality and Patient Safety*, December 2012, Volume 38, Issue 12, Pages 560–565

[2] Academic Medical Center Patient Safety Organization, Safety Culture and Risk Reliability in Health Care, *Exploring the Dynamics of Safety Culture and Organizational Resilience*, 2017, Harvard Medical Institutions Incorporated.

[3] Simon, Walker. *Why Curiosity is and Essential Leadership Skill We Should All Develop*, www.simonwalker.org blog post, 5/20/2018.

[4] Laiteerapong, Neda; Huang, Elbert. *J Gen Intern Med.*, 2015 Jun, 30(6), 848–852.

[5] *Merriam Webster Dictionary*, https://www.merriam-webster.com/dictionary/curiosity.

[6] May 23, 2018 http://www.ihi.org/resources/Pages/Tools/5-Whys-Finding-the-Root-Cause.aspx.

[7] Toussant, John S; MD Ehrlich, Susan. MD, MPP, Five changes Great Leaders Make to Develop Improvement Culture, *NEJM Catalyst*, August 7, 2017.

[8] *What is Appreciative Inquiry*, https://www.centerforappreciative inquiry.net/more-on-ai/what-is-appreciative-inquiry-ai, November 1, 2018.

[9] A Positive Revolution in Change: Appreciative Inquiry, D Cooperrider, *Case Western Reserve University* and D Whitney, *The Taos Institute*, http://www.tapin.in/Documents/2/ Appreciative%20Inquiry%20-%20Positive%20Revolution%20in%20Change.pdf.

[10] Boysen, Phillip II. MD, MBA, FACP, FCCP, FCCM, Just Culture: A Foundation for Balanced Accountability and Patient Safety, *Ochsner J.*, 2013, Fall, 13(3), 400–406.

In: Fundamentals of Leadership ... ISBN: 978-1-53615-729-1
Editors: S. P. A. Stawicki et al. © 2019 Nova Science Publishers, Inc.

Chapter 11

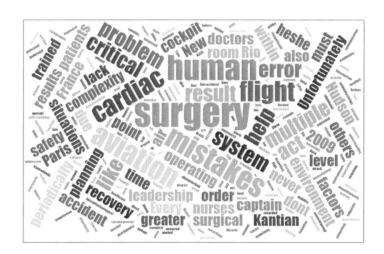

AVIATION AND CARDIAC SURGERY: REVIEW OF THEIR RELATIONSHIPS. IMPLICATION ON COMPLEXITY THEORY AND ETHICAL CONSIDERATIONS

Roberto Battellini[1], MD,
Michael S. Firstenberg[2], MD, FACC, FAIM
and Mauricio Perez-Martinez[3], MD

[1]Cardiac Surgery, Hospital Italiano de Buenos Aires,
Buenos Aires, Argentina
[2]Cardiothoracic and Vascular Surgery, The Medical Center
of Aurora and Rose Hospital, Aurora, Colorado, US

³Department of Surgery, Swedish Medical Center,
Denver, Colorado, US

ABSTRACT

The cardiac surgery operating room is an environment characterized by a high degree of complexity with respect to human-technological and human-human interfaces. Both aviation and surgery, in order to live in these environments, require integrated strategic planning. Leadership is crucial, and the lack of the latter can obstruct the "situational awareness" necessary for the prevention of mistakes and for recovery in critical situations, like in the case of Air France Flight 447 which crashed into the Atlantic Ocean on June 1, 2009 while traveling from Rio de Janeiro (Brazil) to Paris (France) [1]. Given that aviation is more advanced than surgery in the resolution of communication and leadership problems, many believe that among other surgeons and pilots, that transferring the systems from the first to the second helps substantially to approach its international security standard, even if it does not solve the problem in its entirety. In the following article, after analyzing two particular examples, we discuss similarities and differences between both activities; and we propose, thanks to the analysis of the literature, a foundation for understand. Good leadership recognizes problems, prevents and recovers from them, mainly without looking for blame.

Keywords: aviation industry, cardiac surgery, medical error, safety systems, zero error incidence, six sigma

1. INTRODUCTION: WHAT IS COMPLEXITY?

The Chaos Theory is a denomination shared by various sciences that deal with complex dynamic systems which are very sensitive to the variations in the initial conditions. Small variations within these conditions may implicate a significant difference in the behavior of the system, making prediction impossible [2] (Figure 1).

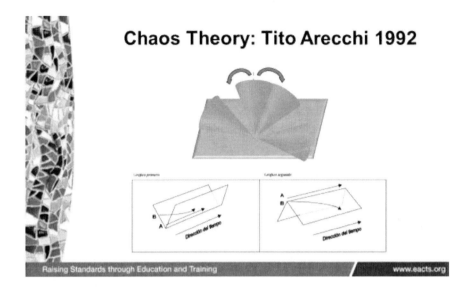

Figure 1. Above: Poincare assured that little changes in the initial conditions can produce big changes towards the end. Below: Tito Arecchi 1992: small variations at the beginning can produce a totally different trajectory. Example: a tear in the aorta while cannulating a patient to initiate cardiopulmonary bypass, retrograde cardioplegia that does not enter the coronary by sliding the catheter, etc. [2].

In 1984, Perrow published his theory on "Normal Accidents", exposing the complexity of interaction, where catastrophes are inevitable in complex systems that are intimately related. He predicted that in these scenarios mistakes can happen in many ways and are impossible to predict. The failure of a single component can have multiple consequences downstream, for example the complex patient that suffers various cycles of medical mistakes. In these systems there's few possibilities of substituting or reassigning personnel due to the high level of specialization, closed personal communication and decreased comprehension of some processes [3]. According to Sigston, there is a point in any self-regulating organization, that once a level of stability is surpassed, it results in the collapse to the next hierarchical level. Close to, or when reaching this point, a change can happen that within itself is insignificant, but in a system it could lead to a massive, fast and disruptive transformation. This, which can be applied to the pathophysiology of carcinogenesis, can also be relevant for other topics within healthcare, per example, forgetting to give heparin to initiate extracorporeal circulation, causing total thrombosis of the circuit resulting in death of the patient. If we think in complexity, we would be able to solve problems that escape linear thinking. This prior statement coincides with the modern analysis of accidents: they are a result of an alignment of conditions and events, each single one necessary but none of them sufficient by themselves. If there can be mistakes within a system, it is complex. Even more, it is frequent that the best people commit the worst mistakes due to an excess of self-confidence (Psychological Complexity) [4].

2. PART 1: COMPLEXITY IN AVIATION AND MEDICINE: THE UNCERTAINTY OF FLIGHT AND SURGERY

As an introduction, the following two stories exemplify how the individuals did not comprehend the existing complexity due to a lack of a systemic focus.

1. Flight AF 447/2009 Rio to Paris: During this transatlantic flight, a storm formed ice crystals on the airspeed gauge (Pitot Tube), causing the autopilot to disengage. The two young pilots in charge, not fully understanding the problem, acted asynchronously and did not ask for help on time. At the last moment, the captain realizes the problem; unfortunately, it is too late. This accident was later explained through the black box recordings [1].

   While analyzing this horrible catastrophe, it is notable how the intense psychological stress, which also occurs in cardiac surgery, tended to obstruct the part of the brain responsible for creative thinking. Immediately relying in the familiar, well-practiced, and usually ineffective protocols. The mistake resided in part because of the difficulties in communication between machine and man: the pilots were not trained for that eventuality (a stall alarm).

Aviation and Cardiac Surgery

Dynamic decisions in not fully understood critical situations require non-linear thinking.

2. A Patient in Cardiac PACU (Post-Anesthesia Care Unit). Back in the 1980's, a surgeon from the US donated to a local institution in Argentina a series of pressure cuffs that compressed IV fluids to 300 mmHg. These were used to purge the catheter used for blood draws from an arterial line. Previously, the pressure cuffs used only compressed to 170 mmHg. The nurses used this pressure to periodically flush the arterial line in order to prevent thrombosis. Every time the plastic sachet was half empty, the nurses would open it and let air in to provide volume and put on the cuff again. An accident never occurred due to the previous low-pressure system. After the introduction of the new models, there was a series of patients who underwent operations requiring cardiopulmonary bypass (CPB) and then, post-operatively, transferred to recovery, that once they were awake and neurologically intact, they were extubated. In these patients, after the blood was drawn for the arterial blood gases and subsequent flushing of the line, they started experiencing seizures, and in a few, coma. The directors of PACU, thinking in a linear manner, thought the root cause was in an inappropriately managed CPB or an inadvertent flush of air in the heart. It was not until they hired an external investigator, similar to the Line Operations Safety Audit in the aviation industry, to perform a comprehensive investigation [5]. What was observed was that the introduction of this new method of flushing the arterial lines introduced IVF fluids to such a high pressure that it surpassed the pressure in the aortic arch and injected air into the carotids.

"When you change the way you look at things, the things you look at, change."

Max Planck 1918

2.1 Complexity in the OR

The Cardiac Surgery OR is an environment characterized by a high level of complexity with respect to the human-technological and human to human interfaces. These surgical procedures require coordinated efforts with multiple groups of people, all working under stress and time limitations (the longer the time the heart is static to fix a defect, the higher the mortality). The main, sophisticated technological factor is the extracorporeal circulation (ECC), in which both the coagulation cascade and the immunological interaction between blood and the plastic lines intervene, always unpredictable. The composition of the OR team is continuously changing, unlike the teams in the aviation industry, which can bring serious communication deficiencies going in and out of the ECC. Whether is low flows, complete cardiac arrest or flushing the heart, a minimal mistake can serious adverse events that can even lead to a coma.

It is known that cardiac surgeons make a life or death decision every 10 seconds during an operation. The majority would be in agreement that 75% of the outcomes are attributed to making the correct decisions and 25% in surgical technique. Surgeons should permanently maintain a conscience of the situation at hand, in other words, the degree of accuracy in which perception follows reality (situational awareness) [6].

Other sophisticated technologies that require similar control to that of aviation is ECMO (extracorporeal membrane oxygenation), which permits prolonging the ECC for various days outside of the operating, and "Cell Saver" blood conversation systems. It is because of these technologies that bloodless (i.e., without the need for transfusions) surgeries have been possible, even heart transplants and complex re-operative surgery. The transesophageal echocardiogram permits to control step by step the functional outcomes of off-pump heart surgery (i.e., cardiac surgery without the use of cardiopulmonary bypass or ECC) - it is the situational awareness, like flight controllers in aviation that enable such complex procedures. Let us imagine the process of a heart transplant, and we will be convinced of how complex it can be.

Aviation and Cardiac Surgery
237

By the end of the 1990's modern technologies emerged like the video-assisted robotics and combined endovascular techniques that are performed in hybrid operating rooms with intraoperative radiology. The actions of a team influence the necessities and functions of the others. All members of the Team should work in coordination having the same goal and technological interphase. Once again, a miscommunication can be catastrophic [7, 8].

2.2. Similarities and Differences between an Airplane and the Cardiac OR: Leadership in Both

Both environments need integrated, strategical planning, with interdisciplinary microenvironments of professional development. Cardiac Surgery and the corresponding anesthesia practice in an OR with a "open door" to many people; aviation, on the other hand, practices inside a cockpit that are closed to the influence of other individuals.

The personnel in an airplane is usually smaller than that of a cardiac surgery OR: in a transatlantic flight three pilots fly in the cockpit, while in cardiac surgery 10 to 15 people from different specialties intervene during a case (surgeon, assistants, technologists, perfusionists, nurses, anesthesiologists, etc). It has been estimated that around 100 individuals intervene in a complete perioperative period [6]. The teams involved are heterogeneous, even in their ways of communicating, however the complementation increases because of the subspecialties of skills involved. As the number of people involved increases, the complexity of their interactions also increases; the intricacies of inter-human relationships grow exponentially and not linearly, and therefore potentially reducing the quality of leadership [9]. The lack of leadership can impede recovery from mistakes in critical circumstances. Cardiac surgery is "Aviation and something more": human beings are more complex than an airplane, and they don't have a complete instruction manual.

Both fields require intense focus to be able to navigate a crisis or emergency situation, often with little information. Treating complications and emergencies can be compared to flying in a storm – an unpredictable scenario that most pilots avoid. Cardiac surgeons frequently encounter these situations, aortic ruptures and dissections are common examples. In the specialty of cardiac surgery there is a lot of unpredictability, and in cases of surgical emergencies, you have to fly, even with bad weather. This is a fundamental difference when compared to aviation, even though emergencies can always appear midflight. An example of excellence in leadership in aviation is the conduct of the pilots of US Airways flight 1549 "The Miracle on the Hudson" in which an Airbus A320, after taking off from LaGuardia Airport in New York struck a flock of Canadian geese. This resulted in a catastrophic engine failure and the need to land emergently in the Hudson River on January 15, 2009. The captain trained all his life for an eventuality that might never happened to him, the predictability of the unpredictable: landing in water [10].

In the cockpit, the pilots' functions are usually superimposed, to a certain degree (they allow substitution), in the OR it should be that way, however because of administrative and economic issues, this is not always the case. If the plane falls, the pilot falls with it. In commercial aviation there's multiple lives at risk; in surgery, there's only one (usually). Accidents in aviation are public, highly noted and generate public demands for investigation and repairs. As a result, economic resources to investigate these incidents are more available, while in iatrogenic adverse events, it is completely the opposite [7]. Safety in medicine is considered a priority for some people in medicine, but is not considered an obligation for all [11].

In aviation, safety is the priority, and a safe landing, in which everyone walks away, is the only acceptable solution. For surgery, there's a broad spectrum of acceptable outcomes, most of time determined by the initial condition of the patient. It is important to remember that patients are different biologically, disease processes differ, and even sometimes we perform surgery on patients on the brink of death, not even knowing their initial condition. This scenario does not occur in aviation, where you always know your initial condition, and if they are not favorable you can simply cancel or delay the flight – or, at least in the setting of icy conditions, take the time to prepare and optimize for the journey as long as necessary to ensure a good outcome. While the concept of "optimization" exists in surgery, sometimes it is the unfavorable conditions that drive the need for urgent or emergent surgery – thereby, by definition, defining a situation of increased risk. Probably the closest analogy in the aviation world, is a plane taking off in the middle of a hurricane to prevent damage and loss of life from existing conditions in which the risk of remaining on the ground is greater than the risk of leaving – although, such circumstances are extremely rare.

2.3. Translational Culture from Aviation to Cardiac Surgery

2.3.1. Culture of Safety: In the Air and in the Operating Room

The science of human factors, a prominent cornerstone in the aviation industry [12], has not yet found its place in Medicine; but it could still profoundly change the comprehension and execution of the decisions made in surgery [13]. Looking for the factors that are unpredictable or complex that relates both, specifically - human error - which often defines complexity. It drives to mistakes due to unexpected or misunderstood problems, if they exceed the cognitive capacity of the individuals or the Team [1]. In this day and age, in both medicine and aviation, society does not want to give room to mistakes – the concept of a learning curve does not exist, nor despite its crucial historical importance, is barely acknowledged. Pilots, much like physicians, and especially surgeons, are expected to be perfect as soon as they complete their "simulation" training. But, experience and judgment develop and mature over time. This had entrusted doctors with the burden of understanding and dealing with the disease. Although it is known that they are human, new technological wonders have created an expectation of absolute perfection. Patients, who have the comprehensible necessity of considering their doctor infallible, have colluded (agreed) with these to deny the existence of the error and reject the uncertainty. However in medicine this has to be tolerated, since paradoxically, only uncertainty is definite [14].

Of course, the paradox in this concept is that while "pilot error" is often the final variable in most airline crashes, surgeons often be blamed for poor outcomes, despite the under-recognized reality that they often have very little influence on the final outcome other than helping to guide a patient through an operation or hospitalization in which hundreds of providers have some impact on the final outcome. The closest analogy in the aviation world is recognizing the safe landing of a flight is determined by everyone from the baggage handlers, the ticket agents, to the flight attendants – and, of course, the mechanics.

Considering the error theory, there are authors who, like Fabri, assert that most of these are cognitive in nature [15]. Others, like Wiegmann, who analyze similar systems, propose that an error results from the disruptions of surgical flow provoked by miscommunications, external distractions, and failure of surgical equipment [16].

The culture that the aviation industry has in terms of safety is definitely something that could easily translate into surgery. The impossible to reach safety rate of the aviation industry (0.017/100,000 flights/year in the US) seduces the need for translation to healthcare. Especially with the medical institutes of the US estimate that yearly around 44,000 to 98,000 people die because of medical mistakes [17]. The report of not just accidents, but also of "near misses" is key in this. The CHIRP program (Confidential Human Factors Incident Reporting) permits the reporting of non-punitive human mistakes and near misses [18, 19]. This has been extrapolated to surgery with good results [11]. Helmreich, a psychologist dedicated to the study of human factors in aviation and surgery, has observed multiple surgical procedures in which he recorded many situations in which communication and team work are suboptimal, parallel to those observed in the cockpit. Rogers, an anesthesiologist and also a pilot, suggested that we do not let ourselves be seduced by moving unviable systems in a different environment [20]. On the contrary, Gaba, also a pilot and a pioneer of simulation in medicine, thinks that if concepts and practices from aviation cannot be transferred directly, it is possible and necessary for appropriate translation and adaptation [20].

Also, there is an existing observational audit translatable to the OR: LOSA or Line Operations Safety Audit, also a project of Helmreich [21] – see the following link for details (www.psy.utexas.edu/psy/helmreich/nasaut.htm). LOSA consists of an audit where expert observers sit down in the cockpit of normal flights to assess threats to safety, mistakes and their handling. These audits identified an average of two threats and two mistakes per flight. More than half of the mistakes where due to violations of already established rules – and finding that was somewhat unexpected.

2.3.2. Simulations

In aviation, every major incident is followed by a simulation of its causes to avoid a subsequent event, becoming a part of training. Moreover, there is a redesign of all equipment involved. In surgery, complications are considered habitual, and apart from being discussed extensively, they are not reported; most of the time due to fear of personal or professional repercussions or false sense of elevated (or need to preserve) self-esteem. In aviation, the simulators constitute a structured part of training, and surgery is catching up thanks to this. The pilots practice without risk, and they learn to develop strategies to recover from a mistake. They don't fly in airplanes in which they did not have extensive simulation training in first – and to which they are periodically and objectively re-tested. In cardiac surgery, as in other areas of surgery, there are multiple instances in which a surgeon has to operate for circumstances in which he/she has not trained due to multiple reasons – the least of which, unlike flying in which a pilot can always abandon a flight, once an operation is started and the patient is placed on cardiopulmonary bypass, it is difficult to turn back without fixing the problem(s) at hand. Unfortunately, the complexity of biologic systems is almost impossible to simulate for now. These don't offer the same amount of realism that an aviation simulation would, despite extensive and growing literature attempting to simulate "real world" critical medical/surgical events. We can comfortably say we are still in very early and primitive in the field [22]. The future of surgical education is hybrid simulators between plastic materials and biologic organs. The sphere in which the greatest achievements in training have been obtained is in emergencies involving cardiopulmonary bypass – in part due to the mechanical nature of the technology [23, 24].

2.3.3. Sterile Cockpit Protocol

In commercial and military aviation, a compulsory protocol of a "Sterile Cockpit" was instituted during periods of high mental demand – specifically, during takeoff and landing. During a "Sterile Cockpit" there are standardized protocols for communication, language and call-back in order to decrease ambiguity. In 2010, Wadhera et al. translated these concepts to the Mayo Clinic, defining eight critical events during cardiopulmonary bypass, implementing the NASA Task Load Index, and decreasing significantly any potential opportunities for miscommunication [25]. Emphasis was made on communication during key actions, like clamping and unclamping of the aorta (i.e., intentionally stopping and re-starting the heart in a manner that limits myocardial injury and, all the while, maintaining adequate oxygenation blood flow to the remainder of the body). The authors concluded that unlike aviation, in cardiac surgery there's no exact time that can be conveniently defined as the main high risk or stress period for the whole team. In Figure 2, from Wadhera, the difference in mental demand in the OR according to the NASA TLI is demonstrated. However, unlike aviation, in cardiac surgery, high-stress situations are different for each component of the team at different times of the procedure. Also, cockpits are not equal: in an airplane it is closed and there's no intervention from the public; in the OR, the door is continuously opening and closing which permits entry and exiting.

Wadhera suggests that effective communication should be structured by defining periods of high mental tension and transferring the sterile cockpit concept to the operating room. The surgeon has to have more creativity than a pilot, not being able to put "autopilot", since a good "landing" (or weaning, to use the technical term) from cardiopulmonary bypass depends mainly on what has been repaired in the heart during the "surgical flight". Wadhera made emphasis to focus in critical events during the procedure rather than on defined periods: Heparinization/ starting CPB/

Aortic Clamping/ Cardioplegia/ Flushing / Stopping CPB. Interestingly, the cultures of operating rooms are often such the surgeon who insists on total silence during such key periods if often view negatively almost in a manner similar to flight attendants not understanding the need for pilots to singularly focused on landing an airplane and being unaware of the consequences of what happens if the plane does not land safely. In fact, most "bad outcomes" after surgery rarely occur in the operating room, even though operative events might initiate the path of a downward spiral that manifests much later in the Intensive Care Unit and often far away (in both time and distance) from those involved in the key triggering events.

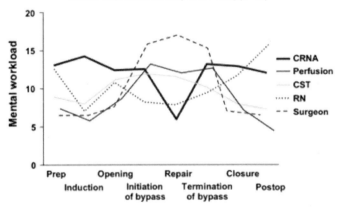

Source: *J Thorac Cardiovasc Surg* 2010;139:312-9

Figure 2. Results of National Aeronautics and Space Administration Task Load Index *(NASA TLX)* show widely divergent cognitive workload measures during course of typical case. *CRNA*, certified registered nurse anesthetist; *CST*, certifies surgical technologist; *RN*, registered nurse; *Prep*, surgical preparation; *Postop*, postoperative.

2.3.4. NASA Model "Threat and Error" Applied to Cardiac Surgery

Hickey suggested considering each operation like a flight. He analyzed 524 flights/patients. He found 763 preoperative "threats" (atypical morphology, multiple lesions, comorbidities) in 72% of the patients (flights). Only 51% of these resulted in an error. In the remaining 257, he observed 430 errors in proficiency or judgment. In 173 (67%) of these, the mistakes were consecutive. Of those, in 60% (n=110; 21% of total), subsequent cycles of additional errors occurred. These cycles containing multiple errors were associated with surgical complications including death in 1.3%. The conclusion is that one unsolved error drives further cycles of errors and dangerous complications [26]. This coincides with the "Swiss Cheese" theory that is also parallel to the nuclear industry disasters (i.e., Chernobyl) and NASA flights that ended in tragedy (Challenger) [27]. In respect to medical mistakes, Hickey mentions that our profession has been stubborn on its focus, instead of adopting a systemic solution we have epitomized that of personal attacks, that at the same time discourages reporting and inhibits the investigation of systemic conditions that produce or result in an error that otherwise could be fixed – unless, of course, such "errors" can be directly attributed to the obvious actions (or inactions) of a single individual. He concludes that two thirds of errors are consecutive and a fifth of the patients suffer cycles of error that are associated with complications [26]. However, a pilot that crashes his plane – even if he/she survives – probably does not get to fly again, while the surgeon who experiences an intra-operative death is often expected to resume operating as if nothing adverse has occurred. Not to mention the rarely of the term "co-pilot error" when describing airline crashes and the potential similarities to medicine in which many providers have some impact on an eventual outcome.

2.3.5. Mission Analysis: "Crew Resource Management"

In the early 1980s, due to several aviation disasters, the concept of "CRM" or "Crew Resource Management" was developed in the United States to improve performance and promote safety [28]. These strategies to improve safety and teamwork can be translated to surgery [6]. In "Briefing and debriefing in the Operating Room using fighter pilot crew resource management", McGreevy suggests two steps. In the first part, or Briefing (instructions), the military pilots explain in advance to their squad not only what they are going to do or expect what will happen, but what could happen and the measures to be taken in each case. In cardiac surgery, an example would be, if immediately after sternotomy a patient would become unstable, how to immediately initiating CPB would be considered or performed. The "debriefing" (reflection) is a wave of introspection similar to brainstorming about what went as expected or not – especially when such discussions involve equipment issues or a formal acknowledgement of those events that "went well" as opposed to those that did not. This is in order to avoid repeating mistakes (not to mention, praising good or effective Teamwork) but also suggesting a role in inducing a positive cultural change. In 2017, Powell-Dunford made a search in PubMed using the terms: Aviation, CRM, and patient safety. This search concluded in 22 relevant manuscripts [29]. Cardiac surgeons are described by McGreevy in 2007 as the fighter pilots of Medicine [30]. A key element in this process (rather than emphasizing the glamorous 'movie star' concept) is to identify mission objectives, benefiting from military CRM. Perhaps the most important thing is to emulate aviation by incorporating surgical specialty services in human factors and psychological aspects in patient safety [11]. Investigation is essential in medicine; curiously, it has been historically specific to diseases and not to the study of errors, which are involved across diseases and specialties. Finally, video and autopsies in cardiac surgery would be the equivalent of black boxes in aviation – and yet, fewer and fewer autopsies are being requested, let alone performed, out of fear of finding something that the surgeon could have or should have done differently or better. The paradox is akin to trying to learn to be better when we prefer to not know the answers to the questions of why something did not go as planned.

3. Part 2: Bioethical Analysis: Is It Possible and Should We Attempt to Reduce Human Errors in Cardiac Surgery while Imitating Aviation?

3.1. Background and Theoretical Framework

The human error is an added product of human activity, and it can result in an unintentional chain reaction of tragic events. Even back in 100

A.C., the Latin proverb would say: "Errare Humanum Est" – translated into the commonly used term – "to error is human". The modern concept of medical error arises mainly after the theories of Popper in 1967. His main school of thought was that knowledge grows by accumulation. Acknowledging mistakes and discarding old and wrong theories will provide a larger opportunity for growth. In "Conjectures and Refutations" [31] he referred to science, but a prior joint article with McIntyre in 1983 [32] includes a powerful comment: "we must learn from mistakes, and how to look for them." "Mistakes will help the scientist grow in terms of knowledge. Each one owes their enrichment thanks to others' criticism, and being reasonable is to be prepared to listen." Learning only from personal mistakes would be a long and painful process, and of unnecessary cost to patients. Experiences must be stored in such a way that doctors learn from the mistakes of others. We should not feel loss of self-esteem or shame to comment on mistakes to others. This philosophy is followed in Aviation, but why is it not the same in medicine? In 1990 James Reason [33] extensively studied the human error in nuclear centers such as Chernobyl and the Challenger tragedy (also discussed above). In 1994 [34] Mary Sue Bogner translated this knowledge to human error in medicine and that was the starting point for a tsunami of literature in the topic. The notion of malpractice-error is changing and also the guilt paradigm of the doctor due to the fact that in the majority of times variables not related to patients and procedures can be involved in certain deaths. In 1996, Marc de Leval asked about the role of human factors in medical outcomes [35, 36], and recalling Chernobyl, he postulates that a negative outcome can be observed and investigated as an accident. With the report, *to err is human, building a Safer Health System (IOM report 1999)* [37] there are no more excuses not to include this issue in hospitals and forcing the designing processes of care in order to avoid error.

Cardiac Surgery can be considered a complex social and technical system [38, 39] that assimilates that of high-risk businesses, such as the aerospace industry. The etiology of surgical errors is deeply enrooted in the effectiveness of teamwork. As discussed above, Wiegmann and colleagues postulated in 2007 that disruptions in team work was the only independent predictor of surgical errors [40]. Now a days, medical mistakes account for the third leading cause of deaths in the United States [41]. These issue are just being recognized, but hard to imagine being 'new', just in 2001 Carthey and de Leval [39] recognized that reporting critical incidents and near misses based on taxonomies of human error was in childhood stages in the field of Cardiac Surgery – while the rest of medicine was even less mature. After Makary published his work, the questions started to be asked: "why not investigate what aviation can teach us in order to reduce surgical mistakes?"

3.2. Our Proposition from Kantian Ethics

In "Fundamental Principles of the Metaphysics of Morals", Kant states: [42] "You may want your maxim to become a universal law". We start to think what the good surgeon or the patient would like regarding the analysis and prevention of medical errors; which, as a human being, should be understood by all? This is reaffirmed by the position "To err is human, building a safer health system". It is a categorical imperative. Kant says it when he writes: "The imperative says, what possible action for me is good, and represents the practical rule in relation to a will". "The categorical imperative declares the action objectively necessary in itself ..." We must put ourselves in the place of the patients in general: would they want the services of a surgical "Team" to have a "Situational awareness", controlling errors and disturbances of the flow during a procedure? Every rational man (or woman) would speculate that, like cockpit checklists, he/she could help. Summing up the Kantian thesis, the moral value of an act is not related to the result of it, but is valid if it is done or conducted from a sense of duty or obligation. *Thus, a surgical error should be forgiven if there was ample pre-operative planning and care by the surgeon, regardless of the final result.* In fact, doctors have no obligation to results provided the system and processes are in place and function effectively to mitigate against such events – much like how airplane crashes are becoming less frequent and are more and more being considered "never events". Extrapolating Kant to our day, we should try to prevent all errors, and in case of committing them, communicate them. In this Robert C. Mavroudis agrees, in an article referring to Kantian ethics and surgery in 2005 [43]. Society should defend the medical profession and not instigate or lead negative changes. This is how we come to the Platonic idea of virtue, which applies to society in its entirety. Physicians cannot be required to be more virtuous than the society from which they come. The extreme of this concept is reflected in the views of some that if a surgeon is not directly responsible for at least "some" deaths, then he/she is not giving enough patients the opportunity to extent their life in the face of challenging and complex problems.

3.3. From Utilitarian Ethics

The English school of Utilitarianism bases its moral on the utility or result of an act before the motive. John Stuart Mill, disciple of Bentham, emphasized that the quality of "The Good" result matters. For him, "The Good", widely constructed, is not only the good of the particular individual but that of the entire society. Mill insisted on the principle of equality, "what ultimately gives happiness is the sense that one was a good person who acted in accordance with his conscience by treating others well" (also in Mavroudis 2005) [43]. Thus, utilitarian ethics would also be in favor of doing everything possible to reduce human error in medicine. If the good has more weight than the bad, the act would be morally correct. Some believe that perhaps a combination of Kant and Stuart Mill would represent the ideal: an act well motivated by a Kantian imperative, with an acceptable result (Mill), and correctly communicating the results to the patient (Kant), and if there were future errors, rescue them (Kantian imperative and Millerian utilitarianism).

3.4. Other Ethics

Santo Tomas de Aquino says, in "Bioética", by Diego Gracia, p. 211 [44]: "The good of the people is more important than the good of one man". "He who seeks the common good of the multitude, consecutively seeks his own particular good". It would seem that Miller took it from Santo Tomas. This justifies this proposal, given that through research in aeronautics, by means of translation, it will be possible to reduce the incidence of errors in the operating room.

In the "Emilio" by Rousseau, it states: "Historical societies are the consequence of a BAD social contract, but it is not said anywhere that it is not possible to build a new society on a GOOD social contract" [44]. Would this new contract be one of goodwill, where doctors learn from our mistakes and we can communicate them without fear? (McIityre and Popper, 1983) [32].

3.5. Comment

Although it is universally known, as mentioned above, that "Errare humanum est", reinforced by the "To err is Human" of the NHI, 1999 [37]. The standard of medical practice has evolved to the point where only perfection seems to be accepted by the public, as people are impressed by the current safety in commercial aviation. This also seems to be the opinion of the press. This feeling was instilled in medical surgeons through medical school and residency. The science of human error is not taught during the curriculum in medicine, students are allowed to believe that error is avoidable and that every mistake is error – and a concept informally emphasized in some training programs that despite their actions, inactions, and co-morbidities, patients should not be held accountable for their own outcomes. Surgeons do not have the power to control all results, even in intensive care units. Mavroudis reported in 2005, 1.7 errors were committed per day per patient in an intensive care unit in the USA [43]. Therefore, it is a "categorical imperative" to prepare comparative works of this type. Not doing it would be, according to Banja, entering a medical narcicism [45] and making us believe that we are all perfect. For the public, cursing to the individual is more emotionally satisfying than blaming institutions, but this is not the way to be better [33].

SUMMARY AND CONCLUSION

1. Both, cardiac surgery and aviation develop in complex environments.
2. Given the more heterogeneous human environment, added to the greater number of personnel involved in the operating room and the greater biological variability of the human being, the possibilities of error in cardiac surgery are more unpredictable.
3. Aviation has become more methodical and systemic to solve safety issues, and there are various reasons for that: the pilot's life is at risk, tragedies are public and there are more resources to investigate – not to mention the consequences, both in terms of lost of life and the financial costs (direct and indirect) of a crash are substantial. Nevertheless, aviation accepts the inevitability of an error – but still strives to avoid them.
4. Physician tend not to recognize error or fatigue, and together with patients make a pact to acknowledge this. Systems must be put into place to recognize and appropriately manage both. Unlike how pilots are restricted in their work hours and conditions, the surgeon/hero is often a martyr to endless work hours in extremely adverse conditions. As a society, medicine must overcome this cultural barrier.
5. Adopting the systems from aviation and translating them to surgery gets everyone closer to a standard and culture of safety, even though it does not solve the whole problem. Research on human factors, especially the psychology of safety, has a very important role that we must develop, enlarging the "islands of excellence in a sea of invisible faults".

REFERENCES

[1] *AF 447 Final report* 2012: www.bea.aero/enquetes/flight.af.447/ rapport.final.en.php.

[2] Arecchi FT. Coherence, complexity and creativity: the dynamics of decision making. In: *Decision theory and choices: A complexity approach* 2010 (pp. 3-21). Springer, Milano.

[3] Perrow C. Normal Accidents: living with high risk technologies. New York basic books 1984. En: *Human error*, Reason 1990. Cap. 7 Latent errors and systems disasters.

[4] Bogner MS. *Human Error in Medicine.* Erlbaum publishers, New Jersey 1994.

[5] Helmreich RL. *Line Operations Safety Audit.* www.psy.utexas.edu/ psy/helmreich/nasaut.htm.

[6] Marvil P, Tribble C. Lessons from crew resource management for cardiac surgeons. Editorial. *The Heart Surgical Forum* 2017;20(2) Epub April 2017.

[7] Bogner MI, Helmreich RL, Schaefer HG. Team performance in the operating room. In: Bogner M, ed. *Human Error in Medicine.* Hillsdale, NJ: Laurence Erlbaum 1994.

[8] ElBardissi AW, Wiegmann DA, Dearani JA, Daly RC, Sundt TM. Application of the human factor analysis and classification system methodology to the cardiovascular surgery operating room. *Ann Thorac Surg* 2007;83:1412-9.

[9] Pendharkar P, Roger J. An empiric study of the impact of team size on software development effort. *Inf Technol manage* 2007;253-62.

[10] Eisen LA, Savel RH. What went right: lessons for the intensivist from the crew of US Airways Flight 1549. *Chest* 2009;136:910-7.

[11] Kapur N, Parand A, Soukup T, Reader T, Sevdalis N. Aviation and healthcare: a comparative review with implications to patients safety. *Journal of the Royal Society of Medicine Open.* 2015;0(0): 1-10.

[12] Schappell S, Wiegmann D. The human factor analysis and classification system. HFACS levels. *Human Factors* 2007;49:227.

[13] Eltorai AS. Lessons from the sky: an aviation-based framework for maximizing the delivery of quality anesthetic care. *J Anesth* 2018 Feb23 doi: 10.1007/s00540-018-2467-y Epub ahead of print.

[14] Simpkin A. Tolerating uncertainty-The next medical revolution?. *NEJM*; 2016: 375:1713-15).

[15] Fabri PJ, Zayas-Castro JL. Human error, not communication and systems underlies surgical complications. *Surgery* 2008;144:557-65.

[16] Wiegmann D, ElBardissi AW, Dearani JA, Daly RC, Sundt TM. Disruption in surgical flow and their relationship to surgical errors: an exploratory investigation. *Surgery* 2007;142:658-65.

[17] Helmreich RL. On error management: lessons from aeronautics. *BMJ* 2000;320:781-785.

[18] Eidt JF. The aviation model of vascular surgery education. Presidential address. *J Vasc Surg* 2012;55:1801-1809.

[19] Rogers J. Have we gone too far in translating ideas from aviation to patient safety?. *BMJ* 2011;342:c7309.

[20] Gaba D. Have we gone too far in translating ideas from aviation to patient safety? *NO. BMJ* 2011:342:c7310).

[21] Helmreich RL. On error management: lessons from aeronautics. *BMJ* 2000;320:781-785.

[22] Feins R. Simulation-based training in cardiac surgery. *Ann Thorac Surg* 2017;103:302-21.

[23] Riley JB, Winn BA, Hurdle MB. A computer simulation of cardiopulmonary bypass: version two. *J ExtraCorpor Technol* 1984;;16:130-136.

[24] Stevens LM, Cooper JB, Raemer DB, Schneider RC, Frankel AS, Berry WR, Agnihotri AK. Educational program in crisis management for cardiac surgery teams including high realism simulation. *J Thorac Cardiovasc Surg* 2012;144:17-24.

[25] Wadhera R, Hendrickson-Parker S, Burkhart HM, Greason KL, Neal JR, Levenick K, Wiegmann D, Sundt T. Is the sterile cockpit concept applicable to cardiovascular surgery intervals or critical events? The impact of protocol-driven communication during cardiopulmonary bypass. *J Thorac Cardiovasc Surg* 2010;139:312.

[26] Hickey EJ, Nosikova Y, Pham Hung E, Gritti M, Schwarz S, Caldarone C, Redington A, Van Arsdell GS. National Aeronautics Space Administration "threat and error" model applied to pediatric cardiac surgery: error cycles precede 85% of patient deaths. *J Thorac Cardiovasc Surg* 2015;149: 496-507.

[27] Reason JT. *Human Error*. Cambridge University Press 1990.

[28] Ricci M. Is aviation a good model to study human errors in health care?. Editorial. *Am J Surg* 2012;203:798-801.

[29] Powell-Dunford N, McPherson MK, Pina JS, Gaydos SJ. Transferring aviation practices into clinical medicine for the promotion of high reliability. *Aerosp Med hum Perform* 2017 May 1;88(5):487-491.

[30] McGreevy J. Briefing and Debriefing in the operating room using fighter pilot crew resource management. *J Am Coll Surg* 2007;205:169-76.

[31] Popper KR. Quantum mechanics without "the observer". In: *Quantum theory and reality* 1967 (pp. 7-44). Springer, Berlin, Heidelberg.

[32] McIntyre N and Popper KR. The critical attitude in Medicina: the need for a new ethics. *BMJ* 1983:287:1919-23.

[33] Reason J. *Human Error*. Cambridge University Press, 1999.

[34] Bogner MS. Human Error in Medicine, Lawrence Erbium 1994.

[35] de Leval MR. Human factors and surgical outcomes: A Cartesian dream. *Lancet* 1997;349: 723-25.

[36] Marc de Leval: *The Edgar Mannheimer Invited Guest Lecture,* Congreso Aleman de Cirugía Cardíaca. Dresden 1967.

[37] Kohn LT, Corrigan JM, Donaldson MS et al. *To err is human. Building a safer health system.* Institute of Medicine, Washington DC, National Academy Press 1999.

[38] De Leval M; Carthey, J; Wright D, Farewell V, Reason J. Human factors and cardiac surgery: a multicenter study. *The Journal of Thoracic and Cardiovasc Surg* 2000; 119:661-72.

[39] Carthey J, De Leval M, Reason J. The Human factor in cardiac surgery: errors and near misses in a high technology medical domain. *Ann Thorac Surg* 2001;72:300-5.

[40] Wiegmann DA, El Bardissi AW, Dearani JA, Sundt TM. Disruptions in surgical flow and their relationship to medical errors: an exploratory investigation. *Surgery* 2007; 142:658-6512.

[41] Makary, M; Daniel, M. Medical Error-the third leading cause of death in the US. *BMJ* 2016; 353:2139.

[42] Emmanuel Kant. *Fundamentación Metafísica de las costumbres*. Ed Porrúa, México 1990, trad. Francisco Larroyo, 7a ed. Pág. 28.

[43] Mavroudis RC. "Should surgical errors always be disclosed to the patient? *Ann Thorac Surg* 2005;80: 399-408.

[44] Thomasma DC. Clinical Bioethics in a Post Modern Age. In: *Clinical Bioethics* 2005 (pp. 3-20). Springer, Dordrecht.

[45] Banja, John. Medical errors and Medical Narcissism. Sudbury, Mass, Jones and Bartlett, 2005.ISBN 0-7637-8631-7 Commentary in: *N Eng J Med. Book Review* 2005;353:324.

In: Fundamentals of Leadership ...　　ISBN: 978-1-53615-729-1
Editors: S. P. A. Stawicki et al.　　© 2019 Nova Science Publishers, Inc.

Chapter 12

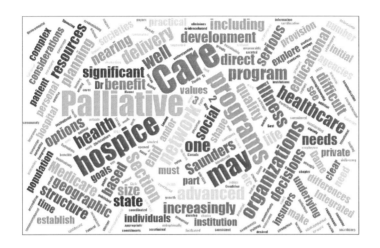

SETTING UP A HOSPICE AND PALLIATIVE CARE PROGRAM AT A UNIVERSITY HEALTH NETWORK: TURNING CHALLENGES INTO OPPORTUNITIES

Ric Baxter[1], John R. Interrante[1], Gregory S. Domer[2], Timothy Oskin[2], Michael S. Firstenberg[3] and Stanislaw P. A. Stawicki[4],*

[1]Department of Palliative & Supportive Care, St. Luke's University Health Network, Bethlehem, Pennsylvania, US

---

* Corresponding Author's E-mail: stawicki.ace@gmail.com.

2Department of Surgery, Heart & Vascular Center, St. Luke's University Health Network, Bethlehem, Pennsylvania, US
4Department of Research & Innovation, St. Luke's University Health Network, Bethlehem, Pennsylvania, US
3Department of Surgery (Cardiovascular), Medical Center of Aurora, Aurora, Colorado, US

Keywords: hospice, organizational excellence, palliative care, program development, program leadership

ABSTRACT

Our population is aging at an unprecedented rate, with approximately 8,000 "baby boomers" entering Medicare daily. As health-care advocates, it is our charge to care for all patients with compassion, respect and yet maintain sustainability. Despite the tremendous advances in both acute and chronic disease management and therapies, the unescapable truth of the end-of-life and eventual mortality remains unchanged. Recognizing the amount of resources that are often invested in an attempt to alter the natural history of this "end-stage" – including potentially or inherently incurable disease or unsuccessful/futile attempts at therapy – Hospice and Palliative Care programs (HPaCP) are becoming more and more important in helping both patients and their families navigate through the end-of-life process. While such initiatives do not inherently imply that providers are "giving up", they serve to recognize that not all interventions are successful and sometimes the focus of care needs to change from one of curative intent to one of providing comfort, dignity, and emotional support during the final days of one's life. Establishing programs for HPaCP can be both arduous and challenging at many levels, including the need for dedicated administrative structures which might differ from existing disease management Departments, the presence of potentially substantial organizational knowledge gaps, the possibility of provider resistance regarding the roles and importance of Palliative Care in the co-management of dying patients, regardless of expected outcomes or life-expectancies. The purpose of this chapter is to highlight the key concepts and steps necessary to establish a successful HPaCP within a health-care system – including the emphasis on disease-specific management – such as oncology, cardiovascular or pulmonary medicine. The authors' primary goal is to make the process of establishing a HPaCP easier to understand and follow, thus lessening the burden of potential challenges and any associated frustrations. We also outline a systematic approach to effectively turn those challenges into opportunities, and ultimately successful programmatic implementations.

1. INTRODUCTION

Hospice Care was introduced to the United States by Dame Cicely Saunders during her visit and lectures in 1963 [1, 2]. Dame Saunders was a nurse, a social worker, and a physician who started St. Christopher's Hospice in Sydenham, outside of London [3, 4]. She elevated the concept of truly holistic and interdisciplinary care for the provision of patient and family centered care [5-7]. She also taught the concept of *total pain,* postulating that components of pain and suffering include physical, emotional, psycho-social and/or spiritual domains [1]. In 1973, at the Royal Victoria Hospital in Montreal, Canada, Dr. Balfour Mount opened a "palliative care ward" based on the work of Dr. Saunders [8]. This was the first official use of the term and led to the development of Palliative Care services at Royal Victoria Hospital and McGill University [9].

In 1982, the U.S. Congress created the Medicare Hospice Benefit (MHB) under Medicare part A and published the Conditions of Participation for Hospice under Medicare [10, 11]. More recently, the growth in the utilization of hospice services exceeded 130% [12]. As of 2010, hospital-based Palliative Care programs are present in 67% of all US hospitals with $\geq$50 beds (85% of hospitals with more than 300 beds, 54% of public hospitals and 26% of for-profit hospitals) [12, 13]. There continues to be significant variability among HPaCPs – both quantitatively and qualitatively – with significant differences depending on geographic regions, facility or hospital size, etc.

In this chapter, we will explore components of HPaCPs with an attempt at understanding the underlying forces that shape individual programs. Cost versus benefit will be strongly considered, especially in the context of HPaCP in a University Health Network setting. The first section will examine hospital and network structures with a focus on system and component needs as well as resource availability (both internal and external). The second section will explore some of the options for sustainable HPaCPs – how they are structured and supported. The third section will raise the question of establishing the goals underlying program development, looking at personnel, patient, institutional, community, and educational needs. Finally, the fourth section will look at some ancillary considerations in the development of particular programs and specialized entities such as an Ethics Committee, training/fellowship development, etc., as well as intentional growth planning.

2. WHO DEFINITION OF PALLIATIVE CARE

Critical to the understanding of how to develop HPaCP is a clear definition of what "Hospice and Palliative Care" actually represents. As such, the World Health Organization (WHO) defines palliative care as an approach that improves the quality of life of patients and their families facing the problems associated with life-threatening illness, through the prevention and relief of suffering by means of early identification and impeccable assessment and treatment of pain and other problems, including physical, psychosocial, and spiritual spheres [14].

Palliative care [14]:

- Facilitates relief from pain and other distressing symptoms.
- Affirms life and regards dying as a normal/natural process.
- Intends neither to hasten nor postpone death.
- Integrates the psychological and spiritual aspects of patient care.
- Provides a support system to help patients live as actively as possible until death.
- Offers a support system to help the family cope during the patient's illness, as well as during the bereavement process.

- Uses a team approach to address the needs of patients and their families.
- Helps enhance quality of life, and may also positively influence the course of illness.
- Preferably applicable early in the course of illness, in conjunction with other therapies that are intended to prolong life, including those investigations needed to better understand and manage distressing clinical complications.

3. SECTION ONE: DO WE NEED TO DO THIS? IF SO, WHY?

In 2015 the Institute of Medicine (IOM) published its landmark report, *Dying in America* [15]. This important work clearly recognized and identified current and future needs of our increasingly large elderly population (e.g., approximately 8,000 new "baby boomers" entering Medicare daily) as well as an increasing complexity of healthcare issues and an increasingly diverse population [15]. Currently, a relatively small proportion (~10%) of the population account for approximately 70% of health-care expenditures [16], potentially contributing to widening disparities and maldistribution of resources. In addition, it is increasingly recognized that the care provided for this population may be unwanted, suboptimally coordinated, and lacking in continuity [17, 18]. In summary, the 5 recommendations promulgated by the *Dying in America* report are [15, 19, 20]:

1) Government-based health insurers and care delivery programs as well as private health insurers should cover the provision of comprehensive care for individuals with advanced illness who are nearing the end of life.
2) Professional societies and other organizations that establish quality standards should develop guidelines for clinician-patient

communication and advance care planning that are measurably actionable and evidence-based.

3) Educational institutions, credentialing bodies, accrediting boards, state regulatory agencies, and healthcare delivery organizations should establish the appropriate training, certification, and/or licensure requirements to strengthen Palliative Care knowledge and skills of all clinicians who care for individuals with advanced serious illness who are nearing the end of life.

4) Federal, state, and private insurance and health-care delivery programs should integrate financing of medical and social services to support the provision of quality care consistent with the values, goals, and informed preferences of people with advanced serious illness nearing the end of life.

5) Civic leaders, public health, and other governmental agencies, community-based organizations, faith-based organizations, consumer groups, health-care delivery organizations, payers, employers, and professional societies should engage their constituents and provide fact-based information about care of people with advanced serious illness to encourage advance care planning and informed choice based on the needs and values of the individual.

As can be seen above, there is clear delineation of the need for prioritizing Palliative Care with clear and concise recommendations for all the potential stakeholders. At the same time, the established model of hospital-based health-care is being closely scrutinized and increasingly focused on delivering optimal services to this important and vulnerable patient population [21-23]. As we move forward with an ever sharper eye on costs, producing desired results without sacrificing quality will be both challenging and necessary. Palliative Care providers are well positioned to navigate the increasingly complex process of change, including bridging some of the most difficult gaps [6, 24-27]. The IOM report is also careful to delineate the critical need for primary Palliative Care provided by all physicians (especially primary care practitioners, cardiologists,

Setting Up a Hospice and Palliative Care Program ... 261

oncologists, pulmonologists, etc.) Expert/consult level Palliative Care should be a well-defined, limited resource as the current national demand far exceeds supply [26, 28]. However, despite all of these initiatives, there exist tremendous educational gaps and learning opportunities surrounding the roles of HPaCPs – especially in the context of end-of-life issues and the administrative aspects of how the health-care system can, appropriately and with dignity, allow patients to die [29]. From the perspective of setting up and/or strengthening a Palliative Care program, specific approaches toward initial evaluation and subsequent implementation steps are outlined below:

3.1. Systems Assessment

What is your system? Structurally, organizationally, and functionally
- Size of your institution, including both primary and satellite facilities.
  - Full-service hospitals
  - Associated long-term care facilities (LTAC's)
  - Rehabilitation centers/facilities
  - Specialty centers – out-patient surgery, orthopedic, etc.
  - Hub-spoke referral affiliated hospitals to tertiary care hospitals/centers of excellence.
  - Religious affiliations and mandates
  - Hospital charters that may impact patient care at end-of-life
- Are you practicing within a network of multiple hospitals merged into one network/entity? Is it a truly integrated, multi-site network?
- Is your organization for-profit vs. not-for-profit?

What is the composition/character of your medical staff and organizational leadership?
- Physician-driven with separation from administration.
- Physician and Administration in partnership.

- System-owned practices? Primary Care and Specialty Care driven?
- What is the percentage of independent physicians?

What is your institutional culture?
- Evaluate your Mission Statement.
- Evaluate your organizational and departmental Hospital Consumer Assessment of Healthcare Providers and Systems (HCAHPS) [30] results.
- What are your employee satisfaction scores? How about employee turnover or retention?

What role do Advanced Care Practitioners play in your system?
- Determine the degree of participation/contribution, both clinically and non-clinically.
- How are Advance Care Practitioners integrated into the health-care delivery platform?

What is your overall patient capacity?
- What is the facility/hospital size? Number of beds?
- What is the number and configuration of your specialty units/facilities including Pediatrics? How developed are the operations/interoperability?
- What is the geographic area covered? Do resources match the actual or anticipated need?

What out of hospital services exist within the network?
- Hospice? If so, in-patient, out-patient, or both?
- Home health? How about telemedicine capabilities?
- Are there patient care navigators?
- Does your institution have physical/occupational/speech therapy capabilities/services?
- What transportation services are available to patients/providers/ visitors?

Setting Up a Hospice and Palliative Care Program ... 263

- Is there a well-developed community health infrastructure?
- Existing clinics, including facilities and staff, need to be considered.

3.2. Needs Assessment

- What is the overall patient capacity?
- What is the number of admissions (per facility); How about Emergency Department (ED) visits (per facility)?
- What are the recent mortality statistics, both for the regional population and for the health-care facility?
- What are the recent "length of stay" and other health-care resource consumption characteristics of the organization?
- Finally, what are your institutional HCAHPS results [30]? And what types of relevant quality measures (Palliative consultation utilization; Percentage of POLST [31] completions)?

3.3. Community

- What is the overall population size? What are their demographic characteristics?
- What is the percentage of insured vs. uninsured patients in the community?
- What faith-based groups are able to participate in local or regional collaboratives?
- How well are local alternative lifestyle groups [32] incorporated into the overall health-care fabric?
- What resources are available to provide necessary services for veterans and other populations? How about other psychosocial and cultural considerations? [33]

3.4. Education

- Is there an institutional affiliation with a medical school?
- Are there any graduate medical education programs (e.g., residencies or fellowships)? If so, is Palliative Care one of the areas of training being offered to potential applicants? How well are these programs incorporated or integrated?
- Does your institution provide nursing education? How about advanced practice education, such as PA/CRNP program?
  - This is especially relevant in the context of specialty training – such as oncology or cardiovascular/heart failure medicine disciplines.
- Consider other additional areas of education of high importance include social work, pastoral care, and other forms of education

3.5. Available Resources

3.5.1. Internal

- Evaluate hospital-owned or affiliated resources and infrastructure.
- Are there appropriate board certified providers at the institution/network? This should include both physicians and advance practitioners
- What is the availability of social work services/support? How about nursing availability and support?
- Finally, what is the availability and support provided by chaplain/spiritual services?

3.5.2. External

- Utilize well-established resources, such as the Center to Advance Palliative Care (CAPC) [34]:

- Palliative Care focus, with the goal to distance from "hospice" and re-frame towards "living".
- There may be additional costs involved in institutional participation.
- American Academy of Hospice and Palliative Medicine (AAHPM) [35]:
  - This organization is more Palliative Care focused, with emphasis on academics and evidence-based standards.
  - Great resource for networking, including a robust annual meeting of experts.
- National Hospice and Palliative Care Organization (NHPCO) [36]:
  - This organization is more focused on hospice-related topics, with an industry lobbying component.
  - Member-based organization, with more robust support provided to non-physician members.
  - There is strong interdisciplinary education.
- Local and State-Wide Organizations:
  - Provider local support, networking, and lobbying.

4. SECTION TWO: OPTIONS – WHAT COULD THINGS LOOK LIKE?

Following a multi-variable, thorough assessment of programmatic needs and resources, one must make important decisions about the structure of the program that is to ultimately take shape. Of note, it is critical to understand that the initial "idealized" concept of a program may not fully reflect the final state. Rather, one must be ready to make sacrifices and show the utmost degree of flexibility on matters that require compromise and team building [37, 38]. There are many options and models to choose from or emulate. Multiple programs can trace their origins to their local environment and resources, based upon diverse sets of circumstances – what has existed before; who is the champion; what are the practical and pragmatic realities of one's situation? Some key initial considerations include:

1. *Hospice to Palliative Care:* Strong/robust hospice program that supports palliative care and contracts with the hospital system.
2. *Hospice and Palliative Care:* Integrated network with home health and hospice as integral parts of the network structure.
3. *Palliative Care; Hospice:* Palliative Care as a direct part of the network structure with independent hospices that may or may not have direct contractual arrangements.

The decisions regarding the above options may become complex and far reaching, with practical, cultural, ethical, geographic, social, religious/spiritual and political implications [33, 39-43]. Close association between hospice and palliative care programs may facilitate smoother transitions and earlier referrals; however, there may be confusion and anxiety about some of the inherent differences that exist between hospice and palliative care – sometimes making it more difficult to facilitate earlier palliative care referrals if patients and/or providers see palliative care as a direct extension of hospice and death. At the same time, complete separation of the programs may increase the difficulty of providing the full educational experience of learners such as residents and fellows.

4.1. What's in a Name?

Will the newly formed unit be called a Palliative Care or Palliative Medicine (Division, Section, or Department); or alternatively will you try to "soften" the image: Supportive Care, Palliative and Supportive Care? This may be one of the most personal and most difficult decisions that may benefit from input by various departments from around the institution, such as oncology, marketing, administration, and very importantly your own staff. How do you see yourself, both in terms of role and overall function?

Setting Up a Hospice and Palliative Care Program ... 267

How do you want to market your service, both internally and externally? What are the costs/benefits/risks of each option? As Palliative Care becomes more accepted and discussed, this may become less of an issue, but it can be a good philosophical starting point: *Who are we?!*

4.2. Alignment

Where will the new structure exist within the organization? One option is to become a division or section of an existing department (family medicine, internal medicine, primary care, oncology, hospice, VNA/Home Health/Community health, etc.). At the same time, hospice tends to be an independent department. There are structural (infrastructure and resources) financial, administrative, political, and credentialing implications to the ultimate decision. Although being only a small part of a larger entity may lead to only limited impact or influence, one should have a clear understanding of the importance of the overall functionality to multiple components of the whole, as well as to the reasons for the final decision.

From a leadership perspective, if the leader of HPaCP is being brought into the organization from the outside, as much of the structural and other considerations should be negotiated and leveraged "up front", with appropriate assurances from the organization regarding the commitment to implementation of said plan(s). If the prospective leader is already a part of the system, he or she will likely already be defined by one's own credentials, internal alliances and a network of champions within the organization. Decisions regarding alignment are often pragmatic and "in the moment"; however, significant amount of analysis and careful thought should be given to the question of where one wants to be within the next 5-10 years, and what alignment will get that individual to their goal. The subsequent sections will discuss some of the more commonly seen alignment possibilities, focusing on how each option affects the overall dynamic of the HPaCP within the organization.

It is also critical to the success of a program to identify and engage those individuals (or potentially, groups) from other areas of medicine to help champion the development of a program. Especially given the role of such programs in areas like cancer and end-stage heart failure, hopefully key leaders or champions from those areas can help partner with Program Leaders to support Hospice and Palliative Care initiatives. Such "external" support – especially when partnered with potentially non-traditional champions (i.e., local religious, business, or community leaders) can be invaluable in lending support and credibility to an area of health-care that is often met with resistance, skepticism, and fear.

4.3. Family Medicine/Geriatrics

If one's primary board certification is Family Medicine and/or Geriatrics, Hospice and Palliative Care specialization may seem like a very natural fit. For example, the Residency Review Committee for Hospice and Palliative Medicine Fellowship training resides within Family Medicine as the primary specialty [44]. Thus, in the absence of additional training, it will be more likely for community-based physicians, as opposed to hospital-based providers, to take full advantage of available Hospice and Palliative Care services. At the same time, it may be challenging for providers with Family Medicine background to garner political and financial support from those who operate primarily in the inpatient setting, thus requiring some degree of negotiation and the ability to clearly delineate the practicality and benefits of Hospice and Palliative Care services within larger organizational frameworks.

4.4. Internal Medicine

There may also exist a natural alignment if one's primary credentials are in Internal Medicine, with the likely gravitation (and increased access) toward hospital-based services. There will also be the possibility of synergy with Internal Medicine residents who are universally required to have at least some Hospice and Palliative Medicine clinical experience. At the same time, one might trade off the affinity for in-patient services for community based-resources, resulting in greater distance and potentially some degree of isolation from Hospice and Home Health services. It will also be critically important to cultivate strong relationships with surgical services.

4.5. Oncology

There are many reasons to align a Palliative Care program with Oncology [45], including:

- High volume/percentage of Palliative Care referrals.
- National Comprehensive Cancer Network (NCCN) guidelines.
- American Society of Clinical Oncology (ASCO) recommendations and guidelines.
- American College of Surgeons (ACS) requirements.

To become truly competitive, comprehensive cancer programs must incorporate Palliative Care services into their structure and function. Yet, there seems to be a persistent (and largely invalid) perception that Palliative Care is equivalent to "hospice, death, and giving up" [46, 47]. A compromise is often reached with a simple change to "Supportive Care" or "Palliative and Supportive Care." Oncology fellowship training requires substantial exposure and experience with Palliative Care. Physically (and conceptually) embedding Palliative Care within Oncology - especially in the outpatient clinic setting will likely facilitate more effective and efficient utilization of Palliative Care services [48]. The potential negative side of full alignment with Oncology is the impact on other disease categories and service lines, potentially limiting the full growth and development of Palliative Care on a system-wide basis.

4.6. Cardiovascular/Pulmonary

There is a growing recognition of the role of HPaCPs in the management of many cardiovascular and pulmonary problems – especially end-stage heart or pulmonary failure [49-53]. Recognizing the importance of HPaCP in the management of patients with end-stage heart and pulmonary disease, and the successes of integrating HPaCP into the management of cancer patients, several major cardiovascular and pulmonary societies have issued position papers in support of such activities [49-53].

Given the many challenges in managing patients with advanced heart or lung failure, especially in the context of growing high-technology, resource intensive options such as transplantation, ventricular assist devices, and high-risk catheter-based interventions and the emphasis on reducing hospital admissions and readmissions in this complex group, integrating HPaCP into existing patient flow pathways has become a required mandate for heart failure programs [54]. Because of the close relationships between heart and pulmonary failure programs (including transplant and mechanical ventricular assist initiatives) and the goals of hospice and palliative care, it is both logical and appropriate that HPaCPs be closely aligned with Departments/Divisions of Cardiology or Pulmonary & Critical Care. As discussed below, another reasonable option is to also consider non-aligned clinical units that have bi-directional overlap in leadership and representation with other many major clinical disciplines – both adult and pediatric [Figure 1]:

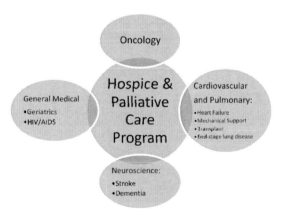

Figure 1. Potential areas of substantial overlap between Hospice and Palliative Care Programs and other clinical Departments/Divisions/Sections.

Setting Up a Hospice and Palliative Care Program ... 271

4.7. Non-Aligned Independent Department

Establishing a Department of Palliative Medicine may represent an ideal approach to the potential options and compromises listed above. This requires support at the highest administrative levels as it may necessitate changes to institutional by-laws. Among benefits of this option is the ability for the department leader to have a true peer-level relationship with all other clinical service line leaders/chiefs, thus increasing the opportunity to have the HPaCP involved throughout the institution and provide support for the required cultural transformation. Administrative and budget support must accompany department development. For institutions with pre-existing HPaCP structure(s), the development of a formalized department may need to take a form of a long-term goal. Individuals being invited to come and start a program may have the opportunity to incorporate this into the initial contract negotiations. However, if such opportunity is not entertained at the outset, political and other institutional pressures may make the consolidation of existing HPaCP structure(s) into a non-aligned independent department very difficult.

5. SECTION THREE: SETTING GOALS AND VISION FOR GROWTH

Charles von Gunten, MD, PhD, and the Editor-in-Chief of the Journal of Palliative Medicine recently wrote an editorial highlighting the truly central role of Palliative Care within our health-care system [55]. After reading this important contribution, one is tempted to ask, "What were Dr. von Gunten's aims?" Reflecting on this question, one inevitably arrives at the conclusion that regardless of the size of the venture, a well-planned execution will help ensure successful implementation. Establishing goals will also speak to how one chooses to establish your process, with important considerations given to: (a) Patient/families; (b) The community; (c) The institution; (d) Hospice integration/relationship; and (e) Education.

If sufficient resources and support exist to establish HPaCP, then the function of the Board of Directors (or equivalent decision-making/advisory body) would assist in defining goals in mission statements and vision documents. Clarity around who has ownership and responsibility for the goals may also be helpful. Early focus on measurements of progress and success will be critical, including the attention to quality and performance metrics. Quantitative data will be critical when advocating for necessary resources. The challenge is most often to stay sufficiently pragmatic to work within the realistic resource limitations while being visionary and gently pushing the boundaries of what the institution is capable of doing. Another question is that of leadership style/approach, which was discussed in greater detail in other parts of this book. Will one be cautious and wait to see what others do, or will one look to lead and be proactive with creative approaches to changing the face of the institution [55].

6. SECTION FOUR: MISCELLANEOUS CONSIDERATIONS

When approaching the building of HPaCP, both from conceptual and practical standpoints, several important considerations must be mentioned. Neglecting to address these considerations may result in lack of important synergies and/or drivers for progress, and may lead to unforeseen crises that will be due to systemic design exposed to latent errors [56]. We will now present an itemized discussion of these important points.

6.1. Ethics Processes/Committees

Will you take an active role in your institution's ethics process? Is there an established Ethics Committee? If so, will you assume leadership or merely participate?

6.2. Fellowship Training

How quickly will you move to establish a Fellowship training program? Long-term staffing and workforce realities will likely push you in this direction. Are there any other Fellowship programs that could synergistically contribute? For example, a Geriatrics Fellowship may integrate well with Hospice and Palliative Care Fellowship. It will be important to develop a good working relationship with the institution's Graduate Medical Education program.

6.3. On-Call Requirements

Balancing staff morale and burnout against patient and institutional needs can be a difficult task. While providers may feel the need/desire to preserve work-life balance and not be available 24/7, institutional credibility and acceptance may be impacted if critical services are not reliably provided as advertised. Consequently, a careful game plan must be put into place, including appropriate cross-coverage and setting appropriate expectations regarding what is reasonably possible at any level of provider/staff availability.

6.4. Research

Clinical research is essential in moving the field forward, especially if the new program is to leave a noticeable local, regional, and national footprint. A well-established research process will increase recruitment, both of patients and new providers. Increasing number of providers express interest in academic/scholarly pursuits, and thus the ability to provide them with an outlet for their scientific expertise and creativity will be viewed as beneficial and may enhance the competitiveness of the new program. At the same time, one must ensure that there is clear delineation of expectations and adequate resources provided to the faculty, including sufficient time to allow for meaningful research projects without compromising clinical patient care duties.

6.5. Focus on Growth

One must work within the stated mission and goals of the newly established program. At the same time, one must also align programmatic priorities and goals with one's institutional culture. To drive growth, it is best to utilize objective metrics that provide logical and undeniable need for further support of the program, both in terms of financial and non-financial resources. Finally, it is critical to resource the program for growth in a proactive, and definitely not reactive, fashion. Reactive approaches will erode trust and credibility within the team.

6.6. Resilience

As a program leader and administrator, one must be mindful of the individual goals and needs of your faculty and staff. One must constantly strive to foster internal compassion, empathic approaches, wellness, and resilience. Without a comprehensive plan in this important domain, burnout and brain drain may well follow [57, 58].

CONCLUSION

HPaCPs have seen tremendous growth since their formal introduction in the early 1970's. Because of the aging population, the need for such programs continues to grow. HPaCPs provide a multidisciplinary team approach that focuses on patients, families and the care provider to provide social, emotional and practical support. Although organized programs are found in the majority of large US hospitals, we must keep pace with the increasing need through continued implementation of HPaCPs throughout the community. The process begins with the understanding of one's own unique health-care resources and culture and identifying the needs of the communities we serve. One must then bring together governmental and private sector insurers, as well as civic leaders to crystallize a clear and concise plan of providing optimal and sustainable care to this inherently vulnerable population. Through active participation of all stakeholders and multidisciplinary collaboration we can fulfill our responsibility and "close the loop" in providing truly comprehensive hospice and palliative care to both our patients and the communities we serve.

REFERENCES

[1] Saunders, D.C.M. and D. Clark, *Cicely Saunders: selected writings 1958-2004*. 2006: Oxford University Press.

[2] Clark, D., A special relationship: Cicely Saunders, the United States, and the early foundations of the modern hospice movement. *Illness, Crisis & Loss,* 2001. **9**(1): p. 15-30.

[3] Alvarez, L.A., *A policy analysis on the Tax Equity and Fiscal Responsibility Act of 1982. 2011,* California State University, Long Beach.

[4] Muscat, J.A., The Hospice Movement. *Maltese Medical Journal,* 1997; **9**(2):14.

[5] Connor, S.R., et al., Interdisciplinary approaches to assisting with end-of-life care and decision making. *American Behavioral Scientist,* 2002. **46**(3): p. 340-356.

[6] Papadimos, T.J. and S.P. Stawicki, The death of Ivan Ilych: A blueprint for intervention at the end of life. *International journal of critical illness and injury science,* 2011. **1**(2): p. 125.

[7] Bennahum, D.A., The historical development of hospice and palliative care. *Hospice and palliative care: Concepts and practice,* 2003: p. 1-11.

276   *Ric Baxter, John R. Interrante, Gregory S. Domer et al.*

[8] van Riet Paap, J., *Quality indicators to facilitate improvements in the organisation of palliative care for people with dementia or cancer in Europe*. 2016, Radboud University Nijmegen.

[9] Wilson, D.C., I. Ajemian, and B.M. Mount, Montreal (1975)-The Royal Victoria Hospital Palliative Care Service. *Death Studies,* 1978. **2**(1-2): p. 3-19.

[10] Mahoney, J.J., The Medicare hospice benefit—15 years of success. *Journal of Palliative Medicine,* 1998. **1**(2): p. 139-146.

[11] Marrelli, T.M., *Hospice & Palliative Care Handbook: Quality, Compliance, and Reimbursement.* 2018: Sigma Theta Tau.

[12] Meier, D.E., Increased access to palliative care and hospice services: opportunities to improve value in health care. *The Milbank Quarterly,* 2011. **89**(3): p. 343-380.

[13] Goldsmith, B., et al., Variability in access to hospital palliative care in the United States. *Journal of palliative medicine,* 2008. **11**(8): p. 1094-1102.

[14] WHO. *Noncommunicable diseases and their risk factors: Palliative care.* 2018 December 18, 2018]; Available from: https://www.who.int/ncds/management/palliative-care/en/.

[15] Tulsky, J.A., Improving quality of care for serious illness: findings and recommendations of the Institute of Medicine report on dying in America. *JAMA internal medicine,* 2015. **175**(5): p. 840-841.

[16] Bodenheimer, T., High and rising health care costs. Part 1: seeking an explanation. *Annals of internal medicine,* 2005. **142**(10): p. 847-854.

[17] den Herder-van der Eerden, M., et al., How continuity of care is experienced within the context of integrated palliative care: A qualitative study with patients and family caregivers in five European countries. *Palliative medicine,* 2017. **31**(10): p. 946-955.

[18] Kapo, J., L.J. Morrison, and S. Liao, Palliative care for the older adult. *Journal of palliative medicine,* 2007. **10**(1): p. 185-209.

[19] Meghani, S.H. and P.S. Hinds, Policy brief: The Institute of Medicine report Dying in America: Improving quality and honoring

individual preferences near the end of life. *Nursing outlook, 2015.* **63**(1): p. 51-59.

[20] Unroe, K.T., M. Ersek, and J. Cagle, The IOM report on dying in America: A call to action for nursing homes. *Journal of the American Medical Directors Association, 2015.* **16**(2): p. 90-92.

[21] Fine, P.G., *The Hospice Companion: Best Practices for Interdisciplinary Care of Advanced Illness.* 2016: Oxford University Press.

[22] Gregory, A., *Invisibility of the older person as a partner in health care.* 2016.

[23] Blacker, S., et al., *Charting the Course for the Future of Social Work in End-of-Life and Palliative Care.*

[24] Berwick, D.M., T.W. Nolan, and J. Whittington, The triple aim: care, health, and cost. *Health affairs, 2008.* **27**(3): p. 759-769.

[25] Truog, R.D., et al., Recommendations for end-of-life care in the intensive care unit: The Ethics Committee of the Society of Critical Care Medicine. *Critical care medicine*, 2001. **29**(12): p. 2332-2348.

[26] Adolph, M.D., et al., Palliative critical care in the intensive care unit: A 2011 perspective. *International journal of critical illness and injury science*, 2011. **1**(2): p. 147.

[27] Papadimos, T.J., et al., Diagnosing dying. *Anesthesia & Analgesia*, 2014. **118**(4): p. 879-882.

[28] Cohen, M.S., et al., Patient Frailty: Key Considerations, Definitions and Practical Implications, in *Challenges in Elder Care*. 2016, InTech.

[29] Dalvin, M., J. Aultman, and M.S. Firstenberg, Surgical residents and palliative care, hospice care, advance care planning, and end-of-life ethics: An analysis of baseline knowledge and educational session to improve competence. *International Journal of Academic Medicine*, 2018. **4**(3): p. 284-288.

[30] Zusman, E.E., HCAHPS replaces Press Ganey survey as quality measure for patient hospital experience. *Neurosurgery, 2012.* **71**(2): p. N21-N24.

[31] Lee, M.A., et al., Physician orders for life-sustaining treatment (POLST): Outcomes in a PACE Program. *Journal of the American Geriatrics Society,* 2000. **48**(10): p. 1219-1225.

[32] Cloyes, K.G., W. Hull, and A. Davis. Palliative and End-of-Life Care for Lesbian, Gay, Bisexual, and Transgender (LGBT) Cancer Patients and Their Caregivers. In *Seminars in oncology nursing.* 2018. Elsevier.

[33] Periyakoil, V., Psychosocial and cultural considerations in palliative care. *Oxford American Handbook of Hospice and Palliative Medicine and Supportive Care,* 2016: p. 245.

[34] CAPC. *Center to Advance Palliative Care.* 2018 December 8, 2018]; Available from: https://www.capc.org/.

[35] AAHPM. *American Academy of Hospice and Palliative Medicine.* 2018 [December 8, 2018]; Available from: http://aahpm.org/.

[36] NHPCO. *National Hospice and Palliative Care Organization.* 2018 [December 8, 2018]; Available from: https://www.nhpco.org/.

[37] Michan, S. and S. Rodger, Characteristics of effective teams: a literature review. *Australian Health Review,* 2000. **23**(3): p. 201-208.

[38] Yukl, G. and R. Lepsinger, *Flexible leadership: Creating value by balancing multiple challenges and choices.* Vol. 223. 2004: John Wiley & Sons.

[39] Rosenberg, J.P., *A study of the integration of health promotion principles and practice in palliative care organisations.* 2007, Queensland University of Technology.

[40] Cinnamon, J., *Examining the spatial accessibility of palliative care services in British Columbia: recommendations for providing care in BC's rural and remote regions.* 2009, Dept. of Geography-Simon Fraser University.

[41] Donovan, R., *Shifting the Burden: The Impact of Home-Based Palliative Care on Family Caregivers Living in Rural Areas.* 2007.

[42] Goldberg, A.L., *The Seriously Ill Patient's Broken Care Continuum: One Community's Action Response.* 2017, Capella University.

[43] Feild, L., Religiosity and Spirituality at the End of Life. *Challenges of an Aging Society: Ethical Dilemmas, Political Issues,* 2007: p. 74.

Setting Up a Hospice and Palliative Care Program ... 279

[44] ACGME. *Procedure for Processing Hospice and Palliative Medicine (HPM) Program Applications.* 2010 December 8, 2018]; Available from: http://www.acgme.org/Portals/0/PFAssets/Program Resources/120_Procedure_for_Processing_HPM_Applications.pdf.

[45] Temel, J.S., et al., Early palliative care for patients with metastatic non–small-cell lung cancer. *New England Journal of Medicine,* 2010. **363**(8): p. 733-742.

[46] Hinton, J., The progress of awareness and acceptance of dying assessed in cancer patients and their caring relatives. *Palliative medicine,* 1999. **13**(1): p. 19-35.

[47] Bioethics, C.o., Palliative care for children. *Pediatrics,* 2000. **106**(2): p. 351-357.

[48] Albuquerque, K., et al., *Division of Gynecologic Oncology Education Program for Fellows in Gynecologic Oncology.*

[49] Jaarsma, T., et al., Palliative care in heart failure: a position statement from the palliative care workshop of the Heart Failure Association of the European Society of Cardiology. *European journal of heart failure,* 2009. **11**(5): p. 433-443.

[50] Goodlin, S.J., et al., Consensus statement: palliative and supportive care in advanced heart failure. *Journal of cardiac failure,* 2004. **10**(3): p. 200-209.

[51] Allen, L.A., et al., Decision making in advanced heart failure: a scientific statement from the American Heart Association. *Circulation,* 2012. **125**(15): p. 1928-1952.

[52] Gore, J.M., C.J. Brophy, and M. Greenstone, How well do we care for patients with end stage chronic obstructive pulmonary disease (COPD)? A comparison of palliative care and quality of life in COPD and lung cancer. *Thorax,* 2000. **55**(12): p. 1000-1006.

[53] Edmonds, P., et al., A comparison of the palliative care needs of patients dying from chronic respiratory diseases and lung cancer. *Palliative medicine,* 2001. **15**(4): p. 287-295.

[54] Braun, L.T., et al., Palliative care and cardiovascular disease and stroke: a policy statement from the American Heart Association/

American Stroke Association. *Circulation,* 2016. **134**(11): p. e198-e225.

[55] von Gunten, C.F., World Domination. *Journal of palliative medicine,* 2018. **21**(1): p. 2-3.

[56] Helfat, C.E., et al., *Dynamic capabilities: Understanding strategic change in organizations.* 2009: John Wiley & Sons.

[57] Tolentino, J.C., et al., What's new in academic medicine: Can we effectively address the burnout epidemic in healthcare? *International Journal of Academic Medicine,* 2017. **3**(3): p. 1.

[58] Wernick, B., et al., Brain drain in academic medicine: Dealing with personnel departures and loss of talent. *International Journal of Academic Medicine,* 2016. **2**(1): p. 68.

In: Fundamentals of Leadership ...
Editors: S. P. A. Stawicki et al.

ISBN: 978-1-53615-729-1
© 2019 Nova Science Publishers, Inc.

Chapter 13

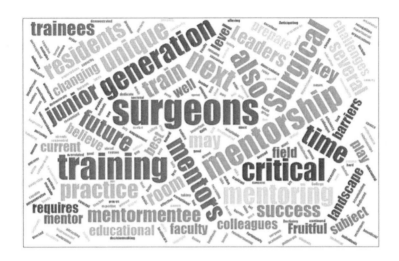

TRAINING THE NEXT GENERATION OF SURGEONS: LEADERSHIP FOR MENTORS AND MENTEES

Alexander P. Nissen[1,2], Juan B. Umana-Pizano[1], Jacqueline K. Olive[3] and Tom C. Nguyen[1,4,]*

[1]Department of Cardiothoracic and Vascular Surgery,
University of Texas Health Science Center Houston,
McGovern Medical School, Houston, Texas, US

---

* Corresponding Author: Tom C. Nguyen, MD, FACS, FACC, Director of Minimally Invasive Valve Surgery, Associate Professor of Cardiothoracic Surgery, 6400 Fannin St, Suite 2850, Houston, TX 77030, Phone (713) 486-5139, E-mail: tom.c.nguyen@gmail.com.

²Department of Surgery, San Antonio Military Medical Center, Fort Sam Houston, Texas, US
³Baylor College of Medicine, Houston, Texas, US
⁴Memorial Hermann Heart and Vascular Institute, Houston, Texas, US

ABSTRACT

Surgical training is a unique time-honored tradition that must also be adaptable to a changing practice landscape in order to prepare future generations for success. We believe mentorship provides an exceptional opportunity for those in practice to train and prepare junior colleagues and residents for challenges that lay ahead, and to be future leaders themselves. Here we outline the necessity for mentorship in training future generations of surgeons, as well as current barriers to mentorship. A fruitful mentor-mentee relationship requires active engagement from both sides, and will evolve with time. We also explore key leadership opportunities for both mentors and mentees alike.

Keywords: career, collegiality, education, graduate medical education, mentorship, surgical training

1. INTRODUCTION

In healthcare, surgeons are frequently viewed as natural leaders, and each may be uniquely driven to lead on a societal, institutional, departmental, or individual level. On an individual level, the importance of surgical leadership through mentoring cannot be overstated. Fruitful mentor-mentee relationships allow for important transmission of critical training to the next generation of surgeons, and may also assist in recruiting the best and brightest to the field. Emphasis on the importance of mentorship in training the next generation of physicians and surgeons has been lauded since Osler [1] and Halsted [2], and here we offer leadership lessons learned for mentors and mentees from our perspective within the field of cardiothoracic surgery. While our subspecialty may represent only

Training the Next Generation of Surgeons   283

a portion of the larger medical community, the central messages of this chapter remain broadly applicable across disciplines. Before moving further it is best to offer a definition for mentorship as it applies within this chapter. While varying definitions may abound, for the sake of clarity, we would tend to agree with the definition of a mentor used in a recent systematic review by Entezami and colleagues as "a senior member of a field who guides a trainee in personal, professional, and educational matters" [3]. Mentorship and fruitful mentor-mentee relationships are crucial to be a successful leader, and we hope to outline lessons learned for both mentors and mentees in this chapter.

2. BARRIERS TO MENTORSHIP

Mentorship is a critical responsibility for physicians to train the next generation, but if effective mentoring were easy, everyone would be doing it. There are several key barriers that may de-incentivize seasoned physicians and surgeons from taking up this calling. The first key barrier is time. Surgeons have a very limited amount of free time daily to dedicate to mentoring a trainee or junior colleague. Time spent operating comes at an even higher premium. As pay for performance metrics and other outcomes-based methods for reimbursement become more widespread, this can frequently be reason for faculty to grant less resident autonomy in the operating room and instead perform substantial portions of cases themselves. Recent data demonstrate a gap between faculty and resident expectations and actual resident autonomy in common cardiothoracic surgical procedures, in part due to these constraints on time and efficiency in the operating room [4]. This diminishes time spent teaching technical aspects of surgery to trainees. Accumulated experience in this paradigm will lead residents to be as good at observing as they are at operating. While we clearly agree with efforts to improve patient care, one must be cognizant of the degree to which changes in the daily practice of faculty may distance trainees from direct patient care.

Faculty also suffer from decreased incentives to mentor [5]. Within academic medicine, revenue is generated primarily through clinical productivity and research, with few incentives for educational accomplishments. Coupled with this model of success, we remain limited in our ability to quantify time and effort spent on educational and mentoring endeavors. While it is unlikely that financial remuneration for mentoring will change significantly in the near future, as physicians we must better support colleagues who provide such excellent mentorship, with deserved recognition and awards.

Finally, being an excellent surgeon does not necessarily translate into being a good mentor or teacher. As with any subject, accumulating expertise in education and mentoring requires familiarity with the subject, dedicated practice, honest self-appraisal, and possibly further training. Fortunately, several organizations have also recognized the woeful lack of educational training among academic surgeons, and responded by offering educational training programs. These include programs from the American College of Surgeons (ACS), and Joint Council on Thoracic Surgery Education (JCTSE) [6], as well as sponsored fellowships and national meeting symposiums.

3. LEADING AS A SURGICAL MENTOR

3.1. Training the Next Generation

Mentorship is key for professional and personal development throughout different stages of training [7]. To mentor junior surgical colleagues or trainees is to take ownership of one's obligation to train the next generation or surgeons. Cardiothoracic surgery as a field faces unique challenges that further highlight this critical concept. Declining rates of trainee interest in pursuing cardiothoracic surgical training [8] have been compounded by a simultaneous decline in suitable jobs for new graduates [9, 10]. These declines are juxtaposed with both increasing prevalence of cardiovascular disease and anticipated retirement rates among currently practicing cardiothoracic surgeons [11, 12]. With these factors in mind, coupled with the limitations posed by the ACGME-mandated 80-hour workweek for trainees, it is critical that we maximize the value and efficiency of training provided to the next generation of surgeons. Mentorship enables experienced surgeons to convey intraoperative decision-making and techniques that cannot be fully demonstrated in any other format but the operating room. Surgical heuristics, pattern recognition, and tissue handling are just a few such examples. Mentors have the unique opportunity to uncover areas of unrecognized weakness in their mentee with the goal for deliberate practice and improvement [13].

Anticipating the changing landscape of cardiothoracic surgery, it is insufficient to focus solely on mentoring current trainees. Leaders should also concern themselves with attracting the best and brightest students and residents to their specialty to ensure its future remains in capable hands. While mentorship assuredly proves beneficial for the maturation of those who have already chosen to pursue cardiothoracic surgery, mentors can also play a vital influence in the eventual specialty choice of junior trainees [14]. For illustration, in surveys of cardiothoracic residents in both integrated and traditional programs, approximately 80 - 90% of subjects cited mentors as moderately to extremely influential on specialty choice [14]. Engaging and mentoring trainees at even earlier stages in their careers, such as the preclinical years of medical school, may be particularly beneficial for retaining the interest of women and other traditionally under-reached groups [15]. While mentors should never coerce a trainee to pursue particular subspecialization, those who serve as role models and demonstrate the aspects of cardiothoracic surgery that are fulfilling, exciting, and rewarding can spark interest for students when exploring our demanding specialty - actions will speak louder than words.

3.2. Teaching Techniques and Judgment

Unique to surgical training is the requirement for learning both dexterous technical skill, and sound clinical judgment. Surgeons are not isolated clinicians, academicians, or researchers, and the best place to simultaneously hone technical and cognitive skills is the operating room. In order to maximize the opportunity for technical teaching, mentors and mentees should meet regularly outside the operating room, discussing in depth the specifics and nuances of a patient's case, considerations for planning and choreography of the operation, as well as pearls and pitfalls for key steps of the case [4]. Certainly, surgeons should pay substantial attention to the steps of how an operation is completed, but we typically give little consideration to how an operation is taught. One response, beginning in 2016, has been the Society of Thoracic Surgeons (STS) "How I Teach It" editorial series as a for-surgeons-by-surgeons collection addressing common cardiothoracic operations to fill this gap [16].

Judgment may seem harder to teach than technical skill, but it is no less important. If technical proficiency can get a surgeon and patient out of a bad situation, it is judgment that prevents one from being in a bad situation to begin with, or at least avoids making an already bad situation worse. For trainees and young surgeons who are hungry to operate, it is perhaps most imperative that mentors impart a sense of when to call for help. Teaching judgment requires much more than mentoring trainees on what one would do in a hypothetical situation. Mentors must also walk the walk. The commitment of a mentor is not a day job from 7:00 – 5:00. If a junior colleague is faced with an acute Type A dissection while alone on call, or a particularly challenging reoperation, mentors should be willing to be there for their mentee. Support during these most trying cases allows mentors to demonstrate the work ethic expected of their junior colleagues, while guiding them towards eventual independence. The success of a mentor-mentee relationship is reflected in the mentee's eventual independence and preparation to lead others and operate in the face of adversity.

3.3. Shortening Learning Curves

Amid external constraints on both mentors and their mentees, every effort should be made to shorten learning curves and prepare junior colleagues and trainees for the future. As recently as a few decades prior, learning curves during accumulation of knowledge and skills were recognized and accepted by both physicians and the public. Rapid progress in clinical outcomes research, patient selection, and an increasingly educated public, paralleled by advances in medical and surgical therapy have all but eliminated tolerance for these learning curves among physicians and patients alike [17]. When the stakes are highest, acceptance of the reality of learning curves is particularly low – and in cardiothoracic surgery, the stakes are always high. Together, these factors highlight the imperative need for skilled and dedicated mentorship of junior surgeons and trainees, should they hope to reach or excel the achievements of their surgical forefathers. On a practical level, as clinicians we all want the best outcome for every patient, and minimizing learning curves allows junior surgeons and residents to provide the highest quality care beginning early in their careers. Lastly, good outcomes will also beget further referrals for experience and growth of a surgeon's practice, which are key for sustained success over a career, while patients ultimately benefit [18]. Mentors should keep in mind that by shortening learning curves for their mentee, they will indirectly impact the care of more patients than one could ever treat alone. For instance, if a surgeon mentors 20 junior colleagues or senior residents during their career, who eventually move on to each perform 200-250 cases annually, the mentor will also have a subtle hand in the care of an additional 4000-5000 patients every year.

3.4. A Mentor's Motivation

A mentor's motivational approach can substantially impact both the short and long-term performance of their mentee. In a thorough review on the subject, Spreier and colleagues [19] describe the three most common motives among leaders and their effects on team performance. Motives were described as 1) achievement, 2) affiliation, and 3) power, with power being subdivided into "personalized power" or "socialized power." Effects of a leader's ego were wrought in their motivational style, and surgeons may frequently have colossal egos, cardiothoracic surgeons being no exception. As surgeons, if we hope to be effective mentors, we must begin with honest self-appraisal of our leadership style, and recognize that effective mentors often must place the needs and goals of the mentee ahead of their own. In turn, this can help mitigate the negative effects of one's ego during the mentoring process.

When studied, leaders primarily influenced by achievement and personalized power were driven to improve their personal performance to exceed benchmarks of excellence [19], and more frequently used leadership tactics that relied on being controlling, micro-managing, coercive, or simply completing tasks themselves without the input of others. While these leaders could achieve short-term success, their teams invariably underperformed in the long-term. In contrast, leaders motivated by socialized power, focused on empowering and persuading those around them, proved most charismatic and capable of getting the most out of their teams. This group used more varied leadership tactics in appropriate situations, for sustained success. These more frequently included mentoring and coaching, offering a vision with clear goal setting, and flexibility.

3.5. Other Areas for Mentorship

Mentoring the next generation of surgeons extends far beyond the operating room. A mentor should aim to adopt the role of coach, sponsor, or connector in the appropriate circumstances [20]. In a recent appraisal of mentorship for cardiothoracic residents and fellows, Stephens and colleagues [21] showed that greater than 80 - 90% of trainees sought networking opportunities, involvement in leadership, and a role model from their mentors. In fact, networking was more frequently desired than technical training among the 288 residents and fellows surveyed. Leaders should anticipate these non-cognitive areas as opportunities for further mentorship, as guidance in any of these realms allows trainees to broaden their expertise and be prepared to lead in the future. Assistance with career advice and work-life balance were two of the most frequently lacking characteristics among mentors. Networking and career planning are key for junior surgeons and trainees to take their careers to the next level in terms of future academic and clinical opportunities for growth after training [22]. It is clear that the next generation of surgeons is keenly focused on both proficiency in the operating room, as well as professional and personal fulfillment while not operating. A strong mentor-mentee relationship also allows senior colleagues to serve as role models, sources for career advice, as well as networking and research opportunities for their mentee. Moreover, demonstrating solidarity with and offering encouragement to mentees are crucial to foster a sense of partnership and bolster mentee's motivation and self-confidence amidst the various challenges of training. "Never miss an opportunity to make students, residents, and junior faculty look good on rounds or conferences," said Kenneth Mattox MD, Professor of Cardiothoracic Surgery at Baylor College of Medicine and Surgeon-in-Chief at Ben Taub Hospital [23]. These nontechnical areas of expertise allow for training well-rounded surgeons ready to lead subsequent generations.

4. LEADERSHIP TRAITS FOR MENTEES

In many instances the mentor may be thought of as a direct or indirect superior of the mentee, based on seniority, experience, faculty position, connections within the field, and/or research funding. Simply put, the mentor may be seen as "in control," and the mentee subordinate. You may be asking, how then could a mentee possibly lead from their role in the mentor-mentee relationship? The position of the mentee is by no means passive, and their relationship with the mentor must be bidirectional. Every bit of effort displayed by the mentor towards the mentee's growth must be matched, if not exceeded, by the effort and fervor the mentee puts forth in order to succeed and grow into a mature and capable cardiothoracic surgeon. The trainee should seek to control their own destiny, clearly define their goals, and, with the aid of a mentor, pursue them vigorously.

Leadership from this subordinate roll is commonly referred to in military parlance as "leading up the chain of command" [24]. The next logical question is, what does it take for mentees to lead up the chain of command? We offer what we believe to be key attributes for mentees to demonstrate, allowing them to lead in their own right.

4.1. Grit

"Nothing in this world can take the place of persistence. Talent will not; nothing is more common than unsuccessful men with talent. Genius will not; unrewarded genius is almost a proverb. Education will not; the world is full of educated derelicts. Persistence and determination alone are omnipotent." - Calvin Coolidge.

Simply put, grit as a character trait represents a combination of passion and perseverance towards long-term goals [25]. Surgical training can be an exceptionally demanding period of time, and daily stresses can cause even high-achieving residents to lose sight of long-term goals. This causes an unfortunate number to quit before realizing the satisfaction and fulfillment experienced through a career spent improving the lives of patients. These stresses are commonly cited as a central cause for attrition rates as high as 20% amongst surgical residents [26, 27]. When examined in populations of surgical residents, higher levels of grit have been associated with higher resident wellbeing and reduced levels of burnout and attrition [28, 29]. Gritty residents are not necessarily those blessed with unique cognitive or technical ability, but those who find the determination within themselves to maximize their success through continued ardor *and* capacity for hard work. Gritty individuals set themselves on the path of long-term goals, maintaining interest over years despite adversity, plateaus in progress, or failure. Notably, nearly half of cardiothoracic surgery residents and fellows report deciding to pursue cardiothoracic surgery before (22.3%) or during (26.0%) medical school [30]. The mentee must demonstrate at least as much investment in their future as their mentor, and demonstrating grit as a

Training the Next Generation of Surgeons 291

surgical trainee is a key component. Demonstration of grit is not brash or boastful, but a sustained commitment proven through daily actions and attitudes. It is this combination of drive and purpose that allow a surgical mentee to show they are worthy of a mentor's invested time and effort towards mutual success. If surgical training is an endurance sport, the gritty resident's advantage is their stamina. Developing grit as a character trait ensures the mentee is focused on important long-term goals even as their relationship with the mentor evolves over time, ensuring the mentee remains a driving force in the pair's mutual successes.

4.2. Goal Setting

Goal setting is critical for a successful mentor-mentee relationship as it forces both parties to give in-depth consideration to where the mentee currently stands, and how to get where they are trying to go. Areas for consideration should include the mentee's current standing in terms of technical, research, teaching, and academic goals. Goal setting should involve outlining tiered levels of achievement. Goals should include 1) "realistic" goals, which would be attainable with deliberate practice and time, 2) "reach" goals indicating those that are achievable but likely difficult, and 3) "dream" goals indicating those which require a combination of extreme dedication from the mentee and an element of luck to become reality. We encourage setting aggressive goals. If the mentee doesn't believe in themselves, who will? Goal setting sessions between mentors and mentees should include discussion of both short and long-term goals. If need be, long-term "dream" goals can be further broken down into critical components to offer achievable milestones along the way, helping to maintain focus on the path to success. Another benefit of thoughtful goal setting is establishing accountability for both the mentee and the mentor. Goals should be detailed and specific, and mentees should not shy away from putting their goals into writing. Revisiting one's goals periodically allows the mentee to assess their progress, recognize areas for improvement, and continue to strive towards these goals. Accountability can also come from regular meetings with mentors to discuss milestones in terms of both dedicated time and practice, and preliminary results of those efforts. Accountability requires honest self-appraisal to be effective, and ensure the mentee remains focused and on their path to success.

Whether explicitly stated or not, mentees should also have the eventual goal of independence. In many ways this independence will likely come about as the culmination of achieving numerous smaller goals along the way. Any mentor-mentee relationship will evolve over time and eventual independence of the mentee allows them to assume a leadership role mentoring their own junior colleagues and trainees.

4.3. Ownership

"Accepting performance feedback and looking at our outcomes is as much about our character as our talent or ability as surgeons." - Richard Prager MD, 2018 Society of Thoracic Surgeons Presidential Address.

Ownership is taken to mean a combination of honest self-appraisal, accepting feedback, and controlling everything that one can control that impacts their success. Ownership entails accepting full responsibility of both success *and* failure when executing tasks and striving towards goals. Ownership begins with honest, introspective, self-appraisal. What are the mentees areas of strength and weakness? What can be done to improve areas of weakness? Is active effort being put forth to attack areas of weakness, and if not why not? This type of introspection and self-critique sets the mentee on a path towards self-determination and maximized preparedness for success. Being prepared will maximize readiness to absorb critical teaching in the operating room, on rounds, in conferences, and likewise readiness to decisively contribute during critical meetings with mentors. Owning one's outcomes, both successes and failures, is also crucial. For instance, after a difficult case one should not only ask themselves what parts they performed well or poorly during, but what they might have been able to do differently to ensure success in the future. For instance, if a case drags on because a key instrument or suture is unavailable, did the resident make sure to alert the scrub nurse of the need for such equipment before the case began? If there were delays in transport, or postoperative handoffs in the intensive care unit, were the appropriate teams notified in order to anticipate the patient's arrival? This mentality can unlock myriad ways for a resident or fellow to take ownership of their patients' outcomes, and quietly lead those around them towards a common goal. This mentality also ensures that after long-term goals are established between the mentor and mentee, that the mentee will be capable of recognizing areas for self-directed improvement along the way. Taking ownership for areas previously felt to be outside one's control requires humility. Rather than being quick to blame others, honest self-appraisal of the effects of one's own actions and attitudes on the team and each step in a patient's care should come first.

4.4. Communication

Effective growth as a mentee requires time spent meeting with one's mentor. During these meetings, in-depth objective feedback and constructive criticism from the mentor can be golden for the mentee, and help unlock unrecognized areas requiring improvement. There is additional learning value from sharing in unspoken interpersonal communication, such as nonverbal cues and body language. However, if in-person meetings are not feasible, since trainees may not have access to cardiothoracic surgery programs or faculty at their home institutions, social media can serve as a valuable tool to enhance and diversify forms of communication and networking, particularly among same-sex mentor-mentee relationships in cardiothoracic surgery [31]. Clear and effective communication from the mentee to the mentor is a must. Mentees must set realistic expectations of themselves and their action items and consistently relay progress and opportunities for growth to their mentors. It is the mentee's responsibility to ensure they share with the mentor all critical information upon which further guidance can be based. This includes tactful communication, maintaining professionalism, and ensuring the mentor has full situational awareness when assessing the progress of the mentee and helping plan future goals. At times the mentee may need to provide constructive feedback for the mentor, or tactfully ask additional questions to better understand the mentor's goals for them and their decision-making process. As mentees become more independent, this style of communication may similarly evolve toward that of shared input and decision-making between colleagues and friends.

CONCLUSION

We believe that mentorship offers unique opportunities for leadership, and is critical to train the next generation of physicians and surgeons. From the perspective of training the next generation of cardiothoracic surgeons, we have examined several lessons learned for both mentors and mentees, as well as critical components for a successful mentor-mentee relationship. Both mentors and mentees have a critical role to play in their own and each other's success.

REFERENCES

[1] Osler, W. On the need of radical reform in our methods of teaching senior students. *Medical News.*, 1903, **82**(49).

[2] Assael, LA. Every surgeon needs mentors: a Halsteadian/Socratic model in the modern age. *J Oral Maxillofac Surg*, 2010, **68**(6), p. 1217-8.

[3] Entezami, P; Franzblau, LE; Chung, KC. Mentorship in surgical training: a systematic review. *Hand* (N Y), 2012, **7**(1), p. 30-6.

[4] Meyerson, SL; Sternbach, JM; Zwischenberger, JB; Bender, EM. Resident Autonomy in the Operating Room: Expectations Versus Reality. *Ann Thorac Surg*, 2017, **104**(3), p. 1062-1068.

[5] Vaporciyan, AA; Yang, SC; Baker, CJ; Fann, JI; Verrier, ED. Cardiothoracic surgery residency training: past, present, and future. *J Thorac Cardiovasc Surg*, 2013, **146**(4), p. 759-67.

[6] Yang, SC; Vaporciyan, AA; Mark, RJ; DaRosa, DA; Stritter, FT; Sullivan, ME; et al., The Joint Council on Thoracic Surgery Education (JCTSE) "Educate the Educators" Faculty Development Course: Analysis of the First 5 Years. *Ann Thorac Surg*, 2016, **102**(6), p. 2127-2132.

[7] Kibbe, MR; Pellegrini, CA; Townsend, CM; Jr. Helenowski, IB; Patti, MG. Characterization of Mentorship Programs in Departments of Surgery in the United States. *JAMA Surg*, 2016, **151**(10), p. 900-906.

[8] Vaporciyan, AA; Reed, CE; Erikson, C; Dill, MJ; Carpenter, AJ; Guleserian, KJ; et al., Factors affecting interest in cardiothoracic surgery: Survey of North American general surgery residents. *J Thorac Cardiovasc Surg*, 2009, **137**(5), p. 1054-62.

[9] Cooke, DT; Kerendi, F; Mettler, BA; Boffa, DJ; Mehall, JR; Merrill, WH; et al., Update on cardiothoracic surgery resident job opportunities. *Ann Thorac Surg*, 2010, **89**(6), p. 1853-8, discussion 1858-9.

[10] Salazar, JD; Ermis, P; Laudito, A; Lee, R; Wheatley, GH; 3rd. Paul, S; et al., Cardiothoracic surgery resident education: update on resident recruitment and job placement. *Ann Thorac Surg*, 2006, **82**(3), p. 1160-5.

[11] Grover, A; Gorman, K; Dall, TM; Jonas, R; Lytle, B; Shemin, R; et al., Shortage of cardiothoracic surgeons is likely by 2020. *Circulation*, 2009, **120**(6), p. 488-94.

[12] Merrill, WH. Preparing the next generation of residents to care for patients with cardiothoracic disease. *Tex Heart Inst J*, 2012, **39**(6), p. 878-9.

[13] Kron, IL. Surgical mentorship. *J Thorac Cardiovasc Surg*, 2011, **142**(3), p. 489-92.

[14] McCord, JH; McDonald, R; Sippel, RS; Leverson, G; Mahvi, DM; Weber, SM, Surgical career choices: the vital impact of mentoring. *J Surg Res*, 2009, **155**(1), p. 136-41.

[15] Foote, DC; Meza, JM; Sood, V; Reddy, RM. Assessment of Female Medical Students' Interest in Careers in Cardiothoracic Surgery. *J Surg Educ*, 2017, **74**(5), p. 811-819.

[16] Kron, I; Yarboro, L. Introducing the "How I Teach It" Editorial Series. *Ann Thorac Surg*, 2016, **101**(1), p. 11.

[17] Cohen, MS; Jacobs, JP; Quintessenza, JA; Chai, PJ; Lindberg, HL; Dickey, J; et al., Mentorship, learning curves, and balance. *Cardiol Young*, 2007, **17,** Suppl 2, p. 164-74.

[18] Raanani, E. Break the vicious cycle: Time for mentorship. *J Thorac Cardiovasc Surg*, 2017, **154**(5), p. 1686.

[19] Spreier, SW; Fontaine, MH; Malloy, RL. Leadership run amok. The destructive potential of overachievers. *Harv Bus Rev*, 2006, **84**(6), p. 72-82, 144.

[20] Chopra, V; Arora, VM; Saint, S. Will You Be My Mentor?-Four Archetypes to Help Mentees Succeed in Academic Medicine. *JAMA Intern Med*, 2018, **178**(2), p. 175-176.

[21] Stephens, EH; Goldstone, AB; Fiedler, AG; Vardas, PN; Pattakos, G; Lou, X; et al., Appraisal of mentorship in cardiothoracic surgery training. *J Thorac Cardiovasc Surg*, 2018.

[22] Pasque, MK. Extreme mentoring in cardiothoracic surgery. *J Thorac Cardiovasc Surg*, 2015, **150**(4), p. 785-9.

[23] Rosengart, TK; Mason, MC; LeMaire, SA; Brandt, ML; Coselli, JS; Curley, SA; et al., The seven attributes of the academic surgeon: Critical aspects of the archetype and contributions to the surgical community. *Am J Surg*, 2017, **214**(2), p. 165-179.

[24] Willink, JBL. *Extreme Ownership: How U.S. Navy Seals Lead and Win.*, Vol. 1, 2015, New York: St. Martin's Press. 285.

[25] Duckworth, AL; Peterson, C; Matthews, MD; Kelly, DR. Grit: perseverance and passion for long-term goals. *J Pers Soc Psychol*, 2007, **92**(6), p. 1087-101.

[26] Longo, WE; Seashore, J; Duffy, A; Udelsman, R. Attrition of categoric general surgery residents: results of a 20-year audit. *Am J Surg*, 2009, **197**(6), p. 774-8, discussion 779-80.

[27] Yeo, H; Bucholz, E; Ann Sosa, J; Curry, L; Lewis, FR; Jr. Jones, AT; et al., A national study of attrition in general surgery training: which residents leave and where do they go? *Ann Surg*, 2010, **252**(3), p. 529-34, discussion 534-6.

[28] Burkhart, RA; Tholey, RM; Guinto, D; Yeo, CJ; Chojnacki, KA. Grit: a marker of residents at risk for attrition? *Surgery*, 2014, **155**(6), p. 1014-22.

[29] Salles, A; Cohen, GL; Mueller, CM. The relationship between grit and resident well-being. *Am J Surg*, 2014, **207**(2), p. 251-4.

[30] Tchantchaleishvili, V; LaPar, DJ; Odell, DD; Stein, W; Aftab, M; Berfield, KS; et al., Predictors of Career Choice Among Cardiothoracic Surgery Trainees. *Ann Thorac Surg*, 2015, **100**(5), p. 1849-54, discussion 1853.

[31] Luc, JGY; Stamp, NL; Antonoff, MB. Social Media as a Means of Networking and Mentorship: Role for Women in Cardiothoracic Surgery. *Semin Thorac Cardiovasc Surg*, 2018.

In: Fundamentals of Leadership ...
Editors: S. P. A. Stawicki et al.
ISBN: 978-1-53615-729-1
© 2019 Nova Science Publishers, Inc.

Chapter 14

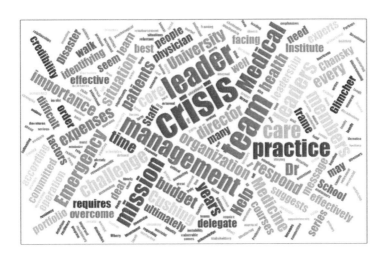

CRISIS LEADERSHIP:
A PRACTICAL PERSPECTIVE

Daniel del Portal[1] and Manish Garg[1,2,3]
[1]Department of Emergency Medicine, Lewis Katz School
of Medicine at Temple University, Philadelphia, Pennyslvania, US
[2]American College of Academic International Medicine,
Philadelphia, Pennyslvania, US
[3]World Academic Council of Emergency Medicine, Dubai, UAE

ABSTRACT

There can be no greater challenge for a physician leader than navigating a health care team through a crisis. A crisis can involve internal or external factors but is best defined as a threat to the core mission of the organization. Effective crisis management requires the health care leader to have planned beforehand, assembling a versatile and trustworthy team that has the emotional intelligence and proper training to respond to a doomsday scenario. Identifying the crisis in real time is critical to the stability of the organization and requires situational awareness in order to respond in a timely and resource-specific manner. When ultimately facing the crisis head on, effective leaders listen to their team while staying committed to the core principles of the organization to guide them to a resolution. Although one may not fathom the next crisis that will challenge the organization, physician leaders can prepare, identify and navigate any crisis with appropriate leadership training.

Keywords: crisis leadership, emergency team management, health care administration, organizational change, physician practice

1. VIGNETTE #1

The medical director of an outpatient medical practice realizes that revenue will fall significantly short of operating expenses. The practice already operates in a lean fashion to minimize expenses, but reimbursement from insurers has been shrinking for years. The medical director writes a long message to staff, titled "Budget Crisis," detailing his decades-long investment in the practice and vowing not to give up, considering he has a great deal on the line and is counting on the practice to be profitable to fund his retirement. He insists that every decision regarding the operation of the practice will now require his approval, so that he can identify wasteful or inefficient expenses. Staff are worried about layoffs, and they fear that patients will face increased wait times for appointments if the practice downsizes.

1.1. Introduction

Leadership is not just steering the ship toward an inviting shore. It is also navigating successfully through a treacherous storm or even shipwreck. Perhaps one of the most renowned crisis leaders was Sir Ernest Shackleton, who in 1914 headed an expedition to Antarctica aboard the ill-fated ship *Endurance*, which became trapped in ice for 10 months before submerging [1]. Nearly a year later, all 22 members of Shackleton's crew had made it safely to land in South Georgia, 1300 kilometers away. Shackleton's indefatigable spirit, selflessness, and ability to motivate his crew even in the most seemingly hopeless circumstances have become the subject of many texts on leadership.

While few physician leaders can claim to have weathered the Antarctic, the health care landscape of the 21st century is anything but tranquil waters. Shrinking reimbursements, physician burnout, and competitive market forces create a baseline instability that leaders must navigate. Additional stressors on a medical team, in the form of family illness or death, budget downturns, and other factors that can threaten normal operation can seem like the proverbial straw on the camel's back. What can a physician leader do when it all seems to be coming undone?

1.2. Defining "Crisis"

Many successful leaders are reluctant to invoke the term "crisis," and prefer to frame situations as "difficult challenges" [2]. While it may seem nuanced, the psychological effect on the leader and on team members can be profound. Framing a crisis instead as a challenge to be overcome suggests that it *can* and *will* in fact be overcome. A leader may privately acknowledge the dire nature of a situation, but announcing a crisis can provoke unnecessary anxiety [3, 4].

On the other hand, in situations where people's lives are endangered such as natural disasters, the severity of the threat should not be understated. Invoking the term *crisis* in these situations can put all levels of leadership on alert and can assist in mobilizing critical resources [5, 6].

Perhaps the best definition of "crisis" is a situation in which the core mission is threatened or compromised [7, 8]. In health care settings where the primary mission is to care for patients, a challenge becomes a crisis when it truly endangers patients by impeding the team's ability to render care.

Whether you are leading through a tough budget cycle or a devastating hurricane, the important thing is to be honest in how you frame the situation. A leader who treats every challenge as a "crisis" will be seen as overly reactionary and lacking resilience, while one who diminishes serious life-altering or life-threatening risks will be ineffective at connecting with vulnerable stakeholders and at mobilizing a proportional response.

1.3. Preparing for a Crisis

1.3.1. Building the "A Team"

According to Dr. Jacob Ufberg, a Professor of Emergency Medicine and residency program director at Temple University Hospital for 15 years, "most of the crisis management comes well before the crisis." He emphasizes the importance of building a leadership team you can trust, through mentoring and identifying each team member's strengths and skills. By cultivating relationships ahead of time, a leader can effectively delegate and rely on the abilities of team members when faced with a crisis.

How do you know you have a team you can trust? "Get to know them socially," suggests Dr. Kathy Shaw, Associate Chair of Pediatrics at Children's Hospital of Philadelphia. "When people let their guard down, you find out their emotional intelligence." Shaw emphasizes the importance of building a diverse, representative team with the emotional intelligence to connect with various stakeholders during a crisis. "Watch how the people you're hiring treat the administrative support staff."

Crisis Leadership: A Practical Perspective

Someone who mistreats your support staff won't be any help to you in a future crisis. You will need a team of people who can identify with and inspire the people in your organization to overcome the crisis together.

Every leader interviewed for this chapter spoke about the importance of trusting and empowering your team during a crisis. Dr. Laurie Glimcher, President and CEO of Dana Farber Cancer Institute and former Dean of Weill School of Medicine at Cornell University, says "If you want to build an 'A' Team, surround yourself with people who are smarter than you are and *don't micromanage them.*" Glimcher, who recalls once facing a public relations crisis in her first week on the job, did not have the benefit of knowing her team for years, but she did know that she was surrounded by incredibly talented individuals whom she respected and who were committed to a shared mission. She did a lot of listening and thanking people as the crisis unfolded and was ultimately resolved.

Dr. Michael Chansky, the longtime Chair of Emergency Medicine at Cooper Medical School at Rowan University, also stresses the importance of teamwork in crisis management. "You can't deal with a crisis alone; you need everyone rowing in the same direction." But while Chansky leans on his trusted team in a crisis, he cautions that in order to maintain credibility with his or her team, a leader cannot delegate everything. "The biggest mistake a leader can make is to turf it. You have to roll your sleeves up, walk the walk. Be aggressive about exerting your power and influence to help the group. Help out personally. You have to be willing to get in the weeds and have credibility with your team by having been in the same position as your colleagues (frequently), and having the same responsibilities that they feel."

1.3.2. Acquiring the Skills

There are many leadership courses, from lectures and seminars to tabletop exercises and disaster simulations, to help prepare leaders to effectively manage crises. Dr. Herb Cushing, the Chief Medical Officer of Temple University Hospital, recommends that every leader learn crisis management and understand how he or she responds to uncertainty. For leaders who are uncomfortable with uncertainty or tend to respond emotionally in difficult circumstances, he recommends a formalized course in disaster preparedness. A series of courses, developed by the Emergency Management Institute within the Federal Emergency Management Agency, allows participants to learn crisis management expertise that can be scaled to their professional leadership needs [9].

1.4. When Crisis is upon You

Cushing likens a crisis to the beginning of a *Mission Impossible* series. "Your mission, should you choose to accept it…" then the self-destructing message. But what next? "Remember the portfolio of experts," he says. The bomb specialist, the SCUBA expert, the pilot, the locksmith… When you need to lead through a crisis, Cushing suggests you consider your own portfolio of experts. The careful team building that you invested in over time will serve you well as you deploy the necessary team members according to their talents.

It is equally important to identify any team members who are a drain on resources without adding meaningfully to resolving the crisis. To understand whether a particular team member will be an asset or a liability, a leader must have an understanding of what the crisis means to all the stakeholders. Realism is key here: despite a commitment to the organization and the mission, most people have competing priorities in their lives. In a natural disaster, the first priority will likely be getting their own family to safety. In a fiscal decline, people may worry whether their own jobs are secure. Will your team members' own needs be met, or are they being asked to defer them?

At the outset of a crisis, it is reasonable to ask team members whether they can help, rather than assuming they will. It shows empathy for their circumstance and reassures them that you have their needs in mind as well. To the extent possible, liberate those who will be distracted by competing priorities, to allow them to take care of themselves first and then engage them once they are able to fully focus on the crisis. Those who return will show a redoubled commitment to helping you.

Crisis Leadership: A Practical Perspective

Cushing notes it is important to recognize whether the crisis is likely to drag on for a long period of time. If so, it is important to gauge your own stamina and well-being. Creating a leadership structure that allows everyone to sleep, eat, and take care of themselves is important, and requires some forethought at the outset of the crisis.

1.5. Communicating during a Crisis

The tone a leader sets can be incredibly influential in times of crisis [10, 11]. Shackleton, stranded in the Antarctic, made great effort to never let his staff see him downtrodden or defeated by the circumstances. He recognized the devastating impact it would have on morale if the crew thought their captain had given up hope. But what can physician leaders say when circumstances out of their control look dire?

Perhaps the most important thing a leader can do during a crisis is to *listen* [12]. Those affected by a crisis want to know that their leader understands what the crisis means to them. Whether this is the potential for job loss or an inability to provide appropriate care to patients, a leader who denies that these concerns exist does so at great peril. Whether or not any individual's fears are justified in a crisis, the leader must appreciate that those fears will likely motivate how that individual acts (or doesn't act) during the crisis. At a time when coordination of efforts is more important than ever, losing the support of your team can create additional dysfunction that only deepens the impact of the crisis.

Spend the time to go on a listening tour. Engaging individuals personally, by asking them how they're doing under the circumstances, can provide useful information about what motivates them and whether they can be counted on to help overcome the challenge at hand. When communicating internally in your organization to stakeholders, let people know that you understand the impact the crisis has on them, and that you have their back.

If external inquiries are received during a crisis, a cautious and informed approach is essential [13]. Dr. Robert McNamara, past President of the American Academy of Emergency Medicine, and Chair of Emergency Medicine at Temple University Hospital advises that "you need to accept what is said, investigate it and never react too quickly." Snap judgments and quick emotional responses can make a leader appear unreasonable and unwilling to be informed. McNamara stresses that effective leaders validate concerns first but do not pass judgment without a careful review of the situation looking at the objective data and speaking as needed with those involved. "It is important to arm yourself with as much data as you can. Sit on your response for a while, revise it a few times, and try to look at it with the eyes of those you are going to send it to."

Clarity is important in a crisis, in both internal and external communication [14-16]. Official statements should be short and to the point. Avoid the temptation to underscore any competing priorities that you face as a leader, and instead focus on acknowledging the dominant concerns and what impact the crisis has. When solutions are not readily apparent, a leader should reaffirm his or her commitment to the core mission. McNamara states that practicing physicians bring a different viewpoint to the table and can speak with authority because they can speak on behalf of patient care as members on the front lines. He believes that physicians need to be involved at the highest leadership levels to ensure the core principles of the hospital are honored.

In health care settings, the primary goal is the commitment to make patient care the top priority. Consequently, one must let all team members know that the leader will not take any action that would endanger patients. One must also emphasize the critical importance of all team members being fully dedicated to fulfilling that mission, as well as committing to preserving the relationships that allow staff to fulfill that mission. Even when specifics are not possible to discuss, hearing these genuine commitments from leaders matters.

1.6. Resolving a Crisis

The way in which a particular crisis is resolved will depend completely on the specific circumstances of the crisis. It would be impossible to create a single blueprint for how to resolve any crisis. The leader will need the input of all relevant content experts and will need to coordinate efforts and to communicate with staff, both by listening and understanding concerns and by reaffirming the commitments that will guide decisions [17-19].

While a leader may need to accept some constraints and new realities when moving beyond a crisis, core principles and expectations should not be sacrificed. A strong leader will look for ways to reinforce the core mission by asking "How can I use this crisis to improve things? How do we make sure this doesn't happen again?" In fact, with many crises come opportunities to lobby for resources, such as additional staff or updating systems. In words attributed to Winston Churchill, "Never let a good crisis go to waste" [20, 21].

1.7. Recognizing the Pitfalls

Let's turn back to the medical director of the outpatient practice at the beginning of our chapter. It is easy to see the mistakes made in managing this crisis. He invoked "crisis" when "challenge" may have been more appropriate and focused on his own fears rather than listening to the concerns of staff. Rather than delegate to a panel of experts, he took the approach of micromanaging all operating decisions, undermining the trust of his team. And he failed to elucidate the principles that would guide his approach to resolving the situation; it appears his motivation is ensuring his own retirement is secure rather than safeguarding the shared mission of patient care. It would be understandable if the staff read the tea leaves and jumped ship, taking jobs at competing practices with more stable finances and a clear commitment to both patients and employees.

1.8. Conclusion: Applying Lessons in Crisis Leadership

Effective crisis management requires appreciation and the appropriate level of involvement (**Figure 1**). If the involvement is too little or too much, the leader runs the risk of poor understanding, disengaged personnel, and a failed preservation of the core principles of the organization. The keys for successful crisis management require foundational work before the crisis, situational awareness to identify a current crisis, and engaged team members during a crisis who understand the organization and support the leadership to crisis resolution and a potential opportunity for growth (**Figure 2**).

NOT INVOLVED ENOUGH	EFFECTIVE CRISIS LEADER	OVERLY INVOLVED
Doesn't acknowledge the severity of a crisis	Acknowledges the severity of a crisis but can frame it as a challenge that will be overcome	Calls everything a crisis
"Turfs" it all	Delegates according to team members' strengths	Lone wolf = will solve it all him/herself
Is absent during critical portions of the crisis	Creates a plan for 24/7 crisis leadership that allows all members to rest and recharge	Tries to manage 24/7 without backup, burns out and becomes ineffective within days
Doesn't invest the time to build an effective team	Knows and respects the team, lets them work	Micromanages the team
Does not listen to concerns of stakeholders	Goes on a listening tour and empathizes with how the crisis could affect stakeholders	Focuses too much on how the crisis will affect the leader personally
Fails to communicate core commitments that will be honored	Reaffirms core commitments and uses these to guide decisions	Betrays core commitments because of personal conflicts

Figure 1. The Continuum of Effective Crisis Management: Involvement to Leadership.

Crisis Leadership: A Practical Perspective 309

Before the Crisis

    Build a Leadership Team You Trust

    Get to Know Your Team Members' Skills and Strengths

    Consider Attending a Disaster Management Course

Identifying the Crisis

    "A Challenge That Will Be Overcome"

    If Life Threats, Call It What It Is - "Crisis" – and Mobilize Resources Early

During the Crisis

    Tap Your Portfolio of Experts

    Ask Who Can Help and Remember Their Personal Needs

    Go on a Listening Tour

    Reaffirm Your Commitments – Back to Core Mission

    Take Care of Yourself, Too

Figure 2. Key Points: A Roadmap for Success in Crisis Leadership.

2. VIGNETTE #2

The medical director of an emergency department in an urban teaching hospital realizes that closure of a nearby community hospital will significantly increase the volume of patients at her emergency department. The volume is already too high and there aren't enough treatment spaces or personnel for the current footprint, let alone the anticipated 20,000 additional patients. The local newspaper has deemed the closure a "catastrophe" and opines that the volume surge to the teaching hospital will be a "crisis of unimaginable peril." The medical director calls a meeting of her operational and educational experts and titles the meeting as a creative opportunity to advance throughput with attention to patient safety and quality. Prior to the meeting she meets with all the ED stakeholders to listen to their personal and professional concerns and, in turn, shares hers. During the meeting, the overwhelming sentiment involves concern for bad patient outcomes due to excessive wait times and the impact overcrowding would have on staff morale and learner education. Several staff fear that the practice environment is unsafe and there are rumblings that they could "work somewhere else where teaching is a priority." The medical director empathizes with her group, validates their concerns, and develops a plan for overcoming the present adversity. She leans on her leaders for creative throughput solutions while maintaining a service versus teaching balance. She demonstrates to hospital leadership how the ideas created from her experts could utilize existing unused space; reduce severe illness walk-outs to maximize safety and capture lost revenue; and pilot educational initiatives involving patient safety and quality. She emphasizes the core commitments of the department as a clinical safety-net hospital with a strong teaching program and she utilizes these concepts to influence hospital leadership to enact her proposed plans. The throughput initiatives work, the training program is lauded for scholarship related to patient safety and quality, and the hospital decides to invest additional resources into the ED by expanding nursing, resident, and staff personnel.

ACKNOWLEDGMENTS

The authors would like to thank the physician leaders who generously participated in interviews and provided insight and wisdom from their experiences.

REFERENCES

[1] Lansing, A. *Endurance: Shackleton's Incredible Voyage.*, 2014, Basic Books (AZ).

Crisis Leadership: A Practical Perspective 311

[2]   George, B. *Seven lessons for leading in crisis.*, Vol. 166, 2009, John Wiley & Sons.

[3]   Bibeault, DB. *Corporate turnaround: how managers turn losers into winners!*, 1998, Beard Books.

[4]   Dweck, CS. *Mindset: The new psychology of success.*, 2008, Random House Digital, Inc.

[5]   Koenig, KL; Lim, HCS; Tsai, SH. Crisis standard of care: refocusing health care goals during catastrophic disasters and emergencies. *Journal of Experimental & Clinical Medicine*, 2011, **3**(4), p. 159-165.

[6]   Zakour, MJ; Gillespie, DF. Effects of organizational type and localism on volunteerism and resource sharing during disasters. *Nonprofit and Voluntary Sector Quarterly*, 1998, **27**(1), p. 49-65.

[7]   Dolnicar, S; Irvine, H; Lazarevski, K. Mission or money? Competitive challenges facing public sector nonprofit organisations in an institutionalised environment. *International Journal of Nonprofit and Voluntary Sector Marketing*, 2008, **13**(2), p. 107-117.

[8]   Bosscher, JL. Commercialization in nonprofits: tainted value? *SPNA Review*, 2009, **5**(1), p. 2.

[9]   FEMA. *Federal Emergency Management Agency: Emergency Management Institute Course Catalog Search.*, 2018, January 16, 2019], Available from: https://training.fema.gov/emicourses/emicatalog.aspx.

[10] Goleman, D; Boyatzis, RE; McKee, A. *Primal leadership: Unleashing the power of emotional intelligence.* 2013, Harvard Business Press.

[11] Kotter, JP. *Force for change: How leadership differs from management.*, 2008, Simon and Schuster.

[12] Goleman, D. Leadership that gets results. *Harvard business review*, 2000, **78**(2), p. 4-17.

[13] Janis, IL. *Crucial decisions: Leadership in policymaking and crisis management.*, 1989: Simon and Schuster.

[14] McDonald, LM; Sparks, B; Glendon, AI. Stakeholder reactions to company crisis communication and causes. *Public Relations Review*, 2010, **36**(3), p. 263-271.

[15] Melewar, T. *Facets of corporate identity, communication and reputation*. 2008, Routledge.

[16] Stawicki, SPA; Firstenberg, MS. Fundamentals of leadership for healthcare professionals. *Health care in transition. 2018, New York: Nova Medicine & Health.* xvii, 269 pages.

[17] Fullan, M. *Leadership for change*, in *International handbook of educational leadership and administration.*, 1996, Springer. p. 701-722.

[18] Covey, SR. *Principle centered leadership.*, 1992, Simon and Schuster.

[19] van Nispen, FK; Scholten, PW. The Utilization of Expert Knowledge in Times of Crisis: Budgetary and Migration Policies in the Netherlands. *European Policy Analysis*, 2017, **3**(1), p. 81-100.

[20] Fuller, S. 'Never let a good crisis go to waste': moral entrepreneurship, or the fine art of recycling evil into good. *Business Ethics: A European Review*, 2013, **22**(1), p. 118-129.

[21] Ryan, C. *The role of crisis as a driver of regional integration: crisis as opportunity*, in *Drivers of Integration and Regionalism in Europe and Asia.*, 2015, Routledge. p. 134-156.

ABOUT THE EDITORS

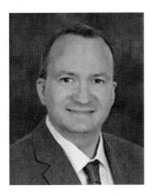

Stanislaw P. A. Stawicki

Dr. Stawicki leads the Department of Research & Innovation at St Luke's University Health Network, headquartered in Bethlehem, Pennsylvania. A specialist in General Surgery, Surgical Critical Care & Neurocritical Care, he co-authored >550 scholarly publications, including 14 books. In addition to important regional, national and international medical leadership roles, he is a member of numerous editorial boards and charitable organizations. His areas of expertise include academic leadership, international health security, medical education, coaching/mentorship, patient safety, traumatology and surgical critical care, injury prevention, and advanced sonography.

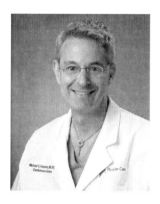

Michael S. Firstenberg

Dr. Michael S Firstenberg is a board-certified thoracic surgeon practicing adult cardiac surgery at The Medical Center of Aurora (Colorado, USA) where he serves at the Chief of Cardiothoracic and Vascular Surgery. He currently holds Adjunct appointments in the Colleges of Medicine and Graduate Studies at Northeast Ohio Medical University and serves on the teaching faculty at the Rocky Vista University. He attended Case Western Reserve University Medical School, received his General Surgery training at University Hospitals in Cleveland, and completed a Fellowship in Thoracic Surgery at The Ohio State University. He also obtained advanced training in heart failure surgical therapies at The Cleveland Clinic. He is an active member of the Society of Thoracic Surgeons (STS), American Association of Thoracic Surgeons (AATS), the American College of Cardiology (ACC), and the American College of Academic International Medicine (ACAIM – for which he is a Founding Fellow). He currently serves a Chair of the American College of Cardiology Credentialing and Member Services Committee as well as being active on several other national society committees. He is the author of well over 200 peer-reviewed manuscripts, abstracts, and book chapters. He has Edited several textbooks on topics ranging from Medical Leadership, Patient Safety, Endocarditis, and Extra-corporeal Membrane Oxygenation – all of which include topics that he has lectured on worldwide.

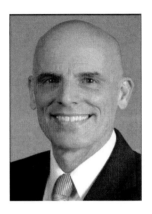

Thomas J. Papadimos

Dr. Thomas Papadimos is a Professor of Anesthesiology and Critical Care Medicine at The Ohio State University Wexner Medical Center, Columbus, Ohio. He also holds visiting professorships at the University of Athens, 2nd Department of Anesthesiology, Attikon Hospital, Athens, Greece and Wenzhou Medical University, 2nd Department of Anesthesiology, Wenzhou, China, and is a retired U.S. Navy officer. He has authored or co-authored over 350 publications. He is a member of many regional and national committees and several editorial boards. His areas of expertise and interest include academic leadership, medical education and mentorship, medical philosophy and ethics, international health, military medicine, epidemiology, aging, and end-of-life decision-making.

INDEX

A

AAHPM, 265, 278
abdicate responsibilities, 59
ability, xi, 4, 7, 12, 15, 19, 20, 50, 53, 54, 55, 58, 62, 79, 89, 107, 112, 114, 115, 117, 120, 121, 123, 134, 136, 140, 144, 145, 158, 162, 165, 167, 169, 171, 172, 175, 177, 206, 208, 220, 268, 271, 273, 284, 290, 292, 301, 302
absolute trust, 15
abstract thinking, 119, 121
academic affiliations, vi, xvii, 197, 198, 199
academic health center, 198, 200, 212, 214, 215
academic institute, 57
academic leadership, 96, 313, 315
academic medicine, 63, 75, 76, 91, 92, 96, 128, 129, 198, 212, 214, 215, 216, 217, 218, 277, 280, 284, 296
academic practice, 198, 204, 216
accept feedback, 116
accepting feedback, 116, 292
accomplishing, 115
accrediting boards, 260
accurate, 7, 21, 98, 157

achieve, 12, 23, 53, 55, 56, 57, 62, 64, 72, 82, 83, 90, 100, 105, 116, 149, 157, 160, 162, 225, 288
achieve a goal, 83, 116
achievement, 14, 31, 60, 287, 288, 291
acknowledge, 55, 250, 301
acquisition, 60
ACS, 269, 284
actions, 5, 9, 11, 30, 69, 85, 116, 154, 165, 237, 242, 244, 249, 285, 291, 293
active participation, 275
acute care facilities, 122
adaptable, 8, 282
additional training, 268
adjust plans, 116
administration, x, 5, 30, 32, 33, 38, 77, 78, 142, 200, 203, 206, 208, 243, 253, 261, 266, 312
administrative, 3, 30, 33, 35, 51, 52, 57, 59, 61, 75, 88, 106, 127, 205, 217, 238, 256, 261, 267, 271, 302
administrative aspects, 261
administrative levels, 271
administrative position, 51, 57, 59, 61, 75
administrative role, 52, 61, 88
administrative roles, 61

318   *Index*

administrative structures, 256

administrator, 56, 57, 135, 203, 209, 210, 274

adult, 35, 132, 270, 276, 314

adulthood, 117

advance, xiv, 9, 31, 45, 52, 56, 75, 98, 107, 123, 140, 205, 244, 256, 260, 262, 264, 277, 287, 309

advance care planning, 260, 277

advance practitioners, 264

advanced care practitioners, 262

advanced illness, 259, 277

advanced practice education, 264

advisory body, 272

advocating, 102, 108, 272

affiliated resources, 264

aging, 134, 188, 196, 256, 274, 278, 315

aging population, 188, 274

alignment, 194, 234, 267, 269

alliances, 135, 198, 212, 267

alternative lifestyle, 263

American Academy of Hospice and Palliative Medicine, 265, 278

American College of Surgeons, 269, 284

American Society of Clinical Oncology, 269

analysis, 31, 41, 43, 44, 46, 75, 87, 92, 124, 125, 140, 168, 178, 182, 190, 223, 232, 234, 244, 245, 247, 251, 267, 275, 277, 295, 312

anticipate, 20, 135, 138, 160, 288, 293

anticipated need, 262

anxiety, 119, 120, 121, 123, 128, 130, 266, 301

apathetic leader, 6

applicant, 23, 46, 52, 55, 56, 60, 62, 73, 264

apply knowledge, 112

appreciative inquiry, 37, 123, 224, 229

approach, xii, 2, 11, 13, 14, 15, 16, 20, 23, 26, 34, 37, 38, 45, 46, 57, 59, 60, 62, 66, 70, 118, 138, 155, 168, 169, 176, 181,

205, 224, 225, 232, 251, 258, 271, 272, 274, 287, 305, 307

appropriate fit, 62

ASCO, 269

assertive, xii, 62, 79, 98

assessment, xii, 107, 125, 180, 192, 258, 265, 296

assistance, 22, 288

assistive steps, 118

assurances, 267

attention, 7, 24, 71, 79, 115, 126, 160, 163, 174, 211, 228, 272, 286, 309

attentional control, xiii, 115, 125

authenticity, 7

authoritarian, 12, 13, 18, 58

authoritarian leaders, 13

authoritarian model, 58

authority, 15, 25, 58, 148, 162, 168, 171, 173, 306

autocratic, 12, 13, 17, 57, 58

autocratic leaders, 58

autocratic leadership, 18, 58

autonomy, 14, 59, 148, 166, 283, 294

Available Resources, 264

aviation industry, xiv, 232, 235, 236, 239, 240

aware, 22, 32, 100, 102, 114, 116

awareness, xiii, 9, 12, 35, 55, 69, 122, 129, 247, 279

B

baby boomers, 188, 196, 256, 259

background, x, xii, 20, 21, 245, 268

background information, 20

behavior, x, 7, 9, 23, 28, 30, 31, 32, 38, 40, 42, 44, 55, 64, 90, 105, 107, 108, 114, 116, 118, 120, 125, 131, 142, 152, 153, 157, 159, 160, 163, 168, 171, 173, 216, 232

behavioral challenges, 2, 26

Index

behavioral characteristics, 11
behavioral issues, 26
beliefs, 46, 55, 56, 68, 74, 119, 160, 173, 174, 178
benefit, v, 10, 13, 16, 30, 67, 68, 74, 85, 87, 89, 90, 100, 104, 108, 123, 138, 140, 156, 175, 180, 186, 191, 192, 211, 257, 266, 268, 271, 276, 287, 291, 303
bereavement process, 258
best interest, 61, 224
bias, 55, 69, 70, 72, 75, 79, 80, 90, 145, 174
bi-directional overlap, 270
big picture, 99, 116, 154
blame culture, 4
blind spots, 9, 35, 90
board certification, 268
board certified providers, 264
Board of Directors, 91, 272
bond between the leader and his/her followers, 18
boundaries, 18, 80
brain, 31, 112, 115, 118, 126, 127, 131, 234, 274, 280
brain drain, 274
brain trauma, 118
brainstorm, 20, 227
bridging, 260
budget support, 271
bureaucratic, 18, 44, 57, 58, 180
bureaucratic leaders, 58
bureaucratic leadership, 18
burnout, xi, 89, 97, 107, 119, 120, 121, 128, 129, 130, 131, 273, 274, 280, 290, 301
business administration training, 51
business model, 20, 51

calm under pressure, 114
cancer, 131, 221, 268, 270, 276, 278, 279, 303

cancer patients, 270, 278, 279
candidates, 19, 23, 50, 54, 56, 62
capacity, 51, 69, 112, 125, 140, 148, 156, 158, 168, 173, 193, 211, 239, 290
CAPC, 264, 278
cardiac surgery, vii, xiv, 153, 158, 180, 182, 183, 231, 232, 234, 236, 237, 238, 239, 241, 242, 243, 244, 245, 246, 250, 252, 253, 254, 314
cardiologists, 260
cardiovascular, 2, 67, 92, 213, 251, 252, 256, 257, 264, 269, 279, 284
care delivery programs, 259
care provider, 106, 114, 202, 274
career, 6, 51, 52, 61, 70, 75, 77, 78, 82, 83, 88, 97, 98, 102, 105, 106, 119, 120, 126, 145, 161, 167, 189, 216, 217, 282, 285, 287, 288, 290, 296, 297
Center to Advance Palliative Care, 264, 278
central executive, 115
certification, 209, 260
Chairman of surgery, 53
challenges, vii, x, 3, 6, 9, 23, 63, 100, 104, 112, 118, 135, 142, 144, 148, 161, 165, 168, 170, 180, 187, 189, 190, 199, 213, 215, 216, 217, 255, 257, 270, 277, 278, 282, 284, 289, 301, 311
challenging, xiii, xiv, 51, 114, 116, 136, 170, 187, 208, 224, 248, 256, 260, 268, 286
champion, 266, 268
champions, 267, 268
change, vi, xiv, xv, xvii, 5, 9, 12, 23, 24, 26, 30, 31, 32, 33, 37, 44, 46, 56, 59, 64, 70, 72, 80, 84, 86, 90, 96, 98, 105, 108, 109, 112, 125, 134, 135, 137, 143, 144, 146, 148, 149, 153, 159, 161, 170, 171, 173, 185, 186, 187, 188, 189, 193, 194, 195, 201, 220, 223, 224, 228, 229, 233, 235, 239, 245, 256, 269, 280, 284, 311, 312
change behavior, 112

Index

change management, xiv, xvii, 134, 188, 220
characteristics, xiii, 6, 12, 17, 20, 54, 58, 112, 114, 138, 152, 263, 278, 289
charisma, 15, 18, 45
charismatic, 12, 19, 45, 58, 59, 288
charismatic leadership, 19, 45
chronic disease management, 256
circumstances, 9, 10, 16, 24, 58, 152, 153, 158, 160, 173, 237, 239, 241, 266, 288, 301, 304, 305, 306
civic leaders, 260
clinical complications, 259
clinical duties, 61
clinical experience, 221, 268
clinical leadership, 96
clinical outcomes, 114, 287
clinical patient care, 51, 274
clinical patient management, 114
clinical productivity, 186, 284
clinical research, 53, 73
clinical role, 55
clinical setting, 56, 108
clinical team, 55, 227
clinician-patient communication, 260
clinics, x, xv, 50, 97, 98, 204, 217, 263
coaching, 8, 34, 36, 75, 100, 122, 123, 132, 167, 288, 313
cognitive decline, 121
cognitive flexibility, xiii, 117
cognitive fluency, 117
cognitive mechanisms, 114
collaboration, xiii, 4, 8, 23, 34, 154, 175, 176, 177, 213, 214
collaborative, xii, 5, 34, 156, 176, 180
colleagues, 55, 56, 72, 78, 87, 97, 107, 168, 204, 205, 246, 282, 283, 284, 286, 287, 288, 292, 294, 303
collegiality, 282
co-management, 256

commitment, 15, 31, 40, 42, 126, 154, 159, 162, 173, 201, 267, 286, 291, 304, 306, 307
committees, 272
common goal, 53, 55, 293
communication, 2, 3, 4, 7, 12, 13, 23, 33, 61, 71, 97, 98, 106, 107, 114, 122, 125, 129, 131, 132, 152, 176, 177, 193, 194, 205, 232, 233, 234, 236, 240, 242, 252, 293, 306, 312
communication skills, 7
communication style, 106, 107, 114
community, ix, xi, xiv, 8, 20, 34, 57, 86, 100, 120, 128, 134, 149, 161, 166, 198, 208, 213, 214, 215, 226, 258, 260, 263, 267, 268, 269, 271, 275, 278, 283, 296, 309
community based-resources, 269
community health infrastructure, 263
community hospital, 57, 134, 208, 213, 309
community-based organizations, 260
community-based physicians, 268
compassion, 130, 256, 274
compassionate, 27, 71, 99, 102
compatibility, xii, 50, 124
competencies, 52, 64, 123
competing priorities, x, 120, 304, 306
competitive, xiv, 29, 41, 64, 134, 141, 204, 269, 301, 311
competitiveness, 215, 273
complacency, 5, 159
complementary behavioral skillsets, 123
complete a sequence, 116
complex cases, 114
complex organizations, 33, 61, 123
complexity, vii, xiii, xiv, xvii, 15, 30, 51, 60, 64, 124, 140, 148, 151, 152, 153, 156, 158, 169, 180, 186, 220, 221, 223, 231, 232, 233, 234, 236, 237, 239, 241, 251
complicated processes, 117
component needs, 258

Index 321

components, 112, 113, 152, 153, 157, 219, 257, 267, 291, 294

composition, 50, 236, 261

comprehensive, xii, 54, 62, 115, 118, 235, 259, 269, 274, 275

comprehensive cancer programs, 269

comprehensive care, 259

compromise, 55, 102, 175, 176, 265, 269, 271

conceptual, 21, 43, 112, 115, 272

conceptual plan, 21

conditions of participation for hospice under medicare, 257

confidence, 6, 10, 11, 17, 19, 62, 74, 78, 79, 144, 226, 234, 289

conflict, x, xiv, 19, 23, 33, 55, 78, 79, 138, 139, 142, 198, 205, 206, 208, 214

confusion, 266

considerations, v, vi, vii, xvi, 49, 57, 58, 62, 98, 147, 231, 258, 266, 267, 271, 272, 277, 286, 291

consistent quality of work, 58

consolidation, 199, 271

constituents, 260

constraints, 25, 36, 51, 55, 283, 286, 307

constructive, 4, 5, 7, 9, 10, 148, 155, 293

constructive change, 5, 7, 10

consumer groups, 260

contact information, 24

continual evolution, 60

continuity, xv, 45, 259, 276

contract negotiations, 271

contributing factors, 60, 198

control, xiii, 13, 25, 33, 58, 112, 115, 118, 119, 135, 136, 141, 142, 166, 172, 177, 200, 202, 203, 206, 213, 222, 236, 249, 289, 292, 305

control over emotions, 118

coordination, 2, 4, 11, 112, 125, 237, 305

core, x, 25, 28, 50, 53, 56, 60, 64, 115, 167, 191, 209, 224, 300, 302, 306, 307, 308, 310

core competencies, x, 50

core values, 56, 167

corrective action, 26

cost, x, xii, 28, 29, 51, 56, 61, 135, 154, 156, 163, 169, 173, 187, 188, 189, 191, 193, 196, 199, 200, 201, 202, 205, 211, 213, 217, 246, 250, 257, 260, 265, 267, 276, 277

cost-effective, 51, 56, 61

cost-effectiveness, 51

counterproductive, 116

course of illness, 259

coworkers, 23, 122, 126, 155

creating a plan, 117

creative approaches, 272

creativity, 13, 22, 24, 58, 88, 158, 162, 173, 226, 242, 251, 273

credentialing, 260, 267, 314

credentialing bodies, 260

credentials, 23, 267

credibility, 9, 33, 55, 65, 268, 273, 274, 303

crisis, vii, ix, x, xv, xvii, 9, 13, 14, 18, 25, 36, 37, 38, 58, 128, 134, 136, 137, 139, 144, 145, 150, 171, 237, 252, 272, 275, 299, 300, 301, 302, 303, 304, 305, 306, 307, 308, 309, 311, 312

crisis leadership, vii, xv, xvii, 299, 300, 307, 309

crisis of autonomy, 25

crisis of control, 25

crisis of leadership, ix, 25

crisis of red tape, 25

critical services, 273

criticism, 116, 246, 293

CRNP, 264

cross-communication, 5

cross-coverage, 206, 273

cultural, 42, 43, 74, 163, 167, 168, 174, 176, 181, 205, 225, 245, 250, 263, 266, 271, 278

cultural considerations, 263, 278

cultural transformation, 271

322 *Index*

culture of curiosity, vi, xiv, 219, 220, 221
curative intent, 256
curriculum vitae, 20
customers, 16, 34

D

dark triad, 26, 47
dealing with stress, 112
death, 3, 28, 39, 85, 234, 236, 238, 244, 254, 258, 266, 269, 275, 276, 301
decision, x, 4, 10, 12, 13, 14, 23, 24, 25, 37, 38, 40, 41, 42, 47, 55, 58, 59, 60, 61, 66, 68, 71, 73, 74, 81, 83, 86, 88, 104, 112, 114, 127, 135, 137, 140, 142, 150, 156, 157, 159, 168, 171, 174, 175, 177, 178, 179, 199, 215, 235, 236, 239, 251, 265, 266, 267, 272, 275, 279, 285, 294, 300, 307, 311, 315
decision making, x, 12, 13, 14, 37, 40, 41, 42, 59, 60, 66, 74, 83, 86, 88, 127, 135, 141, 142, 157, 159, 174, 177, 179, 215, 251, 272, 275, 285, 294, 315
decision-making process, 13, 59, 294
decisiveness, 10
decline, 50, 51, 120, 284, 304
defer decisions, 59
deferential treatment, 26
defining goals, 272
delegate, 17, 88, 302, 303, 307
delegation, 23, 25
delegative leadership, 14
deleterious, 6, 15, 114, 122
delineation of expectations, 273
demand, ix, 33, 65, 159, 203, 209, 242, 261
democratic, 12, 13, 16, 40, 41, 57, 58, 59
democratic leadership, 13, 41, 59
democratic leadership model, 59
demographic characteristics, 263
department, 1, 2, 7, 10, 24, 25, 27, 30, 51, 53, 55, 56, 57, 60, 61, 62, 67, 88, 95, 105, 111, 133, 134, 143, 196, 197, 203, 215, 216, 256, 263, 266, 267, 270, 271, 295, 309, 313, 315
department chairman, 51
department leader, 271
depression, 118, 119, 120, 121, 123, 127, 128, 129, 131, 132
deterioration, 85, 122
development, vi, xii, xv, 3, 14, 25, 32, 34, 35, 36, 39, 43, 45, 46, 48, 60, 64, 66, 74, 76, 78, 83, 84, 85, 93, 95, 96, 105, 109, 123, 124, 126, 146, 162, 163, 164, 174, 219, 237, 251, 257, 258, 268, 271, 275, 284, 295
dialogue, 7, 14, 157, 158, 175, 226
didactics, 123
difficult issues, 7, 9
difficulty, 70, 71, 112, 114, 115, 116, 117, 119, 120, 171, 200, 203, 204, 210, 211, 234, 266
dignity, xi, 80, 256, 261
direction, 8, 12, 58, 98, 134, 201, 202, 210, 273, 303
discipline, 40, 55, 172, 183
disconnect, x, 101, 120
disease management, 256
disease-specific management, 257
disengaged, 20, 307
dismissive, 62
disorder, 118, 131, 136, 145
disregard, 62
dissent, 13, 15, 58
distance, 243, 265, 269, 283
distracted, 116, 304
distractible, 114
distractions, 11, 115, 240
distressing symptoms, 258
distributed leadership, 17, 41
distributed perspective, 17
diverse population, 259
diversification, 27

Index

diversity, xvii, 68, 69, 72, 76, 77, 79, 80, 82, 88, 97, 124, 137, 157, 174, 175

divestment, 25

division, 176, 266, 267, 279

domains of life, 120

downstream, 10, 233

drivers for progress, 272

dual degree-granting, 61

duties, 22, 62, 85, 87, 186, 274

dying, 256, 258, 259, 276, 277, 279

Dying in America, 259, 276

dying patients, 256

dynamic, x, 2, 12, 19, 27, 30, 51, 53, 77, 146, 163, 164, 187, 227, 232, 235, 267, 280

dynamic growth, 19

dynamic interactions, 51

dysfunction, vi, xiii, xvii, 111, 112, 116, 122, 124, 128, 173, 305

dysphoric, 119

E

easily distracted, 115, 116

economic, vi, xiii, xiv, 47, 50, 51, 63, 68, 74, 76, 84, 86, 88, 91, 147, 149, 154, 162, 163, 164, 169, 178, 181, 186, 187, 188, 205, 208, 238

education, 28, 38, 39, 40, 41, 44, 45, 46, 52, 64, 73, 77, 78, 81, 85, 88, 107, 110, 119, 120, 122, 125, 129, 131, 132, 149, 164, 166, 173, 180, 210, 217, 241, 252, 264, 271, 279, 282, 284, 290, 295, 310

educational gaps, 261

educational institutions, 122

educational needs, 258

effective administrator, 51

effective coping skills, 121

effective leader, xii, xiii, xv, xvi, 2, 3, 17, 20, 24, 32, 50, 51, 53, 60, 99, 106, 108, 112, 117, 143, 160, 161, 168, 300, 306

effective leadership, 2, 50, 168

effective planning, 117

effectiveness, xiii, 4, 9, 26, 28, 31, 32, 35, 39, 40, 44, 107, 112, 172, 173, 215, 246

efficiency, 4, 12, 13, 14, 18, 58, 108, 155, 173, 283, 285

effort, 14, 58, 76, 120, 130, 143, 152, 170, 175, 186, 199, 200, 205, 251, 284, 286, 289, 291, 292, 305

eight-step process of change, 5

elderly population, 188, 259

electronic health record, 186, 196

electronic medical record, vi, x, xiv, xvii, 186, 188, 189, 204

embarrassing, 122

emergency, 12, 13, 57, 61, 72, 73, 88, 133, 134, 186, 193, 196, 210, 237, 263, 299, 300, 302, 303, 304, 306, 309, 311

emergency physician, 57

emergency response, 57

emergency situations, 12, 13

emergency team management, 300

emotion, 109, 116, 118, 127, 140, 159

emotion control, 116

emotional, xi, xiii, 18, 35, 39, 45, 47, 50, 53, 54, 65, 66, 80, 89, 97, 99, 101, 107, 108, 112, 114, 116, 119, 121, 122, 129, 140, 144, 145, 168, 256, 257, 274, 300, 302, 306, 311

emotional climate, 122

emotional control, 112, 114

emotional distress, 121

emotional intelligence, xi, 35, 47, 50, 53, 65, 66, 89, 99, 107, 108, 129, 168, 300, 302, 311

emotional life event, 122

emotional responses, 101, 116, 306

emotional support, 256

empathetic leaders, 27

empathic approaches, 274

empathy, xii, 55, 120, 129, 130, 177, 304

empirical observations, 118

324 *Index*

employee, xiii, 2, 7, 10, 12, 13, 15, 16, 17, 20, 23, 26, 27, 33, 35, 38, 41, 42, 44, 46, 47, 48, 50, 60, 63, 65, 69, 70, 80, 123, 126, 141, 162, 165, 205, 206, 208, 262, 307
employee relationships, 15
employee satisfaction, 63, 262
employee success, 123
employee turnover, xiii, 12, 13, 262
employee wellness, 50
employers, 26, 27, 47, 48, 74, 86, 120, 260
empowerment, 32, 44, 51, 65, 74, 89, 109, 158
emulate, 245, 265
end of life, 259, 260, 275, 277, 278
endocrine dysfunction, 121
end-of-life, 256, 261, 275, 277, 278, 315
end-of-life process, 256
end-stage, 256, 268, 270
end-stage heart failure, 268
enforcement of rules, 18
engaged, xii, 17, 22, 59, 86, 164, 193, 308
engagement, 14, 17, 23, 29, 41, 63, 64, 86, 157, 163, 217, 225, 226, 282
enhance quality of life, 259
enthusiasm, 6, 207
enthusiastic, 20, 23, 79, 83, 102
entity, 58, 131, 199, 201, 202, 204, 205, 206, 208, 211, 261, 267
ethical, vii, xiii, 11, 36, 38, 42, 47, 60, 139, 154, 216, 231, 266, 278
ethical nuances, 60
ethics committee, 258, 272, 277
ethics processes, 272
evidence-based, 4, 28, 66, 70, 203, 260, 265
exceptional physician, 51
executive ability, 117
executive dysfunction, 112, 113, 116, 118, 124, 132
executive dysfunction complex, 113

executive function, vi, xiii, xvii, 112, 113, 115, 116, 117, 118, 124, 125, 126, 127, 128, 131
executive functioning, 112, 113, 116, 117
executive teams, 62
expansion plans, 60
expectation, x, 2, 19, 58, 59, 60, 80, 98, 117, 120, 130, 165, 207, 209, 211, 225, 239, 273, 283, 293, 294, 307
expected outcomes, 103, 104, 256
experience, ix, x, xi, xiii, xv, xvii, 4, 5, 6, 8, 12, 17, 20, 24, 27, 28, 29, 34, 53, 55, 56, 69, 70, 78, 81, 82, 86, 98, 103, 112, 117, 120, 121, 129, 134, 142, 143, 144, 162, 166, 193, 196, 212, 213, 215, 222, 239, 244, 246, 266, 269, 277, 283, 287, 289, 310
experienced clinician, 51
experienced leaders, 58
expertise, 3, 9, 126, 160, 164, 166, 169, 186, 273, 284, 288, 304, 313, 315
experts, x, 3, 17, 220, 224, 227, 265, 304, 307, 309
external, 16, 19, 51, 155, 235, 240, 258, 264, 268, 286, 300, 305, 306
external talent, 19

F

facility, 97, 100, 101, 200, 257, 262, 263
faculty, vi, 53, 57, 71, 73, 75, 76, 78, 80, 93, 95, 96, 100, 106, 109, 200, 202, 203, 205, 207, 208, 209, 210, 211, 212, 215, 216, 273, 274, 283, 284, 289, 293, 295, 314
faith-based groups, 263
faith-based organizations, 260
families, 85, 86, 256, 258, 259, 271, 274
family centered care, 257
family medicine, 73, 135, 196, 267, 268
family members, 85, 122

Index

family-like dynamic, 15
favorable outcomes, 60
favoritism, 15
fear, 10, 12, 13, 100, 101, 102, 105, 119, 198, 200, 241, 245, 249, 268, 300, 310
federal, 30, 62, 105, 106, 199, 260, 304, 311
federal government, 62
feedback, xvi, 7, 9, 12, 15, 54, 77, 89, 101, 117, 123, 157, 192, 228, 292, 293
feelings, 9, 55, 120, 123, 140, 160
fellows, 57, 105, 106, 266, 279, 288, 290
fellowship, 53, 57, 61, 105, 258, 264, 273, 284, 314
fellowship programs, 273
fellowship training, 57, 61, 273
fellowships, 264, 284
filtering, 59, 118
final state, 265
financial, xi, xiv, xv, 14, 20, 56, 59, 62, 63, 76, 77, 89, 148, 163, 180, 192, 196, 200, 201, 207, 208, 210, 250, 267, 268, 274, 284
financial means, 59
financial reports, 20
financial strength, 62
financial support, 56, 77, 201, 268
financing, 260
finished product, 114
flexibility, xii, 5, 9, 13, 44, 138, 168, 172, 265, 288
flexible, xiv, xvii, 8, 10, 14, 26, 112, 278
flexing, 17
fluidity, 17
focus, x, xi, xii, xvi, xvii, 4, 11, 27, 50, 51, 58, 68, 69, 78, 99, 107, 112, 115, 118, 122, 129, 139, 173, 192, 193, 214, 234, 237, 242, 244, 256, 258, 265, 272, 274, 285, 291, 304, 306
focus on structure, 58
follower discord, 19
followers, 12, 13, 15, 19, 57, 58, 162, 163, 164, 166, 181

forces, 151, 201, 257, 291, 301
for-profit, 135, 257, 261
for-profit hospitals, 257
foundation, x, 7, 20, 90, 96, 105, 224, 225, 229, 232
four competencies, 53
freedom, 58
frontal lobe, 112, 115, 118, 124
frontal lobes, 112, 118
full commitment, 15
full-service hospitals, 261
function, ix, 27, 111, 118, 124, 126, 127, 131, 132, 142, 150, 153, 154, 199, 227, 247, 266, 269, 272
functional units, 22
functionality, 267
future, xiv, xvi, 8, 20, 23, 34, 52, 53, 56, 60, 65, 83, 90, 97, 104, 108, 112, 116, 117, 119, 149, 151, 154, 158, 161, 171, 179, 180, 196, 199, 200, 201, 205, 213, 214, 226, 241, 248, 259, 277, 282, 284, 285, 287, 288, 290, 292, 294, 295, 303
future needs, 259
future-blind, 117

G

Gage, Phineas, 118, 127
game plan, 273
gaps, 188, 260
general life skills, 123
general population, 118, 119, 127
general surgery residency, 53
genuine, 6, 100, 139, 306
geographic, 199, 257, 262, 266
geographic area, 262
geographic regions, 257
geriatrics, 97, 268, 273, 278
Geriatrics Fellowship, 273
giver, 18
gives up on tasks, 116

326 *Index*

giving up, 102, 256, 269

goal, xi, xvi, 5, 8, 11, 12, 14, 20, 23, 26, 51, 53, 57, 58, 59, 60, 61, 62, 71, 76, 77, 78, 83, 89, 97, 108, 112, 115, 116, 117, 118, 125, 149, 174, 190, 200, 208, 215, 221, 224, 225, 228, 237, 257, 258, 260, 265, 267, 270, 271, 272, 274, 285, 288, 289, 290, 291, 292, 294, 306, 311

goal congruence, 60

goal congruency, 60

goal setting, 116, 291

goals and objectives, 5, 20, 58

good impression, 21

government regulations, 60

governmental agencies, 260

government-based health insurers, 259

graduate medical education, 198, 199, 209, 213, 214, 215, 264, 273, 282

grassroots initiatives, 5

gravitation, 268

greater purpose, 19

group-based strategy, 124

growth, xv, 2, 21, 24, 25, 26, 32, 34, 53, 55, 56, 57, 77, 78, 85, 86, 122, 140, 142, 144, 148, 163, 165, 166, 173, 178, 181, 188, 223, 246, 257, 269, 274, 287, 289, 293, 308

growth and development, 26, 32, 122, 269

growth through coordination, 25

growth through delegation, 25

growth through direction, 25

guidance, 8, 12, 47, 78, 223, 288, 293

guidelines, 70, 259, 269

H

hazardous materials, 18

HCAHPS, 262, 263, 277

health administration, 50, 51, 63

health care administration, 300

health information management, 186

health-care advocates, 256

health-care applications, 112

health-care delivery platform, 262

health-care education, 120

health-care expenditures, 259

health-care fabric, 263

health-care facility, 263

health-care industry, 27, 50

health-care institutions, 5, 27, 51, 76

health-care leaders, x, xiii, xvi, 3, 5, 8, 10, 27, 50, 51

health-care management, 51

healthcare organization, xi, 2, 60, 89, 108, 122, 186, 220

health-care professionals, x, xv, 68, 119, 120, 122

health-care providers, x, 74, 87, 114

health-care recruitment, 50

health-care resource consumption, 263

health-care resources, 275

health-care setting, 4, 114

healthcare system, ix, x, xii, xiv, 2, 4, 5, 51, 56, 86, 89, 91, 96, 109, 110, 186, 195, 219, 256, 261, 271

health-care trainees, 119, 120, 121, 123

heart failure programs, 270

hierarchy, 7, 22, 37, 61

high-impact, 123

high-level communication skills, 122

highly complex, 2, 22, 50

highly skilled, 12, 16, 17

highly skilled workers, 16

high-risk catheter-based interventions, 270

high-technology, 270

hiring, 20, 47, 106, 166, 201, 202, 302

history, 29, 56, 149, 151, 173, 179, 224

holistic and interdisciplinary care, 257

home health, 262, 267

honest, xii, 9, 20, 62, 100, 176, 284, 288, 292, 302

Index

327

hospice, vii, xv, 221, 255, 256, 257, 258, 262, 265, 266, 267, 268, 269, 270, 271, 273, 275, 276, 277, 278, 279
hospice and home health, 269
hospice and palliative care, vii, 255, 256, 258, 266, 268, 270, 273
hospice and palliative care fellowship, 273
hospice and palliative care programs, 256
hospice and palliative medicine, 268, 278, 279
hospice and palliative medicine fellowship, 268
hospice care, 257
hospice services, 257, 276
hospice-related topics, 265
hospital, x, xi, xv, 1, 3, 37, 48, 50, 51, 52, 57, 61, 63, 65, 70, 74, 82, 89, 90, 106, 111, 114, 126, 128, 130, 133, 134, 135, 141, 143, 154, 165, 186, 188, 200, 202, 203, 208, 210, 212, 213, 215, 216, 220, 224, 227, 228, 231, 246, 257, 258, 260, 261, 262, 264, 266, 268, 270, 274, 276, 277, 289, 302, 303, 306, 309, 314, 315
hospital administration, 51, 130, 143, 200, 227
hospital administrator, 51, 61
hospital admissions, 270
hospital charters, 261
hospital consumer assessment of healthcare providers and systems, 262
hospital leadership, 50, 310
hospital services, 262
hospital size, 257, 262
hospital-based, 203, 257, 260, 268
hospital-based providers, 268
hospital-based services, 268
hostile work environment, 26
hybrid model, 198

I

identification, xi, 38, 258
illness, 85, 87, 129, 167, 187, 258, 275, 277, 301, 310
immediate reward, 18
impact, xiii, 7, 20, 22, 30, 32, 36, 40, 41, 44, 45, 48, 60, 65, 69, 76, 85, 89, 96, 121, 129, 131, 136, 148, 149, 164, 168, 169, 177, 186, 189, 191, 196, 210, 216, 240, 244, 251, 252, 261, 267, 269, 278, 287, 296, 305, 306, 310
impersonal model, 58
implement plans, 112
implementation, xiv, xvii, 5, 10, 41, 58, 60, 78, 89, 121, 156, 171, 186, 188, 189, 190, 193, 194, 196, 213, 261, 267, 274
improvement, xiv, 4, 5, 9, 27, 28, 30, 34, 57, 109, 132, 143, 159, 178, 205, 226, 227, 229, 276, 285, 291, 293
improves, 78, 258
impulsive, 114, 115
impulsive behaviors, 115
incentive structures, 25
incentives, 58, 156, 161, 165, 284
inclusion, xii, 51, 69, 80, 109
inclusive, v, xi, 67, 68, 70, 76, 81, 83, 88
inclusive approaches, 68
inclusiveness, xii, 68, 71, 72, 76, 89
incorporated, 145, 228, 263, 264
increasing complexity of healthcare, 259
independent department, 271
independent physicians, 262
individual goals, 274
individualistic, 124, 138
individualized relationships, 19
individuals, x, 2, 6, 12, 21, 26, 27, 53, 56, 57, 59, 60, 72, 113, 115, 117, 118, 121, 123, 148, 151, 152, 158, 163, 164, 169, 173, 175, 187, 193, 194, 195, 205, 206,

223, 225, 234, 237, 239, 259, 260, 267, 271, 290, 303, 305
industrial setting, 18
industry lobbying, 265
influence, 4, 32, 34, 44, 60, 78, 107, 131, 148, 150, 151, 165, 166, 171, 173, 177, 182, 203, 222, 237, 240, 259, 267, 285, 303, 310
information management, 50, 63, 146
informed choice, 260
infrastructure, xiv, 77, 264, 267
in-groups, 15
inhibition, 112, 115, 116, 118, 119
inhibition and volition, 119
initiating tasks, 115
initiation, 115
initiatives, x, 11, 30, 68, 97, 256, 261, 268, 270, 310
innovation, 1, 9, 12, 19, 28, 30, 35, 39, 45, 47, 49, 54, 58, 59, 111, 135, 139, 145, 162, 166, 178, 226, 256, 313
innovative ideas, 21
inputs, 59
inspire, 39, 62, 73, 77, 80, 224, 225, 303
Institute of Medicine, 4, 253, 259, 276
institution, xv, 4, 6, 8, 9, 10, 19, 20, 21, 22, 24, 50, 52, 53, 55, 56, 57, 60, 61, 62, 75, 134, 143, 189, 203, 204, 205, 207, 208, 212, 235, 261, 262, 264, 266, 271, 272, 273
institutional, xii, xiii, xiv, xv, 2, 5, 7, 8, 9, 10, 11, 25, 27, 38, 52, 54, 56, 59, 76, 151, 169, 173, 214, 258, 262, 263, 264, 265, 271, 273, 274, 282
institutional affiliation, 264
institutional behavior, xii, 25
institutional by-laws, 271
institutional change, 2, 7, 10
institutional culture, xiv, 52, 54, 262, 274
institutional goals, 59
institutional needs, 273
institutional participation, 265

institutional pressures, 271
insufficient self-monitoring, 117
insured, x, 263
integrated, 89, 152, 190, 232, 237, 261, 262, 264, 266, 276, 285
integrity, 10, 37
intentional growth, 258
interdisciplinary education, 265
internal, 19, 30, 64, 65, 70, 73, 97, 105, 110, 125, 258, 264, 267, 268, 274, 276, 300, 306
internal development, 19
internal medicine, 30, 64, 65, 70, 73, 97, 105, 110, 125, 267, 268, 276
international reputation, 53
internet, 20, 34, 81, 91, 92, 93
interpersonal communication, 121, 293
interventions, 209, 220, 256
interview, xii, 2, 19, 20, 21, 22, 24, 26, 46, 53, 54, 57, 60, 62, 65, 66
interview preparation, 20
interview process, 19
interviewee, 20, 21, 22, 23, 24, 62
interviewer, 21, 22, 23, 61, 62
interviewing, v, xii, xvii, 21, 23, 49, 50, 52, 57, 60, 62
interviewing skills, 50
intrinsic motivation, 59
introspection, 9, 11, 123, 245, 292
invested, 59, 164, 256, 291, 304
investigate, 62, 238, 247, 250, 306
investment, 12, 16, 43, 290, 300
IOM, 246, 259, 260, 277
isolation, 114, 142, 269

J

job description, 22
job performance, 59
judgment, 55, 172, 239, 243, 285, 286, 306

Index 329

K

key stakeholders, 14
knowledge, ix, xi, xv, 2, 9, 20, 22, 24, 27, 32, 33, 50, 53, 54, 55, 65, 66, 70, 78, 83, 98, 101, 123, 138, 139, 141, 142, 144, 148, 160, 161, 164, 166, 168, 169, 175, 177, 194, 198, 199, 226, 246, 260, 277, 287, 312
knowledgeable, 62, 104

L

laissez faire, 41, 58
laissez-fire leader, 14
latent errors, 272
laws and regulations, 62
leader-follower conduct, 15
leader-follower dynamic, 16
leadership ability, 51
leadership approach, 4, 13, 17, 61
leadership candidate, 20
leadership competencies, 4, 50, 52, 53, 65
leadership culture, 5
leadership development programs, 61
leadership interviews, xii, 23, 50
leadership job interview, 50
leadership model, 12, 13, 16, 17, 60
leadership outcome, 61
leadership perspective, 52, 122, 267
leadership position, v, xii, xvii, 2, 6, 14, 20, 21, 22, 23, 24, 49, 51, 53, 54, 60, 62, 68, 70, 75, 98, 101, 108
leadership qualities, x, 50, 62, 98
leadership role, 13, 16, 17, 19, 51, 53, 56, 61, 76, 96, 98, 100, 108, 167, 292
leadership skills, 88, 89, 96, 106, 112, 161
leadership style, xii, xvii, 6, 11, 12, 13, 14, 15, 19, 23, 24, 40, 41, 44, 51, 57, 58, 59, 60, 65, 97, 99, 134, 138, 139, 168, 224, 272, 288

leadership teams, 51
leadership training, 51, 61, 89, 93, 100, 106, 300
leader-subordinate relationship, 58
leader-team interaction, 14
learning opportunities, 72, 261
length of stay, xiii, 220, 263
let do, 14
let it be, 58
levels of performance, 22
leveraged, 168, 220, 267
licensure requirements, 260
life cycle theory of leadership, 17
life-expectancies, 256
life-threatening illness, 258
like-minded individuals, 56
limited resources, vi, 147, 148, 149, 169, 172, 173
listening, 7, 121, 134, 172, 303, 305, 307
lobbying, 265
local, 21, 75, 105, 108, 168, 172, 235, 263, 265, 268, 273, 309
local environment, 265
logical responses, 116
London, 118, 214, 216, 257
long-term, xiv, 11, 12, 50, 56, 62, 86, 116, 123, 188, 196, 210, 211, 218, 261, 271, 287, 288, 290, 291, 293, 296
long-term care facilities, 261
long-term goal, 56, 62, 116, 271, 290, 291, 293, 296
long-term mentorship, 123
loss of flexibility, 58
loyal, 11, 15
loyalty, 10

M

Machiavellianism, 26, 47
make plans, 117
maldistribution of resources, 259

330 *Index*

malnutrition, 121
management, x, xv, xvi, xvii, 3, 4, 5, 7, 14,
  18, 23, 25, 27, 28, 29, 30, 32, 33, 35, 36,
  37, 38, 39, 40, 41, 42, 44, 46, 63, 64, 65,
  66, 77, 97, 105, 126, 127, 130, 131, 134,
  135, 136, 137, 141, 142, 145, 146, 154,
  166, 170, 173, 186, 189, 196, 202, 205,
  214, 217, 224, 228, 244, 251, 252, 253,
  269, 276, 300, 302, 303, 307, 308, 311
managerial direction, 59
managerial roles, 62
managers, 7, 8, 13, 25, 26, 30, 37, 44, 47,
  63, 162, 186, 195, 311
managing down, 5
managing individuals, 26
managing up, 5
mandate, 270
mandated, 58, 285
many things to many people, 17
marketing, 33, 266, 311
McGill University, 257
MD-MBA, 61
meaning, 7, 79, 82, 87, 162
meaningful research projects, 274
measurably actionable, 260
measurements of progress, 272
medical condition, 123
medical education, 51, 85, 129, 198, 202,
  211, 313, 315
medical education curriculum, 51
medical error, 3, 30, 125, 154, 232, 246,
  247, 254
medical knowledge, 51, 55, 223
medical leaders, vi, 33, 48, 55, 56, 64, 65,
  111, 167, 181, 314
medical leadership, vi, 29, 48, 65, 68, 69,
  111, 167, 220, 313, 314
medical professionals, 114
medical school, 29, 51, 61, 71, 73, 74, 87,
  98, 119, 129, 130, 131, 147, 198, 200,
  201, 202, 205, 206, 210, 211, 212, 213,
  215, 249, 264, 281, 285, 290, 303, 314

medical staff, 134, 143, 220, 261
medical students, 68, 88, 105, 119, 121,
  122, 128, 129, 130, 132, 199, 200, 205,
  207, 209, 211, 218, 296
Medicare, 70, 90, 188, 199, 213, 256, 257,
  259, 276
Medicare Hospice Benefit, 257
Medicare part A, 257
member-based organization, 265
mental health issues, 121
mental health professionals, 119
mental health services, 119, 129
mentoring, 68, 75, 76, 77, 78, 92, 122, 132,
  167, 218, 282, 283, 284, 285, 286, 288,
  292, 296, 302
mentorship, xv, 68, 77, 79, 282, 283, 284,
  285, 287, 288, 294, 295, 296, 297, 313,
  315
merged, 261
metacognitive ability, 123
Mexico, 42, 67, 69, 73, 74, 75, 76, 84, 85,
  86, 87, 88, 89, 91
micromanagement, 14, 142
mindfulness, 115, 120, 123, 125, 130, 132,
  222, 225
mindfulness-based exercises, 123
misinformation, 21
mission, xiii, 11, 20, 21, 22, 79, 155, 160,
  198, 199, 202, 205, 207, 208, 212, 228,
  244, 245, 262, 272, 274, 300, 302, 303,
  304, 306, 307, 311
mission statement, 20, 262, 272
misunderstood, 103, 119, 239
models, ix, x, 3, 11, 12, 29, 34, 87, 155,
  170, 172, 235, 265, 285, 289
modern health-care, ix, xi, xii, xiv, xv, 3, 4,
  5, 27, 124
momentum, 6, 11
mortality, 69, 70, 89, 90, 236, 256, 263
mortality statistics, 263
motivate, 19, 23, 24, 57, 59, 77, 81, 143,
  301, 305

Index

motivation, 6, 31, 41, 45, 55, 165, 166, 228, 287

motivators, 18

Mount, Balfour, 257

multidisciplinary, 3, 124, 226, 274

multidisciplinary collaboration, 275

multidisciplinary team, 226, 274

multi-site, 261

mutual accountability, 5

mutual respect, xii, 59

mutual understanding, 20

N

narcissism, 26, 47, 254

National Comprehensive Cancer Network, 269

national footprint, 273

National Hospice and Palliative Care Organization, 265, 278

natural alignment, 268

natural history, 256

natural process, 258

NCCN, 269

needs, xi, 17, 25, 41, 68, 76, 80, 89, 103, 104, 136, 142, 143, 144, 155, 165, 166, 168, 170, 172, 173, 178, 181, 195, 200, 211, 216, 256, 259, 260, 263, 274, 275, 279, 288, 294, 304

needs and values, 260

needs assessment, 263

neglect, 11, 116

negligent hiring, 2, 26, 47

negotiation, 13, 81, 88, 101, 109, 216, 217, 268

network, vii, xv, 1, 2, 33, 49, 56, 57, 63, 111, 136, 201, 255, 256, 258, 261, 262, 264, 266, 267, 313

network structures, 258

networking, 8, 76, 289, 297

neurodegenerative diseases, 121

neuroscience, 112, 126, 132

new program, 273

new providers, 273

newly founded organizations, 24

NHPCO, 265, 278

nomenclature, 18

non-aligned, 270, 271

non-dysphoric, 119

non-financial resources, 274

non-judgmental, 7, 122

non-judgmental approach, 122

non-physician members, 265

not-for-profit, 261

number of admissions, 263

number of beds, 262

nurse, 32, 63, 142, 145, 200, 209, 210, 221, 243, 257, 293

nursing availability, 264

nursing education, 120, 130, 264

O

objective assessment, 112

objective metrics, 274

objectives, 11, 23, 58, 99, 112, 245

observations, 114, 122, 151

occupations, 18

on-call, 273

oncologists, 261

oncology, 131, 216, 221, 257, 264, 266, 267, 269, 278, 279

oncology fellowship, 269

online, 20, 24, 64, 69, 90, 182

online search, 20

openness, 20, 34, 123

operations, 7, 30, 37, 137, 162, 186, 196, 202, 220, 235, 241, 251, 262, 286

opportunities, vii, xii, 9, 12, 16, 39, 68, 74, 76, 77, 80, 83, 85, 98, 99, 100, 108, 124, 135, 148, 149, 156, 163, 166, 199, 214,

242, 255, 257, 276, 282, 288, 293, 294, 295, 307
opportunity for improvement, 18
optimal performance, 118
optimizing patient care, 61
options, 25, 34, 105, 258, 265, 266, 270, 271
orbitofrontal cortex, 118, 127, 128
organic disease states, 121
organizational approaches, 123
organizational change, 31, 32, 300
organizational culture, 4, 38, 42, 43, 174, 189, 224, 228
organizational design, 123
organizational education, 122
organizational engagement, 51
organizational excellence, 256
organizational frameworks, 268
organizational functionalities, 122
organizational growth, 24, 25
organizational hierarchy, 7
organizational knowledge gaps, 256
organizational leadership, 261
organizational orientation, 53
organizational performance, 37, 40, 51
organizational prowess, 15
organizational resilience, 134, 228
organizational structure, 18
organizational success, 5, 26, 50, 138, 162, 215
organize, 75, 89, 117
organized programs, 274
outcomes, x, xiii, 5, 15, 27, 30, 31, 39, 41, 44, 68, 69, 70, 78, 84, 85, 86, 89, 90, 102, 104, 148, 151, 152, 154, 157, 162, 168, 180, 187, 191, 207, 217, 236, 238, 240, 243, 246, 249, 253, 278, 283, 287, 292
out-group, 15
outpatient clinic, 105, 269
output, 24
ownership, 175, 225, 272, 284, 292, 296

P

pace, 2, 117, 274
pacing, 112, 116, 117
pain, 47, 187, 207, 209, 221, 257, 258
palliative and supportive care, 266, 269
palliative care, 85, 256, 257, 258, 260, 264, 265, 266, 268, 269, 270, 271, 275, 276, 277, 278, 279
palliative care program, 257, 261, 269
palliative care services, 257, 268, 269
palliative care ward, 257
palliative medicine, 266, 271, 276
parent-child relationship, 15
participants, 20, 55, 75, 96, 157, 164, 203, 304
participative, 12, 13, 30, 58, 83
participatory decision-making, 13, 40
partnership, 37, 212, 214, 261, 289
passion, 6, 55, 104, 290, 296
pastoral care, 264
paternalistic, 12, 15, 42
paternalistic leaders, 15, 42
paternalistic leadership, 15, 42
pathological states, 121
patient capacity, 262, 263
patient care, 4, 5, 33, 51, 55, 56, 68, 76, 189, 226, 258, 261, 262, 283, 306, 307
patient care navigators, 262
patient flow pathways, 270
patient interactions, 51
patient outcomes, 2, 27, 28, 70, 114, 131, 310
patient safety, vi, xvii, 2, 4, 30, 34, 50, 51, 61, 63, 114, 125, 135, 219, 220, 221, 225, 227, 228, 229, 245, 252, 309, 313, 314
payers, 260
pediatric, 73, 76, 147, 180, 183, 253, 262, 270, 279, 302
peer-level relationship, 271

Index

peers, 8, 13, 18, 26, 55, 119, 122, 150, 178

people-skills, 54

perception, 43, 44, 200, 201, 211, 236, 269

performance, x, xi, xiv, 4, 14, 18, 21, 24, 25, 31, 33, 37, 38, 39, 40, 43, 44, 48, 58, 64, 74, 78, 116, 120, 123, 124, 127, 128, 130, 152, 159, 174, 175, 177, 182, 192, 196, 209, 213, 244, 251, 272, 283, 287, 288, 292

performance metrics, 272, 283

perpetual cycle, 120

persistence, 3, 11, 55, 170, 290

persistent stress, 121

personal, xi, 9, 12, 15, 23, 37, 55, 56, 58, 69, 71, 77, 78, 79, 80, 100, 109, 112, 116, 120, 123, 134, 140, 143, 144, 175, 177, 195, 223, 233, 241, 244, 246, 266, 283, 284, 288, 289, 309

personal conduct, 116

personal functioning, 120

personal health, 120, 195

personal life domain, 123

personal well-being, 120

personalities, 19, 78

personality, 9, 19, 23, 36, 43, 47, 51, 107, 118, 126, 138, 139, 168

personality changes, 118

personalized baseline, 122

personnel, 66, 122, 125, 200, 208, 209, 227, 228, 233, 237, 250, 258, 280, 308, 309

philosophical, 178, 267

physical, 3, 118, 134, 165, 189, 257, 258, 262

physical injury, 118

physician leaders, 50, 55, 63, 64, 65, 96, 300, 301, 305, 310

physician participation, 51

physician practice, 300

physician satisfaction, 186, 190, 192

physician wellness, 134

physician-driven, 261

physician-leaders, 50, 64

plan, xv, 39, 53, 56, 57, 59, 62, 75, 81, 83, 99, 104, 112, 114, 115, 161, 176, 190, 206, 267, 274, 275, 294, 310

planned decision, 55

planner, 117

planning, 20, 45, 81, 89, 99, 112, 115, 116, 117, 121, 126, 136, 137, 138, 180, 186, 192, 232, 237, 247, 258, 286, 289

planning skills, 117, 138

political, 43, 51, 78, 139, 154, 162, 173, 178, 266, 267, 268, 271, 278

political implications, 266

POLST, 263, 278

poor inhibition, 115

population, xv, 73, 85, 89, 90, 97, 102, 108, 122, 149, 150, 179, 256, 259, 260, 263, 275

population size, 263

populations, 199, 263, 290

position, 2, 4, 6, 8, 21, 22, 23, 36, 51, 53, 55, 57, 58, 59, 60, 61, 62, 66, 73, 97, 106, 108, 155, 162, 167, 198, 203, 205, 211, 247, 270, 279, 289, 303

position papers, 270

positive change, 26, 76

positive reinforcement, 58

practical, v, vii, x, xi, xiii, xv, xvi, xvii, 1, 2, 5, 101, 113, 128, 247, 266, 272, 274, 277, 287, 299

practical standpoints, 272

practical support, 274

practicing health-care providers, 121

pragmatic, 13, 266, 267, 272

preferences, 260, 277

preferred leadership style, 41, 60

prefrontal cortex, 112, 118, 126

prefrontal cortex dysfunction, 118

prefrontal/orbitofrontal regions, 118

preparation, 20, 56, 99, 116, 135, 141, 142, 243, 286

prevent, 51, 85, 86, 87, 116, 124, 125, 144, 199, 219, 222, 226, 235, 239, 248

334 *Index*

prevention, 220, 221, 228, 232, 247, 258, 313

preventive measures, 122

primary care, 3, 97, 106, 260, 262, 267

primary care practitioners, 260

primary credentials, 268

primary stimulus, 123

prioritization, 99, 115, 125

prioritized, 7

prioritizing, 116

private health insurers, 259

private insurance, 187, 188, 260

private sector insurers, xv, 275

proactive, x, 85, 189, 222, 223, 272, 274

problem employees, 26

problem solving, 26, 115

procedural step, 116

procedures, 24, 114, 179, 189, 192, 207, 236, 240, 246, 283

process, x, xii, 2, 13, 19, 20, 26, 30, 31, 37, 41, 52, 60, 97, 99, 107, 114, 117, 119, 137, 142, 154, 157, 158, 162, 163, 164, 166, 169, 171, 177, 179, 186, 189, 195, 207, 219, 220, 221, 222, 223, 225, 227, 228, 236, 245, 246, 257, 260, 271, 272, 275, 288

process of change, 26, 195, 260

procrastinate, 116

product, 16, 20, 24, 87, 225, 245

productivity, 12, 14, 18, 19, 29, 34, 58, 59, 67, 97, 186, 189, 191, 193, 196, 205

professional, v, vi, ix, xi, xii, xiii, xv, xvii, 5, 8, 13, 15, 17, 21, 27, 34, 50, 51, 77, 78, 83, 85, 86, 87, 95, 96, 98, 100, 109, 110, 112, 114, 116, 119, 120, 121, 130, 166, 167, 171, 174, 178, 179, 182, 186, 237, 241, 259, 260, 283, 284, 289, 304, 309

professional advancement, 50

professional groups, 51

professional peers, 121

professional relationship, 13, 50

professional societies, 259

professionalism, 61, 112, 294

program, vi, vii, xv, 53, 56, 57, 60, 61, 62, 69, 70, 75, 81, 88, 89, 93, 95, 96, 97, 100, 101, 102, 104, 105, 106, 107, 108, 109, 122, 146, 188, 190, 192, 196, 200, 203, 205, 208, 209, 210, 213, 218, 240, 249, 252, 255, 256, 257, 260, 264, 265, 266, 267, 270, 273, 274, 278, 279, 284, 285, 293, 295, 302, 310

program development, 256, 258

program director, 53, 57

program leader, 256, 268, 274

program leadership, 256

programmatic implementations, 257

programmatic needs, 265

programmatic priorities, 274

projects, 7, 8, 10, 12, 14, 18, 59, 77, 84, 99, 107, 163, 212

prolong life, 259

promotion, 2, 26, 58, 75, 78, 253, 278

proposed plan, 60, 62, 310

prospective leader, 23, 50, 267

protocols, 24, 57, 205, 227, 234, 242

providing comfort, 256

psychological, 30, 125, 128, 129, 131, 138, 155, 234, 245, 258, 301

psychopathy, 26, 47

psychosocial, 131, 257, 258, 263, 278

public health, xi, 34, 84, 93, 167, 195, 260

public hospitals, 257

publications, 35, 37, 44, 45, 53, 66, 69, 78, 84, 148, 195, 313, 315

pulmonary, 257, 269, 270, 279

pulmonary disease, 270, 279

pulmonary failure, 270

pulmonary medicine, 257

pulmonologists, 261

punishment, 10, 12, 18

pushing the boundaries, 272

Index 335

Q

qualitative, 53, 63, 117, 192, 276
quality, vi, x, xi, xii, xiii, xiv, xvii, 2, 4, 6,
    11, 15, 27, 28, 30, 31, 33, 34, 36, 40, 50,
    51, 53, 55, 60, 61, 62, 63, 68, 70, 71, 89,
    97, 108, 114, 117, 130, 134, 138, 142,
    143, 144, 150, 152, 153, 154, 157, 162,
    164, 165, 167, 169, 173, 177, 178, 191,
    192, 215, 219, 227, 228, 237, 248, 252,
    258, 259, 260, 263, 272, 276, 277, 279,
    287, 309
quality care, 2, 4, 89, 153, 260, 287
quality of care, xiv, 2, 27, 40, 50, 70, 108,
    114, 215, 276
quality of life, 130, 258, 279
quality standards, 259
quantitative data, 272
questions, 20, 22, 42, 46, 66, 74, 97, 135,
    206, 221, 224, 225, 226, 245, 247, 294
quick to react, 116

R

ratings, 114, 125
rational, 55, 117, 156, 157, 247
reactive, 126, 274
readmissions, xiii, 70, 270
re-assign, 27
recommendations, 21, 78, 85, 171, 259, 260,
    269, 276, 277, 278
recruiting, xii, 2, 27, 282
recruitment, 192, 201, 211, 215, 273, 295
referrals, 204, 211, 266, 269, 287
reflect, 9, 11, 23, 62, 112, 120, 159, 265
regional, 21, 57, 263, 273, 312, 313, 315
regional collaboratives, 263
regional population, 263
regional reputation, 57
regulatory agencies, 260
rehabilitation centers, 261

rejection, 10
relationships, vii, x, xii, 2, 8, 12, 21, 38, 55,
    138, 140, 144, 152, 155, 200, 213, 214,
    231, 237, 269, 270, 282, 293, 302, 306
reliability, 64, 114, 124, 222, 228, 253
relief from pain, 258
relief of suffering, 258
religious, xii, 68, 74, 261, 266, 268
religious affiliations, 261
reluctance, 122, 199
reputation, xv, 36, 114, 212, 312
required work, 116
requirements, 22, 33, 106, 186, 193, 198,
    200, 202, 209, 210, 218, 269, 273
research, 1, 4, 16, 20, 21, 23, 34, 36, 39, 40,
    41, 42, 47, 49, 53, 57, 63, 64, 76, 77, 83,
    88, 97, 105, 106, 108, 110, 111, 115,
    125, 126, 130, 131, 163, 165, 177, 181,
    196, 199, 202, 205, 206, 207, 212, 217,
    227, 249, 250, 256, 273, 284, 287, 289,
    291, 313
research process, 273
residency, 51, 52, 61, 63, 89, 135, 208, 209,
    213, 215, 217, 249, 264, 268, 295, 302
residency programs, 51, 209
Residency Review Committee, 268
residents, 57, 60, 73, 74, 105, 106, 187, 199,
    200, 201, 202, 205, 207, 209, 210, 211,
    266, 268, 277, 282, 283, 285, 287, 288,
    290, 295, 297
resilience, vi, xiii, 133, 136, 137, 140, 144,
    145, 146, 274, 302
resilient leadership, xvii, 134, 136, 142
resistance, 110, 170, 189, 256, 268
resource availability, xiii, 258
resource intensive, 270
resource limitations, 272
resources, xiv, 12, 14, 16, 25, 33, 44, 45, 46,
    59, 60, 75, 85, 102, 103, 116, 148, 149,
    153, 161, 168, 169, 170, 173, 188, 212,
    229, 238, 250, 256, 262, 263, 264, 265,
    267, 272, 273, 279, 302, 304, 307, 310

respect, 5, 7, 14, 15, 18, 19, 68, 74, 80, 89, 142, 175, 176, 216, 217, 232, 236, 244, 256
respect for others, 7
responsibility, 3, 7, 13, 21, 22, 25, 28, 54, 61, 62, 68, 70, 86, 89, 93, 99, 105, 118, 139, 166, 167, 171, 202, 272, 275, 283, 292, 293, 303
restructuring, 25
results, 2, 11, 25, 26, 31, 46, 56, 70, 72, 74, 84, 85, 87, 89, 100, 105, 151, 153, 156, 162, 176, 189, 213, 233, 240, 243, 247, 248, 249, 260, 262, 263, 292, 297, 311
retention, 2, 26, 47, 96, 108, 192, 201, 211, 215, 216, 217, 262
rewarding, 27, 285
rewards, 12, 18, 58, 120, 165, 177
risks, 19, 108, 114, 118, 137, 168, 267, 302
risks and rewards, 118
roles, 2, 38, 43, 52, 53, 55, 61, 62, 74, 78, 171, 189, 218, 256, 261, 313
roles and responsibilities, 55, 62
Royal Victoria Hospital, 257, 276
rule restraints, 118
rules and regulations, 58

S

safety, xiv, 4, 18, 30, 44, 114, 137, 142, 149, 154, 219, 221, 222, 223, 225, 228, 232, 235, 238, 239, 240, 241, 244, 249, 250, 251, 304, 310
safety precautions, 18
safety systems, 232
satellite facilities, 261
Saunders, Dame Cicely, 257
scholarly pursuits, 273
scientific, ix, 28, 42, 74, 91, 107, 159, 273, 279
scope of the position, 22
secondary roles, 14

section, 100, 110, 258, 259, 265, 266, 267, 271, 272
self-assessment, 122
self-awareness, 9
self-centeredness, 16
self-directed, 58, 293
self-directed productivity, 59
self-governance, 14
self-improvement, 26, 112, 156
self-improvement cycles, 26
self-monitor, xiii, 112, 114, 117, 122
self-monitoring, xiii, 112, 114, 117, 122
self-pacing, 114
self-regulate, 55, 126
self-regulation, 55, 126
self-reliant, 124
senior leaders, 8
sense of direction, 56
sensitivity, 54, 75, 99
separation, 261, 266
sequence, 54, 117
sequencing, 116, 117
series of steps, 116
serious illness, 260, 276
servant, xvii, 12, 16, 38, 43, 100, 105, 106
servant leadership, xvii, 16, 38, 43
service line leaders, 271
service lines, 269
services, x, 24, 28, 30, 36, 63, 64, 66, 85, 100, 104, 106, 110, 119, 135, 152, 163, 164, 196, 200, 201, 206, 226, 245, 247, 260, 262, 263, 264, 268, 269, 278, 314
set a goal, 116, 117
set-shifting, 115, 117
setting goals, 271
shared decision making, 14
shared goal, 14, 57, 60, 61
shifting between tasks/functions, 112
shifting environment, 117
shifting reality, 115
shortcomings, 124
short-term, 11, 56, 62, 116, 173, 198, 288

Index

337

short-term gratification, 116
significant life event, 123
significant stress, 120
simulated patients, 123
situation, x, 2, 8, 17, 23, 75, 87, 104, 159,
 169, 171, 174, 200, 210, 211, 223, 224,
 226, 236, 237, 239, 266, 286, 301, 302,
 306, 307
situational, 12, 16, 43, 44, 247
situational awareness, 116, 140, 198, 232,
 236, 294, 300, 308
situational leadership, 16, 44
situational scenarios, 123
six sigma, 232
skepticism, 268
skill, vi, ix, xvi, 2, 5, 12, 14, 17, 22, 23, 24,
 27, 36, 46, 47, 48, 53, 54, 55, 61, 69, 71,
 77, 78, 83, 89, 98, 99, 100, 101, 104,
 106, 107, 108, 111, 114, 115, 117, 122,
 132, 136, 138, 141, 143, 144, 161, 162,
 163, 165, 169, 174, 176, 177, 179, 216,
 220, 222, 224, 228, 237, 260, 285, 286,
 287, 302, 303
skill fluency, 123
skillset, 17, 115, 117, 123
skipping, 116, 117
skipping steps, 116
social, vi, xiii, 3, 12, 14, 21, 28, 31, 34, 41,
 44, 45, 51, 55, 65, 69, 71, 74, 78, 84, 85,
 88, 97, 99, 112, 117, 118, 120, 123, 125,
 126, 127, 131, 147, 149, 154, 155, 162,
 163, 164, 166, 169, 172, 174, 182, 188,
 246, 249, 257, 260, 264, 266, 274, 277,
 293, 297
social appropriateness, 118
social equality, 14
social interactions, 117
social life, 117, 120
social media, 21, 71, 293, 297
social scientific inquiry, 12
social services, 260
social signals, 118

social skills, 55, 172
social work, 3, 257, 264, 277
social worker, 3, 257
socializing, 112
societal implications, 122
soft skills, 23, 24, 27, 48
space out tasks, 116
speaking with others, 24
specialized entities, 258
specialties, 51, 70, 73, 125, 210, 217, 237,
 245
specialty centers, 261
specific goal, 12, 23, 116
speech therapy, 262
spiritual aspects, 258
spiritual domains, 257
spiritual spheres, 258
St. Christopher's Hospice in Sydenham, 257
staff, 3, 7, 12, 15, 18, 25, 32, 57, 58, 59, 61,
 101, 102, 105, 106, 110, 134, 138, 143,
 211, 220, 221, 222, 263, 266, 273, 274,
 300, 302, 305, 306, 307, 310
staff availability, 273
staff morale, 273, 310
staffing, 273
stakeholders, xii, xvi, 5, 8, 9, 20, 50, 51, 86,
 122, 260, 275, 302, 304, 305, 309
start a program, 271
state, 2, 9, 32, 44, 52, 62, 67, 73, 91, 106,
 119, 147, 155, 182, 185, 197, 201, 204,
 207, 208, 210, 222, 225, 260, 265, 275,
 314, 315
state-wide, 265
static goal, 18
status quo, 7, 12, 18, 79, 80, 143, 163, 170,
 224, 226
stigmatized, 119
strata of reporting, 22
strategic collaborations, 8
strategic realignments, 5
strategy, xii, 7, 14, 25, 30, 31, 34, 41, 45,
 56, 93, 159, 171, 173, 214

strength, 99, 133, 134, 136, 143, 144, 145, 169, 292

strengths, xiii, 22, 53, 55, 56, 62, 99, 135, 168, 194, 198, 224, 302

stress, 44, 114, 120, 123, 129, 130, 131, 132, 135, 141, 144, 234, 242

stress reduction, 123, 132

stressors, 120, 212, 301

strict hierarchy, 58

stringent rules, 58

structure, 7, 22, 41, 56, 58, 62, 133, 141, 144, 149, 150, 226, 265, 266, 267, 269, 271, 305

structured approaches, 123

styles, 9, 11, 12, 16, 17, 18, 39, 40, 42, 52, 57, 62, 66, 107, 135, 138, 139

subordinates, 13, 26, 47, 58, 59

substance abuse, 121

substance dependence, 123

success, ix, xvii, 5, 9, 12, 16, 45, 50, 52, 56, 59, 60, 62, 74, 76, 77, 78, 79, 84, 106, 109, 137, 138, 146, 157, 158, 159, 161, 162, 173, 175, 195, 199, 200, 216, 267, 272, 276, 282, 284, 286, 287, 288, 290, 291, 292, 294, 309, 311

successful implementation, 271

successful leader, xii, 4, 6, 15, 98, 100, 109, 139, 283, 301

suggestions, 59, 179

supervisors, 7

supervisory relationship, 59

supply, x, 261

support, ix, 5, 9, 11, 17, 26, 56, 60, 73, 75, 76, 77, 78, 81, 104, 120, 144, 156, 163, 164, 167, 169, 172, 178, 195, 199, 201, 202, 203, 204, 205, 208, 211, 227, 228, 258, 260, 264, 265, 268, 270, 271, 272, 274, 284, 286, 302, 305, 308

support system, 258

supportive, 18, 99, 155, 255, 266, 269, 278, 279

supportive care, 255, 266, 269, 278

surgical leadership, 68, 282

surgical services, 269

surgical training, xv, 282, 284, 285, 291, 294

sustainability, xiv, 37, 89, 151, 172, 173, 227, 256

sustainable, xv, 39, 50, 84, 93, 176, 178, 258, 275

symbiotic, 8

synergistic, 8, 21, 36, 37

synergy, xiii, 20, 23, 50, 268, 272

synergy creation, 50

system, x, xiv, 4, 26, 29, 58, 61, 87, 96, 97, 104, 129, 134, 148, 149, 150, 151, 152, 153, 155, 156, 157, 158, 172, 175, 178, 186, 188, 189, 192, 194, 200, 201, 202, 203, 206, 208, 209, 210, 211, 217, 220, 221, 225, 232, 233, 235, 246, 247, 251, 253, 258, 261, 262, 266, 267, 269

system implementation, 186

systematic approach, 225, 257

systemic design, 272

systemic failure, 22

system-owned practices, 262

systems assessment, 261

T

task, 6, 7, 14, 17, 22, 31, 53, 58, 70, 76, 100, 106, 107, 112, 115, 116, 117, 119, 124, 125, 127, 140, 141, 161, 168, 169, 171, 186, 192, 193, 205, 206, 242, 243, 273, 288, 292

task completion, 116

task initiating, 116

task shifting, 116

task-specific attention, 115

teaching experience, 53

teaching hospital, 53, 200, 216, 309

team approach, xiii, 3, 124, 259

team approaches, 3, 124

Index

team building, 11, 123, 265, 304
team decisions, 13
team design, 112
team dynamics, 4, 15, 36, 123
team functioning, 114
team goals, 6
team interactions, 114
team members, 8, 10, 12, 14, 18, 24, 35, 58, 59, 194, 221, 228, 301, 302, 304, 306, 308
team-based care, xii, 3, 30
technical aspects, 26, 283
technical competencies, 26
technical credibility, 15
technical implications, 60
technical skills, 27, 123, 170, 174
technical talent, 124
technical tyrants, 26
technological advancements, 60
technological factors, 51
technology implementation, 55
telemedicine, 262
test anxiety, 120, 130
timeframe, 116
times of crisis, 59, 305, 312
to over-reactions, 116
top talent, 19
total pain, 257
toxic leader, 26
training, vii, x, xi, 4, 27, 29, 32, 48, 53, 61, 62, 63, 65, 68, 70, 71, 74, 78, 83, 85, 89, 100, 101, 107, 108, 125, 137, 144, 145, 161, 163, 164, 167, 192, 194, 198, 200, 201, 208, 209, 210, 214, 215, 222, 224, 239, 241, 249, 252, 258, 260, 264, 268, 269, 273, 281, 282, 284, 288, 290, 294, 295, 296, 297, 300, 310, 311, 314
traits, 5, 6, 22, 23, 38, 43, 50, 53, 54, 65, 107, 108, 145, 289
transactional, 12, 17, 18, 41
transactional leader, 13, 17, 18, 40, 58, 66
transactional leadership, 13, 17, 40, 58, 66

transformational, 12, 18, 30, 38, 44, 66
transformational leaders, 16, 18, 19, 36, 38, 39, 40, 43, 44, 45, 57
transformational leadership, 16, 18, 36, 38, 39, 40, 43, 44, 45, 57
transformational leaderships, 16
transition, xii, 12, 27, 44, 45, 61, 86, 87, 106, 186, 189, 193, 195, 199, 266, 312
transitioning out, 27
transparent, 20, 103
transplant, 236, 270
transplantation, 270
transportation services, 262
trust, 2, 4, 8, 11, 12, 13, 15, 33, 36, 38, 40, 42, 43, 59, 63, 164, 172, 179, 211, 274, 302, 307
trusted advisors, 9
turnover, 12, 15, 16, 42, 43, 126
turnover rates, 16

U

U.S. Congress, 257
unconventional strategies, 19
under stress, 116, 122, 236
under-appreciated, 123
understanding, x, xiii, 2, 4, 5, 18, 20, 22, 23, 24, 53, 55, 56, 60, 62, 63, 69, 89, 101, 114, 118, 125, 129, 144, 148, 163, 168, 171, 172, 175, 205, 214, 216, 218, 226, 234, 239, 243, 257, 258, 267, 275, 280, 304, 307
unexpected circumstances, 117
unexpected outcomes, 112
unforeseen circumstances, 116
unidirectional, 13
uninsured, x, 187, 263
unintended impacts, 10
unique skillset, 51

United States, 50, 150, 168, 176, 182, 186, 187, 195, 212, 217, 244, 247, 257, 275, 276, 295
unrealistic schedules, 117
unrealistic timeframes, 116

V

value, xi, xiii, xiv, xvi, 2, 8, 10, 28, 34, 43, 54, 56, 59, 62, 64, 72, 74, 79, 87, 135, 148, 150, 161, 162, 170, 171, 172, 174, 178, 188, 189, 207, 208, 213, 225, 226, 228, 247, 260, 276, 278, 285, 293, 311
ventricular assist devices, 270
verbal fluency, 115, 117, 127
veterans, 95, 100, 104, 105, 106, 213, 263
vignette, x, 52, 57, 60, 62, 134, 142, 188, 189, 193, 221, 226, 300, 309
vignette-based scenarios, 52
vision, 5, 11, 15, 38, 50, 53, 54, 56, 57, 60, 62, 86, 93, 104, 108, 139, 143, 161, 162, 224, 271, 272, 288
vision documents, 272
vision for growth, 271
visionary, 38, 272
visitors, 137, 220, 228, 262
vocal and facial expressions, 118

W

weaknesses, 22, 53, 55, 56, 62
well-balanced, 124

well-being, 9, 16, 26, 68, 120, 211, 297, 305
wellness, 130, 274
well-planned execution, 271
well-trained, 61, 165
widening disparities, 259
wisdom, 8, 31, 38, 163, 170, 182, 310
wise leader, 26
women, vi, 68, 69, 70, 71, 72, 73, 74, 75, 76, 77, 80, 82, 84, 85, 86, 87, 90, 91, 92, 93, 95, 96, 97, 98, 100, 101, 103, 104, 109, 110, 145, 213, 285, 297
women in medicine, 69, 90, 92, 96
women leaders, 68, 71, 75, 90, 96, 97
work culture, 19
work speed, 116
worker, 18, 141, 142, 225
workflow management, 50
workforce, 17, 164, 208, 215, 273
working memory, 112, 115, 125
working relationship, 205, 273
work-life balance, 117, 273, 289
workplace, xii, 2, 13, 15, 26, 27, 31, 34, 39, 41, 48, 66, 68, 71, 75, 128, 217
workplace bullying, 26, 39
World Health Organization (WHO), 258, 276

Z

zero error incidence, 232

Related Nova Publications

TRANSLATIONAL RESEARCH: RECENT PROGRESS AND FUTURE DIRECTIONS

EDITORS: Francesco Chiappelli, Ph.D. and Nicole Balenton

SERIES: Health Care in Transition

BOOK DESCRIPTION: The chapters in this book highlight the transfer of basic science discovered and cutting-edge developments into clinical applications. Emphasis on continuing research, increasing transparency and accelerating the adoption of translational science into clinical practice is needed to provide the best possible care.

HARDCOVER ISBN: 978-1-53614-598-4
RETAIL PRICE: $230

PANDEMICS: EVOLUTIONARY ENGINEERING OF CONSCIOUSNESS AND HEALTH

EDITOR: Pavel I. Sidorov, M.D., Ph.D.

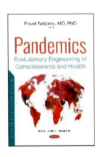

SERIES: Health Care in Transition

BOOK DESCRIPTION: According to WHO, a pandemic is the spread of a disease on a global scale. The globalization of the modern singular world has led to a dynamic development of both communicable and non-communicable types of epidemiology.

SOFTCOVER ISBN: 978-1-53614-274-7
RETAIL PRICE: $95

To see a complete list of Nova publications, please visit our website at www.novapublishers.com

Related Nova Publications

FUNDAMENTALS OF LEADERSHIP FOR HEALTHCARE PROFESSIONALS

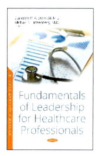

EDITORS: Stanislaw P. A. Stawicki, M.D. and Michael S. Firstenberg, M.D.

SERIES: Health Care in Transition

BOOK DESCRIPTION: Each chapter in this text explores different aspects of healthcare leadership, provides valuable insights into how effective leadership functions, and offers practical perspectives on implementations of theory into practice.

HARDCOVER ISBN: 978-1-53613-620-3
RETAIL PRICE: $195

DEFENSE HEALTH CARE: TREATMENT, PERFORMANCE AND TRICARE

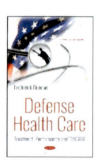

AUTHOR: Frederick Duncan

SERIES: Health Care in Transition

BOOK DESCRIPTION: For over a decade, Congress and DOD have led a series of efforts to address the governance structure of the Military Health System.

HARDCOVER ISBN: 978-1-53615-175-6
RETAIL PRICE: $160

To see a complete list of Nova publications, please visit our website at www.novapublishers.com